Principles and Techniques of
Trauma-Centered
Psychotherapy

Principles and Techniques of **Trauma-Centered Psychotherapy**

David Read Johnson, Ph.D.
Hadar Lubin, M.D.

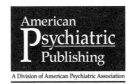

American **Psychiatric** Publishing

A Division of American Psychiatric Association

Washington, DC
London, England

Note: The authors have worked to ensure that all information in this book is accurate at the time of publication and consistent with general psychiatric and medical standards. As medical research and practice continue to advance, however, therapeutic standards may change. Moreover, specific situations may require a specific therapeutic response not included in this book. For these reasons and because human and mechanical errors sometimes occur, we recommend that readers follow the advice of physicians directly involved in their care or the care of a member of their family.

If you would like to buy between 25 and 99 copies of this or any other American Psychiatric Publishing title, you are eligible for a 20% discount; please contact Customer Service at appi@psych.org or 800-368-5777. If you wish to buy 100 or more copies of the same title, please e-mail us at bulksales@psych.org for a price quote.

Manufactured in the United States of America on acid-free paper
19 18 17 16 15   5 4 3 2 1
First Edition

Typeset in Janson Text LT Std and HelveticaNeue LT.

American Psychiatric Publishing
A Division of American Psychiatric Association
1000 Wilson Boulevard
Arlington, VA 22209-3901
www.appi.org

Library of Congress Cataloging-in-Publication Data
Principles and techniques of trauma-centered psychotherapy / edited by David Read Johnson, Hadar Lubin. — First edition.
    p. ; cm.
  Includes bibliographical references and index.
  ISBN 978-1-58562-514-7 (pbk. : alk. paper)
  I. Johnson, David Read, editor. II. Lubin, Hadar, editor. III. American Psychiatric Publishing, publisher.
  [DNLM: 1. Stress Disorders, Post-Traumatic—therapy. 2. Evidence-Based Medicine. 3. Psychotherapy—methods. WM 172.5]
  RC480
  616.89′14—dc23   2015006560

British Library Cataloguing in Publication Data
A CIP record is available from the British Library.

Contents

About the Authors

David Read Johnson, Ph.D., is Co-director of the Post Traumatic Stress Center in New Haven, Connecticut and Associate Clinical Professor in the Department of Psychiatry at Yale University School of Medicine. He was formerly the Unit Chief of the Specialized Inpatient PTSD Unit at the National Center for PTSD, VA Medical Center, in West Haven, Connecticut. He is the co-author (with H. Lubin) of *Trauma-Centered Group Psychotherapy for Women* (Francis & Taylor, 2008), and co-editor (with N. Sajnani) of *Trauma-Informed Drama Therapy: Transforming Clinics, Classrooms, and Communities* (Charles Thomas, 2014), as well as numerous articles on trauma treatment.

Hadar Lubin, M.D., is Co-director of the Post Traumatic Stress Center in New Haven, Connecticut and Assistant Clinical Professor in the Department of Psychiatry at Yale University School of Medicine. She was formerly the Unit Chief of the Specialized Inpatient PTSD Unit at the National Center for PTSD, VA Medical Center, in West Haven, Connecticut. She is the co-author (with D. Johnson) of *Trauma-Centered Group Psychotherapy for Women* (Francis & Taylor, 2008), as well as numerous articles on trauma treatment.

The authors have indicated no competing interests to disclose during the year preceding manuscript submission.

Acknowledgments

We would like to thank our colleagues at the Post Traumatic Stress Center who have helped us develop and refine the ideas presented in this book; in particular, we thank Melissa DeGeso, Angelina Rodner, Rebecca Giagnacova, Linda Berger, Kristin Hale, and Nisha Sajnani. We have drawn inspiration from the clinical work of Judith Herman, Christine Courtois, Bessel van der Kolk, Constance Dalenberg, Sandra Bloom, Lisa McCann, Laurie Pearlman, Kay Saakvitne, Frank Ochberg, Marilyn Cloitre, John Briere, Esther Deblinger, Judith Cohen, Edna Foa, and Terence Keane, among many others. Our gratitude to our clients who have shared their experiences and were willing to journey with us is immeasurable, and it is to their courage and their suffering that we dedicate this book.

Preface

This book is intended for clinicians who wish to conduct a trauma-centered conversation with their clients. Such a conversation includes setting up the proper trauma-centered frame for the therapeutic work, conducting a detailed trauma history, exploring the effects of the various trauma schemas on present-day behavior, handling the inevitable disruptions in the therapeutic relationship caused by the same trauma schemas, and understanding the limits of a trauma-centered approach.

This text has been particularly informed by the work of clinicians such as Judith Herman, John Briere, Christine Courtois, Bessel van der Kolk, Sandra Bloom, Marilyn Cloitre, Lisa McCann and Laurie Pearlman, Judith Cohen and Esther Deblinger, Edna Foa and Barbara Rothbaum, Frank Ochberg, Patricia Resick, Charles Figley, and Constance Dalenberg, and the reader is referred to their books for additional perspectives on trauma-centered treatment. However, none of these excellent texts have examined the process of trauma inquiry in the detail that is presented here. Our intention is to describe the mechanics, step by step, of conducting effective trauma-centered psychotherapy based on imaginal exposure from an in-depth narrative of the client's traumatic experiences.

The purpose of this book is to apply the most up-to-date experience and evidence-based knowledge about trauma and its effects to the psychotherapeutic endeavor. Although our own clinical experience permeates this book, it is not our intention to present trauma-centered psychotherapy as another unique form of intervention or technique. Each of the methods we present has been used by many practitioners over many years; some have been supported by evidence-based research, whereas others have been supported by broad clinical experience. We make no claims that these methods are the only way or the best way to intervene in trauma-related disorders, but they should be readily and widely applicable in clinical practice. At the same time, this book is not intended to be a comprehensive overview of the field or a textbook about all forms of intervention or research about trauma, because several excellent texts are available (Briere and Scott 2006; Courtois and Ford 2013; Foa et al. 2009; Friedman et al. 2007).

The term *trauma centered* is used to distinguish this work from that which is *trauma informed* and, alternatively, *trauma focused*. These terms are not well defined, but basically those interventions that are trauma informed use the knowledge of trauma and its effects but may not directly engage the client in discussion about the traumatic event. Many trauma-informed interventions may emphasize skills training, relaxation, and psychoeducation (Cloitre et al. 2006). Trauma-focused interventions, on the other hand, privilege the discussion and processing of the traumatic event throughout the treatment. In recent years, trauma-focused interventions have tended to be delivered within relatively short-term time periods and, consistent with the trend toward evidence-based practice, to be designed as stand-alone, manualized procedures; these include prolonged exposure (Foa and Rothbaum 1998), eye movement desensitization and reprocessing (Shapiro 1995), cognitive processing therapy (Resick and Schnicke 1993), narrative exposure therapy (Schauer et al. 2011), and trauma-focused cognitive behavioral therapy (Cohen et al. 2006). Many trauma-focused interventions include some form of exposure treatment. The term *trauma centered* is proposed for an intermediate approach where the exploration of the trauma is conducted in the initial phases of therapy and then is utilized as a foundation as the therapy moves into current issues. Thus, the impact of the past traumas on current functioning remains central to the psychotherapeutic work but does not constrict the breadth of exploration as much as a trauma-focused approach must do.

The context within which trauma-centered work takes place is psychotherapy—that is, a helping relationship of relatively lengthy duration (6 months to years) in which clients have some freedom to discuss all aspects of their lives, to gain insights into themselves, and to receive reassurance and support from a professional who gets to know them very well. Despite the trend toward short-term intervention and manualized procedures, psychotherapy and counseling continue to be very widely used in both private and public sectors. This book intends to bring some of the rigor and focus of exposure and cognitive-behavioral treatments into the psychotherapeutic frame, to guide therapists and counselors in conducting effective trauma treatment within the traditional environment of the therapy session. Readers will recognize elements of psychodynamic and client-centered wisdom, as well as cognitive-behavioral and exposure-based perspectives, but hopefully will be left with enough room to integrate the information into their own way of working.

THE TRAUMA INQUIRY

Asking another person about the minute details of a traumatic event is an intimate, intense, and intrusive act. It is not for the faint-hearted. The trauma inquiry should be conducted by a trained professional who is both compassionate and dispassionate. Just as general practitioners of medicine should be able to dispassionately conduct a physical exam, in which the patient disrobes and then is touched on the outside and the inside by the doctor, trauma therapists should be able to proceed with their examination without trepidation, knowing that it is in the service of the client's health.

Despite much public education, many publications and books, and training programs for mental health professionals on trauma, in practice, many therapists hesitate to proceed with more than a cursory inquiry regarding the traumatic pasts of their clients. Many books on trauma focus on the theories of trauma, general themes and issues that might arise during treatment, and general advice regarding challenging situations. There are few basic textbooks that help the clinician through the first session, and then the early phases of the work, examining transcripts of what to say and what not to say in the wide variety of situations that clinicians are likely to encounter. This book intends to accomplish this task, by providing an experience-near rendering of trauma-centered psychotherapy. There is much to learn about the nuances of taking a trauma history and managing the subtle avoidant strategies of the client. Achieving mastery takes training and practice. For example, understanding the difference between the narrative of the traumatic event and the narrative of the client's experience of the traumatic event is very important, because the details of actual events and the victim's perception of these events may lead into different lines of inquiry.

Because many difficulties arise once a trauma inquiry has begun, clinicians frequently abandon the project, either properly, by referring the client to a specialist, or incorrectly, by concluding that exposing the client to his or her memories is too upsetting to the client and therefore unhelpful.

We strongly believe that it is possible to be trained to conduct a trauma-centered psychotherapy effectively and consistently, and our experience with many trainees from a wide variety of fields supports our optimism.

This is a book on technique, not theory. It is appropriate for clinicians who embrace any theoretical orientation, including cognitive-behavioral, psychodynamic, humanistic, and sociocultural. For many clinicians, after conducting their own preferred approach, a time may come when the clinician decides or the client requests to engage in a detailed exploration of the traumatic events. Especially in long-term treatments, which are not uncommon in trauma-related conditions, this moment comes. This book is intended for this moment. Only clinicians convinced that trauma inquiry is to be avoided as a general rule will not benefit from this book. Trauma-centered psychotherapy is not dependent on any one position regarding the causes of posttraumatic stress disorder (PTSD) or other trauma-related disorders. This book does not advocate that clinicians *should* conduct a trauma-centered inquiry, or that it is *essential* for recovery, or that there is more evidence supporting this approach. The scientific data on these issues are not definitive. There are numerous excellent theories based on psychological, neurobiological, and social processes, and the spirited and thoughtful debate in the scientific and clinical communities continues. However, for therapists and counselors who have clients looking across at them every day, waiting for help, one needs to know what to do, specifically. We intend to be specific.

This book describes a method of psychotherapy designed for any person who has had a traumatic event that continues to be troubling, regardless of his or her diagnosis. PTSD is not the only outcome of experiencing a traumatic event, and indeed there are many clients who carry diagnoses of major depression, somatization disorder, dissociative disorder, eating disorder, substance use disorder, or antisocial, paranoid, or borderline personality disorder who will benefit from a careful and thorough trauma-centered psychotherapy.

OUTLINE OF CHAPTERS

Chapter 1 reviews the history of notions of trauma inquiry and illuminates the many contradictions that have existed in the discussion over when, how extensively, and indeed whether one should ask the client about the trauma. For example, ironically, despite widespread scientific consensus that exposure to the traumatic memories is an effective component in trauma treatment, concerns over exposure and the need for safety and containment continue to gain strength in the clinical literature.

Chapter 2 presents four basic axioms of trauma-centered work, upon which the process depends. These are that trauma schemas attempt to reduce the primary emotions of fear and shame, that both client and therapist are actively avoiding these emotions, that the trauma narrative is therefore always in some way incomplete, and that the trauma schemas are personified even if the events were caused by impersonal natural forces. These axioms serve as guides to the treatment and will help ensure success.

Chapter 3 presents the components of establishing a trauma-centered frame with the client, upon which the entire treatment will be based. The trauma-centered frame provides the context and boundaries for an effective therapeutic relationship during the trauma inquiry.

Chapter 4 describes the basic principles of conducting a trauma-centered psychotherapy: beginning the inquiry immediately, personally engaging with the client, and accepting high degrees of emotionality. These clinical principles will guide each intervention by the therapist.

Chapter 5 presents the four main techniques used in trauma-centered psychotherapy, which include getting the details, decoding current behaviors, introducing discrepancy, and disclosing the perpetrator. These four techniques become the fundamental tools the therapist uses to alter the client's trauma schemas. Chapter 6 focuses in detail on the first session and includes numerous transcripts of successful and unsuccessful beginnings. Chapter 7 explains the early phase of the trauma inquiry, and again through transcripts attempts to demonstrate the subtleties in listening for openings in the client's narrative for deeper processing of the memories. Chapter 8 then describes the complex work in the next phase in linking present behaviors to the various trauma schemas.

Chapter 9 examines the inevitable entanglement of the therapeutic relationship with the trauma schemas, with both client and therapist falling into the gap created by the breaking of the empathic connection, and the various anxious maneuvers of both parties to restabilize a highly unstable relationship. Chapter 10 then outlines some of the major considerations for ongoing and long-term treatment. Chapter 11 examines how the therapist is to manage several truly difficult—and unfortunately not uncommon—situations, including dissociative reactions and violence. This chapter will hopefully reassure the clinician that these situations can be successfully managed, for it is in this territory that some clinicians decide to bail out. Chapter 12 illustrates how the trauma-centered method can be applied to clients with dissociative identity disorder, and Chapter 13 addresses work with clients with borderline personality disorder. Chapter 14 describes in detail how the principles and techniques of trauma-centered psychotherapy are applied in groups, and Chapter 15 addresses work with couples and families. Chapter 16 describes some useful adjunctive methods, such as narrative, creative arts, and ceremonial interventions, that can be integrated within a trauma-centered psychotherapy. Chapter 17 examines the clinical challenges caused by the strains on the therapist in trauma work. Chapter 18 discusses the limits to trauma-centered psychotherapy in environments outside of the therapy office, such as the courts, press, and public testimony. Chapter 19 concludes on a personal note.

Study questions are included at the end of each chapter and are intended both to test the reader's comprehension and to stimulate his or her thinking about the issues raised in the chapter.

DEFINITION OF TERMS

Traumatic Event

The *traumatic event* refers to the relatively objective, actual event, as it would have been seen by others or by a videotape. There is never only one objective view of any true event, because each witness perceives the event differently. However, the term *traumatic event* will be used to refer to the actual, real event, such as the Vietnam War, the Holocaust, the rape, the incest, or the surgical error.

Traumatic Experience and Memory

The terms *traumatic experience* and *traumatic memory* refer to how the traumatic event is perceived and remembered by the victim, survivor, or participant. The *traumatic experience* is how the client perceived and felt during the event. The *traumatic memory* is the client's memory of his or her traumatic experience. It is unlikely that a victim of a traumatic event can have an objective view of what happened because, by definition, trauma interferes with the cognitive processing capacity of the individual. However, that does not mean that many or even most elements of the traumatic memory do not match the objective facts of the traumatic event or the traumatic experience at the time. Usually, the client remembers much of the traumatic experience relatively clearly and accurately. The challenge is that it is not possible to determine, within the therapy session, which parts are the objective ones and which parts are the personal ones. Thus, there are built-in discrepancies between the traumatic experience, the traumatic memory, and the traumatic event. Chapters later in the book will examine in great detail how these enduring discrepancies serve as sources of instability in the traumatized person's experience and how they underlie the primary clinical challenges facing the trauma-centered psychotherapist.

Trauma Schema and Neurotic Schema

The term *trauma schema* refers to the set of ideas, feelings, and patterns of behavior that arise *after* a traumatic event and that form the person's adaptation and integration of the traumatic experience. The trauma schema is a form of coping with the injury as well as an active response set that is ready to ward off future states of fear or shame. The schemas will have some elements that parallel or mirror the traumatic experience and some elements that ward off or deny the traumatic experience. For example, the trauma schema that "all men are dangerous" might arise in a woman who was brutally raped by a male friend. The similarity with her experience is that the man who raped her was dangerous and a man. However, the schema when activated will encourage her to avoid contact with all men. This serves to protect her from dangerous men but also from benign men. It turns out that nice men will be more triggering for her because the clear and safely defined boundary of "all men are dangerous" would become ambiguous and unclear if she became intimate with a nice man, who might become dangerous just like the friend who raped her. The trauma schema, therefore, is designed to help her avoid not only danger but also ambiguity and permeable boundaries. It is this ambiguity in a situation, often more than its level of threat, that serves to destabilize the traumatized client's interpersonal world. Thus, it is when she is presented with nice men that her trauma schema will most often be evoked. This dynamic may contribute to the reason that some abused women feel more comfortable around "bad" men, because although they risk insult or injury, the strictly defined boundaries of their trauma schemas are not disrupted.

Trauma schemas are to be differentiated from *neurotic schemas*, which are patterns of thinking that arise from childhood experiences and are further shaped and smoothed out by additional experiences in life. Neurotic schemas differ profoundly from trauma schemas in that at their core, the empathic bridge between self and other is not broken, as it is in the trauma schema. Thus, neurotic schemas that involve the patterns and roles of relationships with parents and siblings, and the conflicts among various aspects of the self-image, are held within the context of a relational bond. Traumatized clients also maintain their neurotic schemas, which is why they are able to relate to others at work or in school or to the therapist at times in a relatively normal manner. Trauma schemas, and the PTSD symptoms that arise from them, are evoked when the person is triggered and usually last for a relatively short period of time. If the traumatic events occur over a prolonged period of time, and at earlier ages, then trauma schemas may become integrated into the client's personality organization and become more enduring, pervasive patterns of thought and behavior.

The trauma-centered psychotherapist is interested primarily in discovering what the client's trauma schemas are, because they are the blueprint from which disturbances in current behavior, as well as symptoms, arise. The traumatic event itself no longer exists; it has passed. The traumatic experience also has passed. The client's traumatic memories can be expanded as more details are remembered, but they cannot be reduced. Only the trauma schemas exist as malleable structures in the mind and body, and therefore they are the targets of treatment.

Primary and Secondary Emotions

Primary emotions are those intense emotional states—primarily fear and/or shame—experienced during the traumatic event. Nearly all traumatic experiences involve some degree of fear, due to the actual or perceived threat of violence to the self or others. In cases of sexual abuse, especially those in which the perpetrator dominates and humiliates the victim, shame may be the strongest emotion. *Secondary emotions* occur as a result of the person's appraisal of the traumatic event afterward and can include a wide range of emotions (anger, guilt, envy, disgust, as well as fear and shame). Both of these forms of emotions will arise in psychotherapy sessions and are often intertwined with each other in complex ways.

With these terms defined, we now invite you to join us on a journey into the world of trauma-centered psychotherapy.

STUDY QUESTIONS

P.1   Match the items:

A. Trauma schema   ___ the objective event

B. Traumatic experience   ___ emotions experienced during the traumatic event

C. Traumatic memory   ___ what the client perceived during the event

D. Traumatic event   ___ how the trauma has impacted the client's view of the world

E. Neurotic schema   ___ pattern of behavior and thinking arising out of major personal relationships

F. Primary emotions   ___ what the client remembers now about the trauma

G. Secondary emotions   ___ emotions arising from appraisal of the trauma after the event

P.2   What is the difference between neurotic schemas and trauma schemas?

CHAPTER 1

The Developing Cultural Context of Trauma-Centered Psychotherapy

This book presents a method for conducting a therapeutic trauma inquiry that is based on the assumption that inquiring about a person's traumatic experience and providing the person with the opportunity to express fully his or her thoughts, feelings, and memories will be productive. This assumption has by no means been generally accepted in our culture, or indeed in any culture, at any time throughout history. In this chapter, we place trauma-centered psychotherapy within its cultural context, both currently and historically.

Psychological trauma is a fascinating area of study and practice that involves political, social, clinical, medical, scientific, moral, and ethical issues. Because psychological trauma lies within a multidimensional cultural context, the topic has garnered interest from many observers from many diverse perspectives.

Society has debated whether it is a good idea to allow suffering people to express themselves freely. At certain times, people are invited to say what is on their mind, and at other times they are told to be quiet. A good part of becoming socialized is learning when one should speak and when one should remain silent. People are urged to speak when they indicate they do not want to, and they are asked to be quiet when they are speaking too much.

The irony of this situation, however, is not lost on victims of trauma, who learn that they are welcome to say just so much about what happened, but not too much.

The dynamic balance between *containment* and *expression* is important in human systems. Society consists of a complex of overlapping, hierarchically integrated systems of social organization: the family, the neighborhood, the school, the church, the town, the tribe, the institution, and the country. Each level of social organization aims in part to contain disorder and ensure continued functioning of the larger system's primary goals of survival and, at the same time, to provide for the expression of needs, ideas, and information that will allow for innovation and improved adaptation to the demands of the environment. Governments need to maintain order but also need to hear from their citizens in order to govern effectively. Society needs to know if its people are suffering so that the problems that led to this suffering can be addressed. In general, higher orders of social organization exert pressure on lower levels of social organization to serve the containment function. Thus, the nation prefers that cities contain their members, and cities prefer that families contain their members, and families prefer that individuals contain themselves. The most effective social organization, whether at the individual or at the national level, is characterized by a dynamic balance between containment and expression, between order and freedom.

Therefore, conflicting pressures have been brought to bear on the trauma victim throughout history, and up to the present day. Some voices call for expression: First, encouraging victims of trauma to speak out about their experience has been viewed as helpful to society at large for identifying important social problems such as child abuse, domestic violence, the plight of veterans, and ethnic and religious persecution. These are the areas of civil rights, litigation, and politics. Second, victims of trauma have been encouraged to speak about their experience as a means of personal recovery, through venting their emotions and thereby desensitizing themselves to their fears. These are the areas of treatment, medicine, and science.

Other voices, however, have emphasized a need for containment among victims of trauma: First, too much airing of distress can lead to greater social disorder, including public turmoil, unnecessary litigation, and even violence. Second, unconstrained airing of distress by individuals may lead to a loss of their ability to function (i.e., work), with subsequent drain on society at large. Third, when the perpetrators are themselves representatives of the society (e.g., parents, teachers, priests, police, elected officials), authority relationships are disrupted. Within the health field, an emphasis on containment is indicated by methods that emphasize regulation, or self-regulation, as opposed to expression, catharsis, or testimony.

Too much containment can lead to the denial of important social problems and to the creation of secrets within social units. On the other hand, too much expression has been associated with increases in disability, malingering for secondary gain, and false accusations. This conflict will be examined in more detail later in this chapter in the subsection "Moral Weakness (Lying and Malingering)." At this point, suffice it to say that when a particular social organization is functioning well and feels comparatively secure, it can afford to allow more expression from its members, whereas when a social organization is under duress and feels threatened, containment is emphasized. In the next section, we explore how the fluctuations in the state of society have affected attitudes toward the expression allowed victims of trauma, both in public settings and in psychotherapy.

PERSPECTIVES ON THE CAUSE OF TRAUMATIC REACTIONS

The history of the concepts of posttraumatic stress disorder (PTSD) and, more basically, trauma is complex and extremely interesting. There has been no dearth of horror, terror, and helplessness in human interaction. Presumably, what are now known as PTSD and other trauma-related disorders have always existed, and states of anxiety, somatization, dissociative experiences, and numbing were likely common throughout history. However, notions of the mechanism responsible for causing these traumatic reactions have been varied and at odds with one another. There are four major perspectives on the cause of traumatic reactions: *character weakness in the victim, responses to social oppression, physical processes,* and *overwhelming arousal* (Table 1–1).

Character Weakness in the Victim

The first and most fundamental explanatory framework can be called *character weakness*. The view that traumatic reactions are due to character weakness on the part of victims is deeply seated in most societies' cultural norms. When a person succumbs to stress, anxiety, or fear due to a horrible event, such as war or a rape or a motor vehicle accident, and is unable to recover within a reasonable period of time, the assumption is that the victim had a preexisting condition of *weakness, lying and malingering,* or *suggestibility.* Some victims of trauma are viewed simply as being physically and/or mentally weak; indeed, phenomenologically it is a common experience that some people seem stronger than others. In contrast, some are viewed as morally weak—that is, they lie or malinger for personal gain. Finally, others are

---

TABLE 1–1.   Causal frameworks for traumatic reactions

Character weakness in the victim

  Because not all victims develop psychopathology after traumatic events, some
  victims must be more hardy (strong, resilient, courageous) than others.

Responses to social oppression

  Interpersonal violence is created, sustained, or tolerated by systemic forces in
  society that privilege certain groups over others. Responsibility for traumatic
  reactions after such violence must be laid upon the perpetrators and the social
  norms that support them.

Physical processes

  Traumatic reactions to toxic stress are mediated by the central nervous system,
  and injuries to that system must be the cause of ongoing chronic symptomatology.

Overwhelming arousal (fear or shame)

  Traumatic reactions are caused by intense emotional arousal that overwhelms the
  person's cognitive capacities to represent the event, leading to a state of
  conditioned arousal that is activated upon reminders of the event.

---

viewed not as uniquely weak or malingering, but instead as being so susceptible to suggestion that they become consumed with fear far beyond what the
circumstances call for. For example, in war, those soldiers who collapse on
the battlefield and can no longer fight may be viewed as weak, as malingering, or as easily suggestible. Treatment for each of these possibilities varies
greatly.

GENERAL WEAKNESS

Until the mid-1800s, one term used for what is now known as PTSD was
cowardice (Babington 1990; Putkowski and Sykes 1999; van der Kolk 2010).
The term *cowardice* is derived from a word that means "one with a tail," and
is signifies subservience as in "to cower, to be cowed." Similar epithets have
been used against domesticated or fearful animals:to *duck* means to lower
one's head, to be a *chicken* is to scramble away from a threat, to be *mousy* is
to be timid, and to run with one's *tail between one's legs* means to be frightened. The symptoms of cowardice in war included refusing to participate
in battle, crying, shaking, and deserting. In general, the "treatment" for this
condition was to be shot. Although the soldier died, the intention was to
dissuade other soldiers from demonstrating similar symptoms. For example, in the waning days of the Civil War as morale was collapsing, Robert
E. Lee employed a rear guard behind each regiment whose orders were to
shoot deserters (Power 1998).

Military leaders all recognize that some people are more hardy than others; indeed military training, such as boot camp, is designed to weed out those recruits who are incapable of handling battle conditions by placing them into simulated battle conditions. Military leaders desire battle-hardened troops rather than those rapidly conscripted against their will to fight. Poorly trained armies have historically had large measures of psychiatric casualties. For example, during the war with Russia in 1808, Sweden had to force thousands of conscripts into battle, and after losing the war, this group of Swedish soldiers was beset by what was termed *conscript sickness*, which was essentially PTSD (Nordstrom 2002). At the end of World War II, as thousands of new, unprepared recruits were sent directly from the United States into intense combat in Europe, the rate of psychiatric casualties skyrocketed to nearly 30% of all casualties within weeks of arrival (Beebe and Apple 1958). Trainers of people seeking stressful jobs such as firefighters, police, and emergency medical workers all employ similar strategies of identifying those individuals who have the fortitude and strength required by the work.

References to victims of trauma as being weak abound in the popular culture: they are commonly asked to "pick yourself up," "pull it together," "forget about it and move on," and "stop complaining." Vietnam War veterans with PTSD were accused of being poorly trained and unmotivated (Lifton 1973); Hiroshima survivors in Japan (the *hibakusha*) were viewed as being bad workers and shunned from employment (Hersey 1985); children who are being bullied are viewed as not being able to stand up for themselves.

This perspective reflects the binary *strong versus weak* and in some measure represents an identification with the perpetrator (who is strong) over the victim (who is weak). Societal derision toward supposedly weaker individuals and groups (which at times have included, for example, Poles, Jews, Africans, and Native Americans) arises from these same sentiments. From the perspective of evolution, being strong rather than weak serves survival.

It seems more parsimonious to explain traumatic reactions as being due to variations in strength among people rather than some complicated medical process of a psychiatric illness such as PTSD. Data that support such a view exist, in that only a portion of people who experience a traumatic event develop PTSD or become disabled, even following horrendous events. In fact, a majority of people appear to weather traumatic events reasonably well after a relatively short period of natural recovery. If two-thirds of people who were raped or experienced severe combat recover within 3 months, then obviously the factor that explains the differences in reaction will be in the individual and not in the event. That factor, previously known as character strength, is now more often termed *resilience*. A great deal of attention and research is now being paid to the nature of resilience (Bonnano 2010; Gonzales

2012). From the point of view of these researchers, the intent is to identify the elements of resilience so that new and improved treatments, or even pretreatments such as refined methods of stress inoculation, can be designed. From the point of view of those who hold a social oppression explanatory model (see "Responses to Social Oppression" subsection later in this chapter), the emphasis on PTSD as an expression of an individual difference takes attention away from the social conditions that give rise to trauma and abuse: if two-thirds of women recover from rape, the sense of urgency in addressing sexism is reduced. The interest in resilience has also engaged those whose explanatory model is physical (see "Physical Processes" subsection later in this chapter), because if a person's resilience lies not in character but in the brain, then the possibility arises of intervening neurologically to strengthen the brain's capacities.

In summary, despite more sophisticated understandings of the causes of PTSD, character weakness remains alive as an explanatory model in the current cultural representations of trauma and victimization.

MORAL WEAKNESS (LYING AND MALINGERING)

A second perspective on the cause of traumatic reactions is that people have moral weakness, as demonstrated through lying and malingering. People lie. People are especially prone to lie if it is in their best interest to lie. People lie, for example, to get themselves out of a dangerous situation, to receive money, to avoid embarrassment, or to stop irritating questions from another family member.

In the history of traumatic reactions, malingering has received the most attention within combat situations, where pretending to be physically unable to return to battle seems an obvious strategy to remain alive. Until World War I, malingering involved the feigning of physical ailments, but once psychiatric ailments were recognized, malingering extended to mental incapacities as well.

Malingering, when viewed as an attempt to get out of harm's way, is explained as another manifestation of character weakness. When malingering is an attempt to gain compensation for an injury, it is viewed as worse: a moral fault. The opportunity for malingering for monetary gain arose in the mid-1800s with the initiation of laws providing compensation for injury. One controversy surrounding malingering began after the creation of railroads, which brought with them accidents and physical injuries. Traumatic reactions that resulted from these crashes and accidents became known as *railway spine* (similar to *whiplash* in today's parlance), which referred not only to physical pain in the spine but also to the idea that the accompanying malaise, anxiety, and disability were due to some injury to the central nervous system (see "Physical

Processes" subsection later in this chapter). An active debate ensued in the late 1800s regarding whether railway spine was a physical injury, a psychological illness, or malingering (Erichsen 1867). Society viewed such complaints—if they lasted more than a few weeks—with a great deal of skepticism. People today receive a similar reaction when they continue to arrive at work wearing a neck collar for weeks following a motor vehicle accident.

Malingering is very damaging to the rights and self-respect of individuals who are truly suffering. Cases of documented malingering and outright deception among a few Vietnam veterans applying for benefits did a tremendous amount of damage to the way the public viewed Vietnam veterans in general. Similar situations occur in cases of false accusations of sexual assault or child abuse. When false accusations, however infrequent, are used to undermine the validity of the truth of traumatic stress reactions, the results can be very damaging. Rather than counter that the number of false claims or reports is actually quite low, a more effective response is to acknowledge that malingering occurs and that it should be properly identified.

Since 1980, when PTSD was officially recognized as a disorder in DSM-III (American Psychiatric Association 1980), courts and juries have awarded victims large amounts of money as compensation, often justifiably so. However, a natural result of such benefit from litigation has been an increasing number of false claims and cases of malingering. The rapidly expanding and highly publicized claims of PTSD in injury cases soon precipitated a counteraction. Organizations such as the False Memory Syndrome Foundation (formed in 1992, http://www.fmsonline.org) sought to protect accused perpetrators of child abuse and developed, in conjunction with the legal profession, increasingly sophisticated legal attacks on the viability of PTSD as a defense.

These false claims and counteractions served to undermine or even eradicate the possibility that legitimate claims of distress or illness could be made. Indeed, some advocates of false memory created the impression that if *any* memory was recovered in psychotherapy, it was likely to be false, because of the implantation of false memories by overzealous therapists. Margaret Hagen (1997), one such proponent, wrote *Whores of the Court: The Fraud of Psychiatric Testimony and the Rape of American Justice*, a demeaning attack on PTSD as pseudo-science and psychiatric fraud, claiming that the entire "PTSD industry" is a self-propelled economically driven effort that views everyone as being traumatized.

Even someone as prominent as Alan Dershowitz (1994) weighed in with *The Abuse Excuse: And Other Cop-outs, Sob Stories, and Evasions of Responsibility*, in which he stated that claims of traumatic disorders will bring down both the economy and democracy. He wrote,

The list of "syndromes" which have been "discovered," "invented," "constructed," or "concocted," as excuses for crime is mind-boggling. They include: battered woman syndrome, Holocaust survivor syndrome, multiple personality disorder, posttraumatic stress disorder, rape trauma syndrome, Stockholm syndrome,…(and included on the same list)…"pornography made me do it defense," "Twinkies made me do it" defense, and tobacco deprivation syndrome. (pp. 18–19).

He criticized the PTSD field for ideas "that encourage people to blame others for their problems" (p. 83).

This disparaging attitude toward trauma victims can be held even when events are well documented. Society may view a victim's expression of pain or injury as being exaggerated and therefore reflective of another agenda: self-interest.

SUGGESTIBILITY (HYSTERIA AND PANIC)

Another variation of weakness as an explanatory model for traumatic reactions is *suggestibility*. Most people are susceptible to suggestion and can easily be convinced of ideas, whether true or not, by demonstrations of authority (Milgram 1974), through specialized methods such as hypnosis (Spiegel and Spiegel 2004), via advertising, or even simply by raising hope, as in the powerful placebo effect (Fabrizio 2008). Indeed, the main claims of the False Memory Syndrome Foundation are that abuse clients are being implanted with memories by their therapists, through leading questions and suggestion. However, suggestibility is much more likely to occur in situations of threat or danger, when both individuals and groups can be sent into panic very rapidly.

Throughout history there have been innumerable incidents of mass panic. Perhaps most relevant to the discussion here is *gas hysteria*, which crippled armies in World War I. Nerve gas agents had just been invented and were used for the first time by both Germany and the Allies. Soldiers were instructed on the signs of being gassed—nausea, racing heartbeat, and trouble breathing—which unfortunately are also symptoms of anxiety. Because nerve gas is invisible, soldiers mistakenly interpreted states of anxiety as having been gassed. Fearful that they would soon die, they dropped their weapons and ran from the front, creating mass retreats. In reality, a gas canister has a very limited effect, harming only people within a few yards of it (Haber 1986). Its major negative effect was to induce panic in the opposing army and cause it to retreat. Because this was true for both sides in the conflict, the collective agreement to ban nerve gas in warfare was achieved in the Geneva Protocol in 1925 (Baker 1925), not only because gas was viewed as a cruel weapon but also because it prevented the generals from conducting the war.

Incidents of mass hysteria continue and are common, though not always widely reported. In 1982, seven people in the Chicago area died after taking pills from bottles of Tylenol that had been contaminated with cyanide, a colorless liquid. Fears rapidly spread that other bottles of Tylenol might also be contaminated. The company first removed all bottles of Tylenol from the shelves of Chicago stores, but this was not sufficient to quell anxieties among the public. A month later, 31 million bottles of Tylenol were removed from all stores in the United States. Eventually, investigators found that only capsules had been poisoned, and the ban was lifted on solid pills.

Each year there are numerous incidents of mass psychogenic illness in schools and workplaces as a result of fears of contamination by unseen toxins or bacteria (Jones 2000). These outbreaks typically cause medical symptoms of the respiratory, gastrointestinal, and circulatory systems, which can temporarily be very debilitating for the victims, although they are often actually symptoms of anxiety.

Panic arising from suggestion is enhanced when people are primed beforehand. For example, merely having people put on a gas mask in a training session will increase the likelihood of their feeling in the future that they have been gassed (Haber 1986). This suggestibility is particularly problematic because it may mean that educating people about a threat beforehand, which is intended to help them prepare, may increase their distress later. Government agencies are hesitant to provide too much information about disasters or other threats for fear of generating unfounded complaints. Disaster planning strategies must take into account the management of a large number of false cases that inevitably clog emergency departments and prevent treatment for truly ill people.

The dilemma is as follows: Educating the public and encouraging them to report child abuse, prepare for disasters, check their houses for radon or carbon monoxide, and identify the signs of PTSD among returning veterans from the Middle East is presumably good public education policy, aimed at lowering the incidence of these conditions. One expects the public to respond by reporting these conditions more often, allowing for better identification. However, an increase in reporting may also be the result of suggestion and lead to the burdening of social agencies with the unnecessary triaging and treatment of false cases. For example, it is possible that bringing greater national attention to the psychological stresses of veterans returning from the Middle East will increase the incidence of reported psychological illnesses in these veterans and referrals for medical care; whether the increase is due to better outreach or to suggestion will likely remain ambiguous.

SUMMARY

The point of view that traumatic reactions are caused by character weakness in its variety of forms remains strong even today, perhaps due to the widespread public interest in trauma. Proponents of this perspective view the mechanism that determines whether symptoms emerge as being within the victim. Recommendations that logically follow from the character weakness perspective are the following: strengthening methods for those whose resilience is low, identification of malingerers, and public education to reduce the incidence of panic and counter the influence of suggestion.

Responses to Social Oppression

The second perspective on the cause of traumatic reactions is that they are the result of oppression by dominant forces, groups, or norms of society. In this perspective, interest in traumatic reactions and the experience of victims is driven by political movements attempting to advocate for the rights of these oppressed classes, which have included women, children, Jews, African Americans, homosexuals, and the poor, among others. The political struggles of each of these classes of people have become attached to an aspect of what is now the field of PTSD: sexual assault and domestic violence, child abuse, anti-Semitism and the Holocaust, racism and postslavery syndrome, homophobia, and neglect. In recent years, bullying (related to school violence) and terrorism have been added to the concerns. Historically, these problems were not initially linked to clinical or psychiatric fields but instead were viewed as social movements. The solutions proposed were not clinical interventions but rather empowerment, public testimony, and civil disobedience. In contrast to the view that traumatic reactions are a form of weakness, which reflects an identification with the perpetrator, the view that traumatic reactions are due to social oppression reflects an identification with the victim.

OPPRESSION OF WOMEN AND CHILDREN

Interestingly, although the history of the diagnosis of PTSD was most influenced by the study of casualties of war among men, a parallel development was occurring in areas related to women and children. From the middle of the nineteenth century to the late twentieth century, rape and sexual assault, domestic violence, and child abuse and neglect, which are now identified as traumatic events, were viewed in the context of civil rights and social action. Nearly simultaneously, the struggle for women's suffrage (right to vote), temperance (prohibition of alcohol), restrictions on child labor, and child protection emerged and interwove with one another. In brief, the fundamental connection among these areas was that women and children were being beaten and abused by intoxicated men.

The years at the turn of the twentieth century leading up to the passage of constitutional amendments 18 (prohibition) and 19 (women's right to vote) reflected a sea change in the cultural context of the rights of women and children. Indeed, the fields of child protection, child guidance, and social work all began during these years. Wayward youths (delinquent boys and pregnant girls) were reconceptualized as children with psychological needs. Although the concept of the battered wife did not emerge formally until the 1970s, the women's movement at the turn of the century was a beginning of its recognition.

During the Great Depression and World War II, American society drew inward toward the need for containment. In the 1960s, however, society began to open up, and culminating events occurred in the civil rights movement for blacks, the women's movement, and the antiwar movement, soon followed by the gay rights movement. This rise in social action provided the environment within which the peer groups of Vietnam veterans (known as "rap" groups) formed, leading to the establishment of the diagnosis of PTSD in 1980. Initially a political movement, the antiwar movement was transformed into an issue for the medical establishment. Similarly and simultaneously, the largely political women's movement supported women's consciousness-raising groups, leading to the opening of battered women's shelters and eventually the recognition that these women were suffering from PTSD symptoms. By the 1980s, *battered woman syndrome* began to be integrated into PTSD; today, sexual and physical assault of women is one of the most prevalent clinical presentations and researched areas within the field of PTSD.

CHILD MALTREATMENT AND ABUSE

Children have likely been sexually and physically abused since the beginning of time. The beating of children must have caused a great deal of personal distress, but generally this was not viewed as a problem until the twentieth century. Freud and Charcot were the first to propose that the hysterical symptoms of adult women might be caused by their sexual abuse as children. So negatively was this suggestion received that Freud eventually abandoned it for the more palpable idea that the hysteria was caused by the women's infantile/unconscious desires for their fathers or other male adults in their childhood.

The history of child protection is also of interest. Arising out of the women's suffrage and prohibition movements at the turn of the twentieth century, and the subsequent formation of the field of social work, child protection and guidance has slowly developed to become one of the most significant components of the field of PTSD.

The child guidance movement had been working independently of the trauma field for over 50 years, with much emphasis being placed on the legal aspects of child maltreatment, such as removal from parents and placement in foster care. Within academia, the field of child maltreatment was also distinct from child psychiatry. Interestingly, not until after the American Psychiatric Association added PTSD as a diagnosis in DSM in 1980 did the work related to childhood maltreatment begin to be integrated into a trauma perspective more generally. With the disruption in family integrity that gripped modern societies in the late twentieth century, child guidance and state agencies began to be empowered to remove children who reported being abused by their parents. The federal Child Abuse Prevention and Treatment Act of 1974 (Pub. L. 93-247) greatly strengthened these efforts by requiring mandatory reporting laws to be enacted in the states. Increasingly, childhood abuse has become a central focus of trauma-based researchers and clinicians. There are approximately 1 million child victims of abuse each year (Children's Bureau 2010), a number that is significantly higher than the approximately 350,000 Vietnam veterans with PTSD (Kulka et al. 1990) and approximately 200,000 rape victims per year (U.S. Department of Justice 2011).

At the cusp of this transition from the problem as civil rights to medical condition, Judith Herman (1981) published *Father-Daughter Incest.* The book received much criticism by a shocked professional audience who could not believe that incest occurred at the frequency the author suggested. By today's standards, the data she reported in her book would be viewed as minimizing the problem. Importantly, however, Herman did not present incest only as a cause of mental distress; she also conceived of it, more fundamentally, as a moral wrong and the basis for supporting women's rights. Herman later emerged as a leader in the PTSD field (Herman 1992).

SUMMARY

Supporters of the social oppression view of the etiology of traumatic reactions emphasize the importance of social advocacy and public testimony in the healing from trauma. Denial and suppression of the stories of these traumatic events are viewed as maintaining the oppressive social order that gave rise to them in the first place, especially when perpetration is conducted by representatives of authority. This perspective embraces the exploration of traumatic experience within psychotherapy but with the caveat that the clients should be encouraged to view the problem not as being within them but instead as having emanated from outside of them in the acts of the perpetrator.

Physical Processes

In contrast to the model of character weakness, which locates the cause in the individual person, and the model of social oppression, which locates the cause in social relationships, the third model locates the cause in physical processes, either external or internal. Throughout the history of the concept of PTSD, observers have often attached the cause of the symptoms to some proximal physical stressor or process (Jones and Wessely 2005). This is due in part to the fact that physical health problems are common sequelae of psychological trauma (Schnurr and Green 2004). However, physical processes also provide a more concrete explanation for the disorder than do the ephemeral psychological processes that only began to be studied and understood midway through the twentieth century.

RAILWAY SPINE

As described previously in the subsection "Character Weakness in the Victim," in the mid-1800s, railway systems were installed. These were by far the fastest mode of transportation yet devised, and as a result numerous railroad accidents occurred that led to physical injuries. In addition to experiencing broken bones and bruises in such accidents, many people began to complain of other symptoms—malaise, anxiety, and loss of control of limbs—that did not resolve in a reasonable amount of time. This condition was labeled *railway spine* because it was assumed that an injury to the spinal cord was responsible for the various nervous system symptoms (Erichsen 1867). Debate raged over the nature of this new condition, and the ultimate conclusion was that it was a form of hysteria.

TROPICAL ASTHENIA

In the late 1800s, scientists such as Louis Pasteur and Robert Koch had established the field of microbacteriology and the role of microorganisms in a range of infectious diseases such as anthrax, tuberculosis, and cholera. The understanding that many illnesses were caused by this new entity, bacteria, which were too small to be seen, permeated society. In 1898, the United States deployed troops in the Spanish American War, and the returning soldiers showed evidence of somatic illnesses. The symptoms included headache, fatigue, loss of appetite, inability to concentrate, vertigo, and irritability (Jones and Wessely 2006). Confused by these symptoms, doctors termed the illness *tropical asthenia* or *swamp asthenia* (*asthenia* being a term for weakness) and hypothesized that it was due to bacteria transmitted to the soldiers when bitten by mosquitoes in the Central American swamps. The prescribed treatment was rest.

SHELL SHOCK

In World War I, soldiers unable to continue fighting reported symptoms of nervousness, fatigue, irritability, loss of concentration, headaches, fainting, mutism, amnesia, and startle responses to hearing the cannon in the distance. This condition, termed *shell shock*, was understood to have been caused by the intense shock wave produced by the new, larger cannons used in World War I, which literally "shook the brain," causing neurological injury within the skull (Myers 1915). By the end of the war, most physicians realized that these were psychological conditions.

GAS HYSTERIA

As described earlier in the subsection "Character Weakness in the Victim," many soldiers in World War I fled the front fearing they had been gassed, when in fact they were experiencing intense fear and anxiety from the battle conditions. Being told they might be gassed by a toxic agent was sufficient for them to make the attribution to this physical cause. Although gas caused only 3% of World War I casualties, it was extremely powerful as a psychological weapon against the confidence of the enemy to fight (Haber 1986).

PERSIAN GULF SYNDROME

In 1990–1991, U.S. troops were subjected to intense experiences in the desert of Kuwait and Iraq. They also were exposed to the fumes from the burning oil wells lit by Saddam Hussein as his troops retreated from Kuwait. When they returned home, many Gulf War veterans began complaining of various symptoms very similar to tropical asthenia, shell shock, and gas hysteria. Many claimed that they had a physical illness caused either by the fumes or by a toxin or bacteria in the desert sands, and the condition was labeled *Persian Gulf syndrome*. This condition has since been assumed to be a psychological response to warfare (Masferrer 1997).

9/11 SICKNESS

After the 9/11 attack, the exposure to smoke and dust from the World Trade Center collapse led many emergency workers and other people to feel that they had been poisoned by toxins from the pulverized computers, building materials, and people. Reported symptoms included nausea, anxiety, fatigue, loss of concentration, physical pains, and headache, with an emphasis on respiratory symptoms (Centers for Disease Control and Prevention 2012). Some concerns about cancer also exist (Lombardi 2006). Fear of contamination was so high that a tanker filled with steel from the World Trade Center was not allowed to unload in Mumbai, India, because of the population's fears that the material was contaminated (Jayaraman and Bruno 2002).

BRAIN DISORDER

In the late twentieth century, scientists developed new radiological methods of examining the brain, including magnetic resonance imaging (MRI) and positron emission tomography (PET), and made significant advances in understanding the neurochemistry of the brain. These developments have led to the current iteration of the physical process model, which views traumatic reactions as caused by the malfunctioning of various neuronal, hormonal, or anatomical systems in the brain, in response to the dramatic surge of adrenaline that accompanies intense fear. Particular attention has been brought to hormonal changes in the hypothalamic-pituitary-adrenal (HPA) axis, as well as neuroanatomical damage to the hippocampus, locus coeruleus, and amygdala (Bremner 1999; Yehuda 2006).

According to this physical process perspective, the potential problem is invisible, hidden inside the brain. By attributing the problem to a physical malfunctioning of the brain, this model also tends to bring attention to the cause of PTSD as being inside the individual rather than resulting from a societal issue, although the model depersonalizes the problem, diminishing blame on both the individual and the perpetrator.

SUMMARY

In summary, physical causes of trauma continue to have power as explanatory models of PTSD. Physical causes are especially likely to be believed when potential exposures involve unseen entities such as bacteria, poisons, gas, or radio waves. These explanations are especially likely in periods after the introduction of a new technology (e.g., railroads, large cannon, nerve gas, PET scan) or new knowledge (e.g., bacteria, neuroscience). In most cases, after the application of various medical or physical treatments has fallen short, psychological etiologies have been recognized.

Overwhelming Arousal

The fourth explanation for traumatic reactions is perhaps the most parsimonious: they are caused by the experience of overwhelming fear or shame. The fact that not all people develop PTSD after a traumatic event is because they experience variations in levels of fear. PTSD symptoms are behaviors conditioned by fear or shame, which are slowly generalized onto other situations not directly connected with the original event. The process is one of distorted learning and of conditioning. This model therefore directs attention to processes within the brain's *cortex*, rather than within the midbrain's limbic structures such as the hippocampus and amygdala.

The single most convincing evidence supporting this model is that through use of methods from learning theory (e.g., exposure, desensitization, cognitive restructuring), symptoms of PTSD can be diminished or eliminated, without the person's character, societal oppression, or brain anatomy being changed. The Institute of Medicine (2007) reviewed all scientific literature on PTSD and concluded that exposure therapy has been shown to be most effective in reducing symptomatology. Desensitization through imaginal exposure is recommended when the person who experienced an event with great fear is continuing to apply that fear to people and situations in the present, as if the initial fear were active. Through exposure to memories of the primary emotions, in a situation where the threat is not present, the person can separate the two states and recondition his or her current behaviors in the absence of fear.

This is very good news, because if traumatic reactions are psychologically caused, they are much more malleable than if they are caused by character, oppression, or anatomy. It is unclear why society has difficulty accepting that intense fear can live on in some persons after a traumatic event. Why do victims of railway accidents, combat, sexual abuse, or 9/11 experience physical pains or other symptoms and not simply say "I was terrified" or "I was humiliated?" Why has it been so difficult for health professionals to recognize that soldiers or battered wives have experienced terror?

The primary reason is avoidance: terror is to be avoided. People would rather hear any other explanation and consider any other proximal cause than the most obvious one—terror—because that one is extremely uncomfortable. People are afraid of the invisible or the unseen, and *fear and shame are invisible. They are also contagious.* This is why society is deeply interested in the containment and avoidance of fear and shame.

The problem with this explanation, however, is that some people who develop PTSD do not report feeling overwhelming emotion at the time of the event (Friedman et al. 2011; Pynoos et al. 2009; Weathers and Keane 2007). First responders, such as police, emergency personnel, and firefighters, may report not having feelings of fear or horror even though over time the stress of being exposed to numerous violent incidents results in symptoms of PTSD, depression, or substance abuse. Emergency workers' training teaches them not to label their reactions as fear or to admit that they were afraid, but enough cases have been documented to show that these individuals may experience fear at the time of an event. In the case of childhood sexual molestation, some victims have reported not feeling in danger or shamed at the time of the event because their perpetrators carefully groomed them and molested them "out of love" without physical violence. Only later, after learning that what happened was wrong, do the victims experience strong emotions of shame, anger, and fear.

Because of these ambiguities, as well as other considerations, the DSM-IV PTSD criterion requiring the experiencing of fear, horror, or helplessness

(American Psychiatric Association 1994) was removed in DSM-5 (American Psychiatric Association 2013). Nevertheless, emotional arousal remains in the DSM-5 criteria for PTSD in the symptoms of psychological and physiological arousal, persistent negative emotions, and irritability (Box 1–1). Ongoing debate about the role of emotion and cognition in the causation of PTSD continues. For purposes of conducting psychotherapy, however, there is little doubt that most clients will present with significant emotional arousal, with both primary and secondary emotions.

Box 1–1. DSM-5 Criteria for Posttraumatic Stress Disorder

Note: The following criteria apply to adults, adolescents, and children older than 6 years. For children 6 years and younger, see corresponding criteria below.

A. Exposure to actual or threatened death, serious injury, or sexual violence in one (or more) of the following ways:

1. Directly experiencing the traumatic event(s).
2. Witnessing, in person, the event(s) as it occurred to others.
3. Learning that the traumatic event(s) occurred to a close family member or close friend. In cases of actual or threatened death of a family member or friend, the event(s) must have been violent or accidental.
4. Experiencing repeated or extreme exposure to aversive details of the traumatic event(s) (e.g., first responders collecting human remains; police officers repeatedly exposed to details of child abuse).

   Note: Criterion A4 does not apply to exposure through electronic media, television, movies, or pictures, unless this exposure is work related.

B. Presence of one (or more) of the following intrusion symptoms associated with the traumatic event(s), beginning after the traumatic event(s) occurred:

1. Recurrent, involuntary, and intrusive distressing memories of the traumatic event(s).

   Note: In children older than 6 years, repetitive play may occur in which themes or aspects of the traumatic event(s) are expressed.
2. Recurrent distressing dreams in which the content and/or affect of the dream are related to the traumatic event(s).

   Note: In children, there may be frightening dreams without recognizable content.
3. Dissociative reactions (e.g., flashbacks) in which the individual feels or acts as if the traumatic event(s) were recurring. (Such reactions may occur on a continuum, with the most extreme expression being a complete loss of awareness of present surroundings.)

   Note: In children, trauma-specific reenactment may occur in play.
4. Intense or prolonged psychological distress at exposure to internal or external cues that symbolize or resemble an aspect of the traumatic event(s).
5. Marked physiological reactions to internal or external cues that symbolize or resemble an aspect of the traumatic event(s).

C. Persistent avoidance of stimuli associated with the traumatic event(s), beginning after the traumatic event(s) occurred, as evidenced by one or both of the following:

1. Avoidance of or efforts to avoid distressing memories, thoughts, or feelings about or closely associated with the traumatic event(s).
2. Avoidance of or efforts to avoid external reminders (people, places, conversations, activities, objects, situations) that arouse distressing memories, thoughts, or feelings about or closely associated with the traumatic event(s).

D. Negative alterations in cognitions and mood associated with the traumatic event(s), beginning or worsening after the traumatic event(s) occurred, as evidenced by two (or more) of the following:

1. Inability to remember an important aspect of the traumatic event(s) (typically due to dissociative amnesia and not to other factors such as head injury, alcohol, or drugs).
2. Persistent and exaggerated negative beliefs or expectations about oneself, others, or the world (e.g., "I am bad," "No one can be trusted," "The world is completely dangerous," "My whole nervous system is permanently ruined").
3. Persistent, distorted cognitions about the cause or consequences of the traumatic event(s) that lead the individual to blame himself/herself or others.
4. Persistent negative emotional state (e.g., fear, horror, anger, guilt, or shame).
5. Markedly diminished interest or participation in significant activities.
6. Feelings of detachment or estrangement from others.
7. Persistent inability to experience positive emotions (e.g., inability to experience happiness, satisfaction, or loving feelings).

E. Marked alterations in arousal and reactivity associated with the traumatic event(s), beginning or worsening after the traumatic event(s) occurred, as evidenced by two (or more) of the following:

1. Irritable behavior and angry outbursts (with little or no provocation) typically expressed as verbal or physical aggression toward people or objects.
2. Reckless or self-destructive behavior.
3. Hypervigilance.
4. Exaggerated startle response.
5. Problems with concentration.
6. Sleep disturbance (e.g., difficulty falling or staying asleep or restless sleep).

F. Duration of the disturbance (Criteria B, C, D, and E) is more than 1 month.

G. The disturbance causes clinically significant distress or impairment in social, occupational, or other important areas of functioning.

H. The disturbance is not attributable to the physiological effects of a substance (e.g., medication, alcohol) or another medical condition.

Specify whether:

With dissociative symptoms: The individual's symptoms meet the criteria for posttraumatic stress disorder, and in addition, in response to the stressor, the individual experiences persistent or recurrent symptoms of either of the following:

1. **Depersonalization:** Persistent or recurrent experiences of feeling detached from, and as if one were an outside observer of, one's mental processes or body (e.g., feeling as though one were in a dream; feeling a sense of unreality of self or body or of time moving slowly).

2. **Derealization:** Persistent or recurrent experiences of unreality of surroundings (e.g., the world around the individual is experienced as unreal, dreamlike, distant, or distorted).

Note: To use this subtype, the dissociative symptoms must not be attributable to the physiological effects of a substance (e.g., blackouts, behavior during alcohol intoxication) or another medical condition (e.g., complex partial seizures).

Specify if:

With delayed expression: If the full diagnostic criteria are not met until at least 6 months after the event (although the onset and expression of some symptoms may be immediate).

Posttraumatic Stress Disorder for Children 6 Years and Younger

A. In children 6 years and younger, exposure to actual or threatened death, serious injury, or sexual violence in one (or more) of the following ways:

1. Directly experiencing the traumatic event(s).
2. Witnessing, in person, the event(s) as it occurred to others, especially primary caregivers.

    Note: Witnessing does not include events that are witnessed only in electronic media, television, movies, or pictures.

3. Learning that the traumatic event(s) occurred to a parent or caregiving figure.

B. Presence of one (or more) of the following intrusion symptoms associated with the traumatic event(s), beginning after the traumatic event(s) occurred:

1. Recurrent, involuntary, and intrusive distressing memories of the traumatic event(s).

    Note: Spontaneous and intrusive memories may not necessarily appear distressing and may be expressed as play reenactment.

2. Recurrent distressing dreams in which the content and/or affect of the dream are related to the traumatic event(s).

    Note: It may not be possible to ascertain that the frightening content is related to the traumatic event.

3. Dissociative reactions (e.g., flashbacks) in which the child feels or acts as if the traumatic event(s) were recurring. (Such reactions may occur on a continuum, with the most extreme expression being a complete loss of awareness of present surroundings.) Such trauma-specific reenactment may occur in play.

4. Intense or prolonged psychological distress at exposure to internal or external cues that symbolize or resemble an aspect of the traumatic event(s).

5. Marked physiological reactions to reminders of the traumatic event(s).

C. One (or more) of the following symptoms, representing either persistent avoidance of stimuli associated with the traumatic event(s) or negative alterations in cognitions and mood associated with the traumatic event(s), must be present, beginning after the event(s) or worsening after the event(s):

Persistent Avoidance of Stimuli

1. Avoidance of or efforts to avoid activities, places, or physical reminders that arouse recollections of the traumatic event(s).

2. Avoidance of or efforts to avoid people, conversations, or interpersonal situations that arouse recollections of the traumatic event(s).

Negative Alterations in Cognitions

3. Substantially increased frequency of negative emotional states (e.g., fear, guilt, sadness, shame, confusion).
4. Markedly diminished interest or participation in significant activities, including constriction of play.
5. Socially withdrawn behavior.
6. Persistent reduction in expression of positive emotions.

D. Alterations in arousal and reactivity associated with the traumatic event(s), beginning or worsening after the traumatic event(s) occurred, as evidenced by two (or more) of the following:

1. Irritable behavior and angry outbursts (with little or no provocation) typically expressed as verbal or physical aggression toward people or objects (including extreme temper tantrums).
2. Hypervigilance.
3. Exaggerated startle response.
4. Problems with concentration.
5. Sleep disturbance (e.g., difficulty falling or staying asleep or restless sleep).

E. The duration of the disturbance is more than 1 month.
F. The disturbance causes clinically significant distress or impairment in relationships with parents, siblings, peers, or other caregivers or with school behavior.
G. The disturbance is not attributable to the physiological effects of a substance (e.g., medication or alcohol) or another medical condition.

Specify whether:

With dissociative symptoms: The individual's symptoms meet the criteria for posttraumatic stress disorder, and the individual experiences persistent or recurrent symptoms of either of the following:

1. **Depersonalization:** Persistent or recurrent experiences of feeling detached from, and as if one were an outside observer of, one's mental processes or body (e.g., feeling as though one were in a dream; feeling a sense of unreality of self or body or of time moving slowly).
2. **Derealization:** Persistent or recurrent experiences of unreality of surroundings (e.g., the world around the individual is experienced as unreal, dreamlike, distant, or distorted).

Note: To use this subtype, the dissociative symptoms must not be attributable to the physiological effects of a substance (e.g., blackouts) or another medical condition (e.g., complex partial seizures).

Specify if:

With delayed expression: If the full diagnostic criteria are not met until at least 6 months after the event (although the onset and expression of some symptoms may be immediate).

CHANGING ATTITUDES TOWARD THE TREATMENT OF TRAUMATIC REACTIONS

The modern notion of traumatic reaction as a psychological event is probably best located at the end of World War II. Since that time, the responses to combat, sexual assault, child abuse, disasters and accidents, and ethnic or racial oppression have been combined and become medicalized within the overarching concept of posttraumatic stress. All of the contradictory streams discussed in the previous sections of this chapter continue to express themselves in an active debate about how best to treat victims of traumatic events. Interestingly, these attitudes have changed dramatically over the past 50 years.

During and after World War II, soldiers' symptomatic reactions to combat were labeled *war neuroses.* This label represented a major advance from earlier descriptions because it identified the traumatic event (war) and indicated that the reactions were psychological in nature (neuroses). Abraham Kardiner (1941) and W. Ronald Fairbairn (1943), among others, were key observers. Influenced by psychoanalytic notions of the unconscious, their view was that the memories of the traumatic incidents were deeply hidden in the unconscious and required strong measures to pull them out. Because of the apparent reluctance of the veterans to discuss their experiences, as well as the disguised form of many of the symptoms (e.g., catatonia, somatic manifestations), great effort and skill were deemed necessary to uncover the underlying events.

During the 1950s, therefore, measures such as hypnosis, sodium amytal injections, and direct interpretations were used in treatment for war neuroses. As late as the 1970s, Lawrence Kolb, a psychiatrist, used sodium amytal to stimulate remembering in war veterans. In one case, presented in a videotape by Kolb, a young Vietnam veteran, while lying on a bed, became overwhelmed with fear and was screaming and wide-eyed as he remembered his combat experience. Kolb viewed this as a therapeutic catharsis aided by the drug, which helped to break through the victim's hard shell of denial and defense that were covering the trauma (Blanchard et al. 1982).

The idea that traumas were deeply buried was also present in early behavioral treatments for PTSD. Notably, Terence Keane and colleagues (1989) showed that *implosive* or *flooding therapy,* an exposure-based method, reduced symptoms of PTSD in Vietnam combat veterans. In this therapy, based on behavioral treatments of phobias, the veteran was presented with an audiotape of war sounds (helicopters, battle sounds, and explosions) while being guided through a script of the memory. The intention was to do this in the most vivid and intense manner possible, to allow habituation to occur. In a videotaped case presented by Dr. Keane, a Vietnam veteran fell out of the chair he was sitting in when he began remembering his event and, dissociated, crawled around to the back of the chair in complete terror, while the voice of Dr. Keane calmly continued to lead him through the memory. This work was based on the process of desensitization rather than catharsis, but the methods were very comparable. Most important, the idea that one had to work hard to break through to the traumatic memory was consistent with the then-current view of trauma.

Extending the work of Keane to women who have been raped, Edna Foa developed a similar procedure, called *prolonged exposure*, in which the client develops a detailed verbal description of the traumatic event and then reads it over and over for an hour for each of nine sessions and listens to a tape of it at home between sessions (Foa et al. 2007). The idea is that intense continued exposure to the traumatic memory, during a state of arousal, will alter the fear schema. As Foa and Rothbaum (1998) stated, "This activation constitutes an opportunity for corrective information to be integrated, and thus to modify the pathological elements of the trauma memory" (p. 85).

Simultaneously, the major figures of the sexual assault and incest field, such as Judith Herman (1992), Christine Courtois (1988), and Mary Harvey, also emphasized how deeply buried their clients' memories were because of their clients' reluctance to speak about their experiences due to the patriarchal society's control over women, and the victims' resulting deep sense of shame. For sexually assaulted women, a highly nurturing therapeutic environment was recommended, which included placing the blame on the perpetrator and continuing to encourage the clients to speak. The goal at this time might be best characterized as "breaking the silence."

The recognition of PTSD in DSM-III and DSM-IV empowered the advocacy movements of women and veterans, and PTSD and trauma soon became a highly popular and energized area for researchers and for journalists, novelists, and filmmakers, among others. Also, significant financial support, attention, and organizational fervor were available throughout the 1980s and into the 1990s.

Changes in the larger culture were also relevant to the transformation in attitudes. Reality television shows and talk shows that emphasized the open discussion of private matters proliferated, and the expansion of the Internet and then social networks challenged traditional notions of privacy. The reactions against so much attention to trauma only stirred up more interest.

By 2000, the dominant belief about trauma—that trauma is barely skin deep and that it could surface with the slightest suggestion—was in direct contrast to that previously held. The development of brief but effective treatments such as *eye movement desensitization and reprocessing* (Shapiro 1995), in which the client thinks about the trauma while tracking the therapist's fingers moving back and forth, or the *counting method* (Ochberg 1996), in which the client thinks about the trauma while the therapist counts aloud to 100, also challenged the idea that trauma treatment necessitates intensive exposure.

Mental health professionals are now less likely to be taught about strong measures such as hypnosis, cathartic treatments, or even intense exposure therapy and instead are taught to ensure client safety, with techniques such as braking, distracting, grounding, and structuring (Briere and Scott 2006). Clinicians are warned against inducing traumatic reenactments and flooding the clients. Whereas only two decades before, trauma was "walled off," it now is a "dam ready to break," "a Pandora's box."

Herman's (1992) advice in her seminal book *Trauma and Recovery*—that remembrance and mourning should follow the establishment of safety—and Marsha Linehan's (1993) premise in her *dialectical behavior therapy*—that traumatic memories should be addressed after the client develops affect regulation skills—also supported a more cautious approach to traumatic inquiry. Interest has also increased in studying resilience, strengths-based treatments, and posttraumatic growth, while less attention is focused on the details of a traumatic experience.

Expressions of concerns about establishing a safe therapeutic environment have increased in recent years to near warnings against engaging with traumatic memories at all. Fears of increased symptoms, drug or alcohol use relapse, or suicidality are often noted (Craemer et al. 2004). Strangely, this trend has occurred even though the most empirically supported forms of PTSD treatment, based on exposure methods, do not require long periods of preparation prior to the initiation of processing traumatic memories. For example, prolonged exposure uses one session, implosive therapy requires two or three sessions, and both the counting method (Ochberg 1996) and eye movement desensitization and reprocessing (Shapiro 1995) often begin in the first session. Clinicians and researchers have found that trauma survivors perceive being in a therapist's office, even for the first time, as safe enough to begin this processing. The danger lies in their memories, not in the external circumstances of the therapy. Despite this contradiction, the trend continues toward greater hesitance in directly addressing the trauma.

CONCLUSION

At the present time in history, the balance between containment and expression has shifted back toward containment. There appears to be greater skepticism about claims of distress over traumatic events and greater hesitance regarding direct inquiry about traumatic experience and its accompanying emotional expression, as well as renewed interest in physical causes in the brain rather than in the psychological experience of fear or shame. Nevertheless, there remains a healthy amount of public expression by victims of trauma, activism about child abuse and other forms of social oppression, and active psychiatric and psychological scholarship devoted to the treatment of trauma.

Mental health professionals have been trained to treat trauma for 30 years: in the 1980s they were asked whether their methods were strong enough, in the 1990s whether the methods were scientific enough, and now whether they are safe enough. The notion that trauma is deeply buried and difficult to access was therefore most likely a result of society's taboos about talking about it. Today's views that trauma is too easily accessed and that treatment should proceed carefully are most likely due to the fact that traumatic events are now more often identified and openly discussed. As noted in the beginning of this chapter, people who are silent are encouraged to speak out, and people who are speaking too much are asked to be quiet.

The conclusion from this historical review of the concepts of trauma and PTSD is that they have been strongly influenced by the changing value systems within the wider culture. This is true because of the moral and legal dimensions of PTSD. The overlap among ethics, law, and psychopathology is highly influenced by varying interpretations by the wider societal culture. Allan Young (1995), in *The Harmony of Illusions: Inventing Posttraumatic Stress Disorder*, makes this point, and although he reiterates that his book is not intended to question the suffering of victims of violence, he essentially proposes that rather than being an objective disease, PTSD is a relative construct that serves the cultural and economic needs of the time.

The simple truth appears to be that society responds best to victims of traumatic events who present themselves as having overcome them. It is these survivors who are believed and offered sympathy. Victims who present themselves as being ruined, disabled, and unable to function are more likely to be viewed as deficient in character or to not be believed.

Even though society's dominant understanding of the nature of PTSD has changed over time, this does not mean that it does not exist as an illness. Traumatic reactions do exist, have existed, and will continue to exist; they have caused tremendous amounts of suffering and disability, burdening individuals as well as society at large. The labels and names may vary, but the descriptions of the suffering have not, as writers as far back as Homer will attest (Shay 1995).

We intend for this book to be a straightforward presentation of how to conduct a trauma inquiry with clients in a psychotherapy context. Given the historical and cultural analysis presented in this chapter, however, some readers may find themselves wondering if it is necessary to spend a great deal of time on the details of the traumatic event, at a high level of intensity, and with so much immediacy. In this sense, trauma-centered psychotherapy will always be considered in relation to the values and norms of its cultural surroundings, which are constantly in transition. Addressing psychological trauma will never be a neutral act. It takes a certain degree of courage in both the client and the therapist to face these tragedies. Ultimately, what should encourage persistence is an abiding commitment to alleviate suffering and to seek a more just and less violent society.

STUDY QUESTIONS

1.1   What are the four main explanatory causes for PTSD?

1.2   When should an individual's experience of trauma be contained, and when should it be expressed?

1.3   What was the difference in the profession's view of trauma prior to 1960 and after 1990?

1.4   Why are treatments such as sodium amytal and hypnosis not used often now for the treatment of PTSD?

1.5   Describe these conditions:

    A. Railway spine
    B. Tropical asthenia
    C. Shell shock
    D. Gas hysteria
    E. War neurosis

1.6   Attribution to physical causes for PTSD tended to follow what developments?

1.7   Why is there a conflict between evidence for exposure therapy and physical causes?

1.8   Why does PTSD present itself so often as a physical malady?

1.9   Do you think that the diagnosis and treatment of PTSD as a medical condition contributes to an avoidance of dealing with the sources of social oppression in our society?

CHAPTER 2

Axioms of Trauma-Centered Psychotherapy

The presentation of trauma-centered psychotherapy is organized in three levels. In this chapter four *axiomatic concepts* are presented that provide a foundation for the work and situate the encounter between the therapist and the client within certain boundaries (Table 2–1). The establishment and maintenance of these boundaries become the trauma-centered frame, without which the interaction is likely to depart from its intended purpose (see Chapter 3, "Establishing the Trauma-Centered Frame"). Second, in Chapter 4 ("Principles of Trauma-Centered Psychotherapy") three basic *principles* that the therapist should apply in his or her clinical interventions are presented. Whereas the axioms refer to the nature of trauma, the principles guide the therapist's behavior. These principles, when followed, concretize the trauma-centered environment for the client, communicating forcibly to him or her that the interaction with the therapist will not be like other therapeutic interactions. Finally, in Chapter 5 ("The Four Main Techniques"), the specific *techniques* that the therapist can use in the moment-to-moment process of trauma-centered work are introduced. These techniques follow from the principles and axioms but are highly specific to particular moments of the therapy. Later chapters present the use of these techniques in treatment.

TABLE 2–1.   Axioms of trauma-centered psychotherapy

---

1. Trauma schemas arise in order to reduce the primary emotions of fear and shame.

    Trauma schemas (patterns of thought and behavior) are activated in the present moment when aspects of the current situation are similar to those of the traumatic event, to protect the person from reexperiencing the painful emotions that occurred during the event.

2. Both client and therapist will be participating in avoidance to some degree all the time.

    Avoidance of traumatic events and experiences is an extremely pervasive process that should be assumed to be operating in each moment in both client and therapist.

3. The client's trauma narrative is always incomplete.

    Because of the presumed operation of avoidance, both during and after the traumatic event, the client's narrative of the event is unlikely to be complete, and therefore the therapist should never imply closure during a trauma inquiry.

4. Trauma schemas are relational.

    Regardless of whether events are interpersonal or natural disasters, victims of trauma will attribute the lack of protection from harm to another person, such as the perpetrator or other people who should have been able to help.

AXIOM 1: TRAUMA SCHEMAS ARISE IN ORDER TO REDUCE THE PRIMARY EMOTIONS OF FEAR AND SHAME

Following a traumatic incident, an individual may feel a variety of emotions, such as sadness, fear, shame, guilt, anxiety, and anger, but fear and shame are the engines of traumatic experience and its sequelae in the clinical arena. *Trauma schemas* are representational structures that develop after a traumatic event in an attempt to stabilize the person's shattered world, and the first and foremost purpose of these schemas is to reduce the reexperiencing of the primary emotions of fear and shame. When a trauma schema is triggered in life or in the therapy session, it is almost always in response to an anticipated moment of fear or shame. In later chapters, we examine the various permutations of what is feared or shameful, but for the purposes of this chapter, it is sufficient to know that in the therapist's journey with the client into traumatic material, fear and shame are what need to be sensed, noticed, and dealt with. Fear and shame are what drive most of the client's and therapist's avoidance. They are what cause therapists to hesitate, withdraw, placate, or lecture.

The implication of the first axiom—that trauma schemas arise in order to reduce the primary emotions of fear and shame—is that the therapist should be on the watch for moments of fear or shame, however minute, and when detected, should move in on them. Moving away from the client's experience of these primary emotions is likely to communicate immediately to the client that the therapist is unprepared for the work that follows, and the client may respond with numerous obstacles, excuses, or challenges for the therapist. The eruption of a client's resistance or challenging behavior is usually a sign that the therapist has just missed an opportunity to address a moment of fear or shame.

Not only should the therapist be an expert in identifying emotional arousal in the client and be able to move toward that experience, but the therapist must do so while demonstrating that he or she has a minimum of fear or shame. The therapist should communicate that he or she is very familiar with this territory and that although the client is terrified, the therapist is not. The therapist may be weathered, even scarred, by previous forays into these jungles, deserts, caves, or fires, but he or she needs to remain calm.

As demonstrated throughout the book, not establishing at the beginning of treatment that the work will be about fear and shame will create the conditions by which the experience of emotion may be viewed as a problem for the client or a mistake by the therapist or a contraindication for the method. Obviously, this first axiom will have significant impact on how the issue of *safety* is characterized. Too much emphasis on establishing safety will create a problem when highly emotional states emerge into the process. It is better to emphasize *risk* than to emphasize safety, and to communicate to the client that the risk is manageable and that the fear can be overcome with the help of the therapist. All growth and learning take place in a state of relative risk; many important, normal developmental tasks, such as learning to ride a bicycle, dive into water, downhill ski, drive a car, or form an intimate relationship, are faced with some trepidation. When children say that riding a bicycle is "too scary," parents do not usually say, "Okay, you do not need to learn to ride a bike." Instead, they say, "With my help, you will be able to ride a bike." When a teenager says he is too scared to ask a friend for a date, parents encourage him to do so. They cannot tell their child that dating is without risk, that it is safe. Similarly, when a client says, early in the therapeutic process, "I cannot do this; going over my trauma is too painful," the trauma-centered therapist does not say that it is okay but rather says, "Yes, there is risk, but you—we—can do it."

As an example, a 30-year-old female client described her rape to her therapist:

> Then he told me to go back into the room, the bedroom, and I knew what he was going to do, I just knew it, and…I…had trouble opening the door…The doorknob was stuck. I was nervous. Anyway, he pushed me onto the bed and raped me. I was out of it, just looked up at the ceiling or something….

From an objective point of view, the therapist might view the rape as the most important and most intense act and therefore follow up with questions regarding the sexual assault. However, the client's narrative broke up, and she showed a spike of anxiety, when she was speaking about not being able to open the door. From the point of view of the first axiom, the therapist should inquire about her not being able to open the door.

> THERAPIST: So tell me more about not being able to open the door.
> CLIENT (*showing heightened anxiety*): I just couldn't open it, I was nervous, it was stupid, it was my own bedroom door.
> THERAPIST: What happened?
> CLIENT: He raped me.
> THERAPIST: No, I mean what happened when you couldn't open the door?
> CLIENT: He grabbed my hair and slammed my head against the door.
> THERAPIST: That is horrible….Did he say something?
> CLIENT: Yeah, he said, "Open the door you f—king bitch, or I'll crack your head open." (*Cries.*)
> THERAPIST: You must have been terrified.
> CLIENT: Yes, I didn't want to die.

The client seemed somewhat prepared for the inevitable rape, although she was not prepared for the physical assault, which surprised and frightened her. The therapist correctly put aside assumptions about what the traumatic event might be and picked up on the obvious signs of arousal and fear in the client's narrative, allowing an approach to the sliver of experience that was terrifying to her.

Trauma-centered work takes place in a state of some risk, some reawakened fear or shame, and the therapist should show equanimity when the client periodically clutches and falls, just as parents do when they allow their child to fall off the bike in the school parking lot.

AXIOM 2: BOTH CLIENT AND THERAPIST WILL BE PARTICIPATING IN AVOIDANCE TO SOME DEGREE ALL THE TIME

To live even a minimally ordered and peaceful life, each person must avoid a myriad of small and large truths; this state is what Janoff-Bulman (1992) and others have called the *assumptive world*. People live in a bubble of illusion, or else no one would get in a car and drive on the highway. Thankfully, people do not know of all the suffering occurring around the world, or in the poor neighborhoods in their own towns, or even in the houses next door. In the therapeutic session, as clients approach talking about what happened to them, they do so only partially, constantly editing the details as they monitor the therapist's reactions, as well as their own. Therapists, meanwhile, can guess at some of the events left out of the clients' descriptions, carefully choosing to ask about only some of those guesses. The world around both the client and the therapist is also steeped in denial and avoidance: The client's family and friends no longer ask or are tired of hearing about the incident, or they do not believe that it happened. The therapist's colleagues and family also have limited capacity to hear about the work. As the many thousands of therapists sit with their clients, listening to the horrors of what people do to each other, the world goes on, seemingly creating more and more injured souls.

The axiom of avoidance suggests that no matter how attentive the therapist thinks he or she is, or how open the client seems to be, both are also avoiding something more. This something, of course, is fear or shame (axiom 1). The client is applying his or her trauma schemas to manage these emotions, the therapist is applying his or her defenses to protect himself or herself, and soon the client and therapist manage to co-create new strategies and new agreements that support the avoidance of the traumatic material. Because these cocreated behaviors are very destructive to the task of trauma-centered psychotherapy, they should be scrupulously identified and disrupted. The most common one is *delay:* "I don't feel up to it today"; "The client needs more time to build an alliance with me"; or "A stressful event or holiday or vacation is coming up, so we should wait." Another is the *warm-up:* "Before we get back into talking about your rape, how are things going?" or "I'd like to know more about your family in general before we tackle your abuse." Another is the *immediate crisis:* "I'd like to talk about it, but I have to discuss what happened last night…it's really terrible" or "Doctor, what am I going to do about my daughter's pregnancy?" Methods of handling each of these situations are discussed in Chapter 4. Nevertheless, this axiom states that both therapist and client will be appreciative of any opportunity to avoid further exploration of the fearful memories, often while believing that what they are doing instead is important, or justified by another, non-trauma-centered, perspective. Because there are indeed many important things to be working on, it is not hard to justify avoidance of the trauma work. If the therapist remembers this axiom, however, he or she will know that both therapist and client are avoiding and perhaps will be able to bring the session back on track sooner. In the end, as clinical transcripts will demonstrate, once the trauma-centered work has begun, *there is nothing else to do but that*. When the client sees that the therapist is capable of standing behind the trauma inquiry, the client's courage is usually bolstered, as evidenced in the following session fragment.

THERAPIST: Good morning, Pete. How are things going?
CLIENT: Not so good. My son got a DUI last night, and we had a huge fight....He ended up storming out of the house, and I don't know where he is now....He won't respond to my phone calls.
THERAPIST: I see. You must be worried.
CLIENT: Well, he's 22, so he's not 6 or something, though frankly he acts like it sometimes. I don't know. I guess he will come home.
THERAPIST: Are you worried more about him being out and not answering your phone calls or drinking and driving?
CLIENT: Both, really.

In a general psychotherapy frame, discussing this incident further would be entirely appropriate, because it seems to be an important aspect of this client's family life. Helping Pete think through how he is going to deal with his son's behavior will be useful. However, if this is a trauma-centered psychotherapy, continuing to discuss this current issue is a form of avoidance. The therapist participates in this avoidance by asking the innocent question "How are things going?," which serves to elicit current issues rather than continue the trauma inquiry. The therapist ignores the client's comment that his son is "not 6 or something," which could be a reference to the abuse Pete experienced when he was 6, as well as the subtle references to his own parent's alcoholism and frequent neglect when they left Pete alone in the house for long periods of time. Breaking into this discussion abruptly and redirecting the client to his past traumas will be impolite at best and disruptive at worst if the overall frame of the work has not been previously established. This issue is addressed in Chapter 3. For the current purposes, this example demonstrates the challenge to the therapist in maintaining the trauma inquiry when other important issues arise.

AXIOM 3: THE CLIENT'S TRAUMA NARRATIVE IS ALWAYS INCOMPLETE

Axiom 3 follows logically from axiom 2, because if avoidance is in effect to some degree, then there are details that have not been shared. The result is that as a clinical rule, the therapist should never assume that closure has been attained, no matter how detailed or explicit the client's telling has been.

As long as the client has pain, or fear, or symptoms, a piece of frightening memory remains lodged inside.

If one thinks about a traumatic experience as a narrative with multiple layers, each one more detailed and explicit than the last, then it makes sense that when telling his or her story to someone else, the client begins with the outer layer first and then reveals more details until the listener indicates belief that he or she has heard the full story. For example, the following statements are all descriptions of the same event: "He messed me up last night." "I was raped." "He pushed me down on the floor and slapped me hard before ripping off my pants and entering me." "As he was finishing, he laughed and said he wanted to push the broomstick all the way up to my throat." At which statement would someone feel they had heard enough? Usually, this is indicated when the listener says, "Yes, that was *terrible!*" and then shifts eye contact or bodily posture. The axiom of incompleteness acknowledges that the last statement about the broomstick is not the end; there is still more. In fact, there is always more. As a result, the trauma-centered psychotherapist often ends sessions with "and I know there is more" rather than "that was quite a lot."

Many therapists conducting trauma inquiries make the mistake of communicating to the client that they have heard the complete story, or at least complete enough. Indeed, they may have heard a lot; however, the worst is among the last to be told. Some clients will reveal new details about a traumatic experience years into their therapy, long after the therapist had made the assumption that the story had been told.

An important ramification of this axiom, which is discussed in more detail in Chapter 8 ("Conducting Ongoing Treatment"), is that when the client goes home after a session and becomes distressed, and then calls the therapist to leave a message that "the session was too upsetting," it is due to details *that he or she did not reveal* rather than those that the client talked about. Therapists often make a mistake at this point by thinking the session covered too much rather than too little and agree to back off from the inquiry. Instead, trauma-centered therapists will explain to the client that they are sorry the client became upset and that it is because no doubt they missed something, a detail perhaps, that the client had wanted to mention.

Similarly, the upsetting details that clients do not mention are sometimes about events that did not happen. It seems sensible that if one had had a bad experience and was asked to describe it, one would speak about what had happened. However, the worst part of many trauma experiences, the ones that carry the most fear, are the moments when one imagines that something even more terrible is about to happen. These are often the parts of the narrative that a client avoids and does not mention. For example, a woman was in a car accident in which she was rear-ended by another driver. She was thrown forward in the car but was completely unhurt. Her infant child was in his car seat in the back seat and was also fine. The car had minor dents. The woman became flooded with posttraumatic stress disorder (PTSD) symptoms in the month after the accident, to the point that she was unable to work. Why? Because when the car was hit and she was thrown forward, a package sitting on the back seat was also thrown forward into the windshield. For a split second, she had the thought that she had not secured her child's car seat, because she had just transferred it from the family's other car that morning, and that the package was her infant. She experienced a brief moment of unbelievable terror over an event that did not happen. She was viewed as being hysterical and overreacting to the accident, and her first therapist viewed her as having a personality disorder. Once this piece of terror was identified and expressed, however, her symptoms ameliorated immediately.

A man became totally disabled after an incident at work in which a container of flammable material spilled and he was hemmed in by it for 15 minutes before they were able to extract him. The fluid never ignited, and he was unharmed. Nevertheless, within a month he became flooded with PTSD symptoms. The missing detail was that 2 months earlier a similar fluid container had burst into flames and killed a worker at the plant, as this man watched helplessly.

A Vietnam veteran had serious and long-standing PTSD symptoms although he had not had any combat experience. He was accused of being a malingerer, but his symptoms were real. Therapists concluded that he might have had childhood trauma instead, but he had not experienced any. The missing detail was that in Vietnam he was a lineman, who sat in a cherry picker, without a weapon, and repaired telephone lines cut by the Viet Cong, while his buddies sat inside the armor-plated vehicle below. The average lifetime of linemen was weeks, because they were easy prey for snipers. Each moment he was up there, he was waiting to be shot. He survived in this job for 3 months. He was never shot at. Nothing happened, except he experienced a state of constant fear. When this story was finally revealed in therapy, the patient said, "I never thought to bring it up." As a result of this understanding, he learned why he was so hyperaroused: "I guess I am always so on edge because I think I am about to be shot." This was his core trauma schema.

When helping clients construct a narrative of their trauma, therapists should be on alert to what is being left out, particularly moments of fear over events that did not happen. Narratives that stick too closely to the events rather than the states of emotional experience may lose their therapeutic effectiveness. As an illustration, compare the following trauma narratives of the same event. The main narrative is presented in regular type; the missing personal reflections of the client not mentioned to the therapist are presented in italic type.

> I was 20 years old, home from college, and driving a taxi at night during the summer. I picked up this guy—oh, he was about 30, had a jacket on, seemed nice enough—and took him to the address he gave me. He asked me to stop in the middle of the street in this residential neighborhood. Suddenly, I felt funny. *I had the fleeting thought, oh no, I'm going to be mugged like I had been before.* Next thing I knew, my head was in my lap, and blood was spurting out of my head. *The flap of my skin had fallen over my eye, so I thought for a second that my eye had been knocked out, and I wondered if it was on the floor of the cab…I didn't want to step on it.* I put my hand on my forehead and looked back and saw him holding a hammer in the air. *The light from a street light was coming in behind him, so he looked like I don't know what…I was terrified…It looked like he was about to hit me again with the hammer…I saw his hand holding the hammer tight…He was going to hit me directly on my skull and kill me or I'd be brain damaged…He seemed deranged. I will never be able to get that scene out of my head, ever.* I cried out, "Don't hit me again! I'll give you my money." And he got out of the car, looking distracted, and then took my wallet. *I tried to give him just the cash in my wallet but he grabbed it…I was so mad that my license was going to be taken…He didn't have to do that.* He threw the wallet to the ground and ran off. I called dispatch, and in a few moments two other taxis came, and they took me to the hospital, where my dad met me. I was okay, because he had hit me on the forehead, so they stitched me up and I went home.

It was the man's terror over the eyeball on the floor, being hit again with the hammer, and the license being taken—none of which had occurred—that most haunted the client, even years later. The important point is that it is useful for trauma-centered psychotherapists to remember that at all times their work is being conducted in a condition of incompleteness.

AXIOM 4: TRAUMA SCHEMAS ARE RELATIONAL

Axiom 4 specifies that trauma schemas involve relationships with other people. People may give names to hurricanes, but no one actually blames a hurricane for its effects. Instead, people blame the town officials who minimized the danger and did not warn the people in time, the police who told the public to stay in their homes when they should have evacuated, the engineers who did not build the levees strong enough, and the fire department that took too long to save people from their flooding houses. Trauma schemas are primarily constructed to stabilize a person once he or she has been pushed off balance by a trigger that serves as a reminder of the traumatic situation or some aspect of it. People are inherently destabilizing influences because of their many degrees of freedom and potential unpredictability. Indeed, the weather shares some of this ever-changing, unpredictable nature, which may explain why people are fascinated by it and carefully monitor it. However, when people prepare for rain and it is sunny, or vice versa, they do not blame the weather; they blame the meteorologists.

It is because trauma schemas are intimately personal and relational, as is the psychotherapy session, that at some point in the therapy, they will be applied to the therapist and his or her behavior. This is discussed in great depth in Chapter 9, "The Gap: When the Trauma Schema Emerges in the Therapeutic Relationship." Because it is rarely obvious which detail in the trauma narrative caused fear or shame (a conclusion that can be drawn from axiom 2 about avoidance), one can never know what type of interpersonal behavior will trigger the use of a trauma schema. For example, a caring or loving response by a foster parent can trigger a disruptive episode for a traumatized child. The words "I love you" may be more destabilizing than an angry or threatening response because those words were used by the incestuous parent just prior to the molestation or because they bring up the promise that the child will be cared for, a feeling that he or she has had many times, only to be greatly disappointed or betrayed.

This fourth axiom implies that the therapist should try to identify interpersonal triggers that set off a trauma schema or distress in a client. When a client's trauma schema is triggered by an impersonal element, such as colors, sounds, smells, time of day, anniversary date, or physical objects, the therapist should inquire further into the interpersonal dimension of this trigger, which often lies just under the impersonal element.

> A businessman was in a train accident in which a commuter train went off the track and the passengers had to be evacuated through the windows of the train car. He had to leave his briefcase behind, and he became enraged when the briefcase was not found and returned to him. Briefcases became a trigger for him. The man did not receive a lot of sympathy about the accident or his lost briefcase, because he was not hurt and people often lose briefcases. On the assumption, derived from axiom 4, that there is a relationship behind the briefcase, the therapist inquired further and learned that 20 years earlier, this man had been in a commuter airplane accident, in which the engines burst into flames and the small plane crash-landed on a frozen lake. The client was in the rear of the plane. The front of the plane was on fire, and the pilots and two passengers were being burned to death. The client had the presence of mind to grab a briefcase and use it to smash a hole in the back of the plane and escape, along with three other passengers. He held onto the briefcase and later discovered that it belonged to one of the dead pilots. Eventually, he was able to send it to the pilot's family. As soon as this link was made, and the client realized that his rage and distress

over briefcases was a derivative of his terror in that plane accident and his feelings about the dead pilot, his symptoms disappeared. The therapist spent some time with the client discussing how his focus on his briefcase was actually a reference to his own fortitude and his gratitude to the sacrifice of the pilot. Without an understanding of the personification of trauma schemas, no protocol to desensitize this client to briefcases or the train accident would be effective.

Even though people cannot be blamed for everything, they typically are. There is an advantage to this clinically, in that if people are to blame, then negotiations can occur, compromises made, dialogues imagined, and repairs made. The impersonal world and its strong natural forces are not open for negotiation; they cannot say "I am sorry," and they cannot be punished or confronted. Thus, in clinical practice, whenever possible the therapist should anticipate and look for the interpersonal elements in the client's narratives and schemas.

CONCLUSION

The four axioms discussed in this chapter are extremely important. In the course of psychotherapy, they are often only intermittently applied, despite therapists' best intentions. These axioms, which are not just theoretical assertions, have direct consequences on therapeutic technique.

STUDY QUESTIONS

2.1   What are the four axioms of trauma-centered psychotherapy?

2.2   What is the major reason for avoidance?

2.3   What are common forms of avoidance in the therapy session?

2.4   If the narrative is always incomplete, what is it that is not included? Why should this matter?

2.5   If the client goes home and becomes upset after the session, what might this mean?

2.6   Why do people tend to view traumatic events in relational terms?

2.7   Who are the most likely people to be blamed for impersonal traumatic events and why?

CHAPTER 3

Establishing the Trauma-Centered Frame

The greatest single error or oversight made by clinicians hoping to conduct trauma-centered psychotherapy is not establishing a trauma-centered frame for the work. If a client enters treatment believing that he or she is going to a general therapist for help with current problems, and then at some point in the treatment, the therapist gingerly suggests that perhaps some of the person's childhood events are important and deserve exploring, or that a rape the client briefly mentioned should be gone over in detail, the client is much more likely to express hesitation, concern, and even outright resistance.

The reason for this reaction is that psychotherapy clients who have been traumatized maintain an awareness of their traumatic events, whether or not they are speaking about them. They usually know how damaging the event was and how much of a burden it has been. When they engage the services of a new therapist, they are not sure whether he or she is going to ask them about the event—much like alcoholics and smokers fear that their general medical practitioner will bring up their drinking or smoking at each office visit. The clients both fear and hope for such questions. When the questions are not asked, the clients proceed with discussing their other issues, but inside they are disappointed. The traumatized child or victim inside them has been overlooked again. Thus, when weeks or months or even years later the therapist finally comes around to asking about the traumatic event, a client may express anger.

This book is intended not only for specialists working with trauma cases, in which the frame is much easier to establish from the beginning, but also for general practitioners who treat a variety of conditions and for clinicians in general mental health clinics or residential treatment centers. The point may come when, for whatever reason, the therapist decides to initiate a trauma-centered inquiry, whereupon he or she needs to establish a trauma-centered frame prior to initiating a change in the treatment.

RATIONALE

What underlies trauma-centered psychotherapy is that *imaginal exposure is the primary therapeutic element in trauma treatment.* After many years of therapeutic innovation and exploration, most studies of trauma treatment have concluded that organized exposure to thoughts and images of the original trauma in a safe, therapeutic setting leads to habituation of the fear response (Foa and Rothbaum 1998; Friedman et al. 2007; Institute of Medicine 2007). Many studies have shown little difference in therapeutic efficacy among a wide range of treatments. The one common therapeutic element among all of these treatments is imaginal exposure. What differentiates these treatments is the method used to interrupt the client's avoidance of this imaginal exposure. For example, in prolonged exposure, direct pressure from the therapist and homework are used to keep the client on task. In eye movement desensitization and reprocessing, following the eye movements is used. In the counting method, the structure of the therapist's counting aloud to 100 keeps the client's focus on his or her memories. Too often, advocates for a particular approach emphasize what is different about their approach and may seek explanations for its therapeutic efficacy from these differences, when instead the therapeutic efficacy is more likely derived from what is common among the treatment approaches: imaginal exposure.

Therefore, in establishing the trauma-centered frame, the therapist will be indicating to clients that during the treatment they will be exposed to memories of their traumatic events, in this case, through the process of psychotherapy and not a set-apart procedure such as prolonged exposure or eye movement desensitization and reprocessing.

There are convincing arguments to support a trauma-centered frame. There is a great deal of evidence that trauma, abuse, and neglect in childhood through adulthood are major contributors, exacerbators, or causes of many mental illnesses (Edwards et al. 2003). The co-occurrence of mental illness and psychological trauma is so overwhelming and common that the trauma history of every new client should be assessed (Kessler et al. 1995). The literature is filled with documentation of inaccurate diagnoses being made because of ignorance of a client's trauma history. Screening for trauma is as important as for suicidality and homicidality, and someday it will be viewed as a standard of practice. Obviously, for any clinician reading this book who is interested in doing trauma-centered psychotherapy, it should be a standard of practice—with every client.

The following is a sample of a therapist's statement used to elicit the agreement of the client in forming a trauma-centered frame:

> So it appears that you have had some significant trauma in your life, including [description of what is known about the traumatic events], and you have suspected, and I also believe, that these events have had a strong influence on your life, both for good and for bad. Although these events occurred quite some time ago, there seems to be evidence that they continue to bother you and that they may in fact be contributing to your current symptoms, such as [name these].
>
> No one enjoys talking about traumatic events, and I know you have felt hesitant to get into the details of your experiences with your family and friends, but I can tell you that the scientific literature has discovered that spending some focused time going over the details of these experiences with a trained therapist can dramatically decrease the degree to which they bother you. I believe that doing this will be helpful to you.
>
> What this means is that we will be spending most of our time going over the details of your traumatic experiences, to a degree that you are perhaps not used to. We will then begin to look for patterns in your current life that appear to be influenced by the ways you adapted to the traumas, so we can unhook them from each other. In this way, we will be separating the past from the present. Along the way, you will no doubt reconnect with how upsetting the event was and become emotional. I expect this, and the reason for this is because what happened to you was indeed terrible and upsetting. Becoming upset will not be a reason for us to stop doing this work or to talk about other things. The reason for this is that by going through this process, you will become much more comfortable remembering and discussing your traumatic events. This is known as *desensitization*. What gets in the way of desensitization is avoidance. For example, you may find that you want to talk about other things instead of the past, and although they may be important, I will have to assume that this might be a way you are trying to avoid remembering what happened. So you will find me curious about whether there is a connection between those new topics and your past traumatic experience.
>
> At times you may also experience me in a similar way to some of the people who were present at the time of the trauma, such as [name them], including even your perpetrator. That is normal for this process, and I will not take offense but instead will be curious about what has triggered your memories.
>
> I do not expect this process to take forever, and in a couple of months we can revisit this plan and see how it has been going. Do you have any questions? Are you willing to begin this process with me?

In addition to this basic interaction, there are a number of other opportunities to enhance the establishment of a trauma-centered frame. In addition to providing a basic rationale for trauma-centered work once therapist and client meet, the therapist can communicate the trauma-centered frame from the moment that the client calls the office, enters the waiting room, and fills out forms.

FIRST CONTACT

The first contact with a client is usually by phone, and in addition to taking basic information and inquiring about the presenting problems and previous treatment, the therapist should ask one simple question: "Have you experienced any highly upsetting or traumatic event in your life?" Most clients will answer this question. Some will have had none and say no. Others who have had a traumatic event will feel uncomfortable and also say no. However, they will know, from this beginning contact, that the therapist is thinking about trauma.

Office Environment

The office environment and waiting room provide an excellent opportunity to set the stage for trauma-centered work. Many therapists, influenced by years of thought about therapy as good-enough mothering or unconditional positive regard, display in their waiting rooms pictures or photos of sailboats or sunrises, pleasant abstract paintings, and upbeat pamphlets about recovery or spirituality. Some keep the environment strictly neutral. Occasionally, clinicians may have brochures or posters about common mental illnesses such as depression or anxiety. Although there is nothing wrong with these sentiments and choices, they do not serve to communicate to the client that the therapist is thinking about traumatic events and is open to discussing them. These pleasant environments communicate that there is time; however, many traumatized clients feel that they are experiencing an emergency.

> A client in his 30s was diagnosed with stage 2 melanoma and was sent to an oncology office, and then to another one for a second opinion. He was terrified of having cancer and very anxious about the possible treatment options. In the first office, he was presented with pastel tones, abstract paintings, and music like Pachelbel's Canon. His association was that he was in a funeral parlor: his own. There was no indication anywhere that this office dealt with cancer. In the second office, there were many brochures with information about the treatment for a variety of cancers, several posters on the wall with somewhat explicit pictures of cancerous organs, and most important a sign

on the wall that said, "It's Us versus Cancer: And we are going to win!" The terrified person/child inside this man was reassured, uplifted, and relieved because he felt deeply that these doctors understood the fear and were adamant about helping. More than finding sympathy and soothing, the client wants help in overcoming the problem.

If the therapist begins by avoiding mentioning trauma on the first contact and further avoids the issue by not having any representation of it in the waiting room, approaching the topic later becomes all the more difficult. Thus, whenever possible, signs related to trauma can be located outside the office, in paintings on the walls, and in literature on the tables. In this way, a therapist communicates consistently that in this office traumatic experience is not feared and will not be avoided.

Forms

It is standard for clients to fill out forms in the office at their first visit. These forms include consent-to-treatment forms, privacy policy forms, and personal information sheets. It is useful to have a reference to trauma on these forms. The consent-to-treatment form should include language that specifically indicates that the content of the therapy will be concerning traumatic or abusive experiences and that some degree of distress is to be expected (see Appendix A). The privacy policy form should include "traumatic events" in the list of items about which the client may or may not choose to release information. The basic information sheet that lists address, doctors, medications, and medical problems should also have a basic list of traumatic events for clients to check off. The result is that even before the therapist meets the client for the first time, the client has been primed to speak about his or her traumatic events.

AFTER TREATMENT HAS COMMENCED

Establishing the Frame

If the decision to work on the trauma occurs well into therapy, then before initiating this work, the therapist needs to establish the frame with the client. This task essentially involves establishing an overt contract with the client about what the therapist is going to do. The first step is to jointly decide that spending some time going through the client's traumatic events will be useful. The therapist can provide the client with the rationale as well as information from the literature. However, the agreement must be mutual. At this point, it will be useful to give the client a revised consent-to-treatment form that specifically mentions that the therapist will be talking about traumatic events (see Appendix A), as well as a revised privacy form that asks whether the client wants the therapist to discuss these traumatic events with anyone else. Then the therapist should provide a checklist of traumatic events for the client to fill out (see Appendix B). The therapist should conclude with a statement such as, "So we have decided to get into what happened to you in more detail. I think this is a good idea and will be helpful to you. It may be difficult at times and upsetting to revisit these memories, but continuing to avoid them is no longer helpful to you. I can only imagine the burden you have had to carry. Shall we begin?" Although many clinicians decide to say this at the end of a session, with the idea that they will begin the next week, this tactic is a mistake. The therapist should present the rationale at the beginning of the session in which the work will begin, or the client's anticipatory anxiety will rise precipitously and the client may back off.

Handling Avoidance

The purpose of establishing a frame for trauma-centered work is to create an agreed-upon boundary around the therapist's activity. The client is allowed to avoid the topic, to skip sessions, to refuse to speak about the trauma, and to minimize it; however, the frame prevents the clinician from doing these things, for when push comes to shove, as it often does, the client will attempt to engage the therapist in a mutual avoidance of the task. With the frame in place, a confrontation may go something like this:

> CLIENT: I don't want to talk about the rape anymore. It's too upsetting. Things are really crazy at home.
> THERAPIST: You don't have to talk about the rape.
> CLIENT: I don't?
> THERAPIST: You don't. You have been avoiding talking about it for a long time because it upsets you. I understand that.
> CLIENT: You do? What do I do now?
> THERAPIST: It seems to me that we've come to the door, and you know that you have to go through the door, but you know that there are a lot of bad things on the other side. You can wait. I can wait. I will wait for you until you are ready.
> CLIENT: What about my problem with my roommate?
> THERAPIST: (*Stays silent and looks gently at the client.*)
> CLIENT: Oh, boy. I have to do this, don't I?

The therapist indicates that the avoidance will be the client's; the therapist's attention will remain on the traumatic story. That is where, psychically, the therapist stands.

A 32-year-old client was referred to a trauma-centered therapist. He was addicted to heroin and currently undergoing methadone treatment. He had had many relapses. He was single, unemployed, and living with his mother. In the first session, he described three absolutely horrendous childhood traumatic events involving domestic violence between his parents, witnessing a murder, and being raped anally by a friend of his father's. The therapist told him he had come to the right place and that he looked forward to working with him on these experiences. The client felt relieved he had spoken about the events and made an appointment for the next week. The next week, however, he called the therapist and said he could not come in because the memories were too upsetting and he did not want to relapse. The therapist said that he understood and that he was always available when or if the client decided in the future to work with him. The client asked if they could meet and not talk about the traumatic experiences, and the therapist said no, because trauma was what he talked to people about. Six months later, the client called again to make an appointment. He came in and gave further details about two of the incidents, which were truly sad and frightening, and explained his early turn toward narcotics. He said he had been doing okay but had been thinking daily about these events. He had driven by the therapist's office every week or so but felt too frightened to come in. He made an appointment for the next week, but he later canceled the session for the same reason: he felt he could not handle talking about the trauma. He liked the therapist and wanted to see him but wondered if they could take it slow, by which he meant not talking about the events much. The therapist again said no, that he was there to talk about these things but that the client should take as much time as he needed before he began. Four months later, the client made another appointment and made it through four sessions before he broke it off again. Three months after that, he again reengaged and continued for eight sessions. He then broke off the treatment for another month, before reengaging and seeing the therapist continuously for several years, working through his traumas and maintaining, even strengthening, his sobriety.

By holding to an established trauma-centered frame, the therapist allows the client to titrate his or her own avoidant strategies but maintains for him or her the hope and optimism that in the battle between Us and Trauma, we will win.

STUDY QUESTIONS

3.1   Why is it important to establish a trauma-centered frame?
3.2   What is the rationale for conducting a trauma-centered psychotherapy?
3.3   What are some effective ways of establishing the frame?

CHAPTER 4

Principles of Trauma-Centered Psychotherapy

In this chapter, we present three clinical principles—of immediacy, of engagement, and of emotionality (Table 4–1)—that serve as helpful guides to the therapist in successfully managing an approach to trauma. These principles are not for psychotherapy in general or, for that matter, for most forms of psychotherapy or clinical intervention. They are specific to trauma-centered work. Once the therapist and client have jointly agreed to engage in this work, these principles should be applied consistently throughout the treatment. These principles are not applicable to those clinicians in a general clinic or a general private practice until the trauma-centered frame has been established.

IMMEDIACY

The principle of immediacy states that inquiries about the traumatic events in the client's life should begin immediately in treatment and that whenever new material arises, it should be addressed immediately. This is an important principle because traumatized clients have been carrying the memories of these horrific events for weeks, months, and often years. Presumably, these memories have been bothering them and have caused multiple problems in their relationships, functioning, and peace of mind. These individuals have been told by numerous people to address the issue, but they have

---

TABLE 4–1.   Principles of trauma-centered psychotherapy

Immediacy

The therapist proceeds with the trauma inquiry as immediately as possible by inquiring about the traumatic events that occurred rather than the symptoms or disorders that resulted.

Engagement

The therapist demonstrates an active, engaged stance that appropriately reflects the horror or shame of the event and conducts the inquiry as if he or she were present in the client's story.

Emotionality

The therapist anticipates and tolerates strong expressions of emotion (grief, anger, fear, shame) in the client and does not attempt to dampen or manage their emergence.

---

delayed or have kept much of it secret and avoided speaking about it. The feelings have been eating them up from the inside, but the associated fears have held them back. Once the clients have agreed to discuss the events, their anticipatory anxiety begins to mount precipitously. If the therapist delays, even a little bit, their anxiety may become too great for them to continue. Like the child who finally climbs up onto the high dive or agrees to have a tooth pulled out, the clients want to get it over with.

According to this principle, in the first session, after saying hello, the therapist says, "What happened to you?" or "I understand you had a terrible experience" or "I understand you were raped by your boyfriend a month ago." At this point, the therapist generally does not ask about how things are going, how the client is feeling, who is in his or her family, or any of a myriad of good questions. These and other demographic questions can be asked later. Occasionally, experienced therapists do not even have to say hello. For example, one client came into the therapist's office and was obviously quivering with anticipatory anxiety. The therapist said nothing, looked at her intently, and nodded his head. She began to cry. He said, "Tell me about it." She did.

The therapist communicates immediately that there will be no delay and no informal pleasantries, that what happened to the person is being taken very seriously, and that the therapist is there to help and, even more than help, to remove the toxins. When the client knows what he or she is preparing for, a therapist's emphasis on safety, on skill building, and on preparation—however reasonable—leads to unnecessary buildup of anticipatory anxiety, and the client may never make it to the trauma exploration. The following case demonstrates the importance of immediacy in a medical situation.

A middle-aged man worries that the pain in his abdomen is cancer. He mentions it to no one, even his doctor, for a year. The pain continues, as does his worry. Finally, in an office visit, he mentions the pain to his doctor, who examines him, reassures him, and says to keep an eye on it. A year later the pain has continued, and the doctor suggests that the patient go to an oncologist for a checkup. The patient now feels more anxious and therefore delays making an appointment with the oncologist. When the pain flares up again, the man finally makes an appointment, which he then reschedules several times. Finally, after several years of worry, he arrives at the oncologist's office for his appointment. The doctor enters the examination room, greets him, and then says, "I know you are very anxious and worried that you might be diagnosed with cancer. I do not want to upset you, and it is important that you feel safe and know how to handle the feelings that will come up if you indeed have a cancer diagnosis. So you and I are going to meet for several months to get to know each other, and you will come to special classes on 'how to handle getting a cancer diagnosis,' and then, when you feel comfortable, I will conduct the diagnostic procedure. How does that sound?"

Few people will find this example credible, because the medical field has established norms that privilege conducting effective treatment over avoiding pain. However, this example is similar to how many mental health professionals handle trauma. The part of the client that wants to avoid discussing the trauma will be relieved, but the part that wants to be helped will feel abandoned. The point is that by the time clients walk into an office where they are expected to talk about their trauma, they are ready to talk about their trauma, even if they are scared.

CLIENT: (*Enters room and sits, looking anxious.*)
THERAPIST (*looking intently at client*): I understand something bad happened to you.
CLIENT: Yes.
THERAPIST: What happened?
CLIENT: Do you mean when I got raped, or what happened when I was a child?
THERAPIST: Which was worse?
CLIENT: (*Pause.*) When I was a child.
THERAPIST (*looking at client*): It must have been bad.
CLIENT (*tearing up*): Yes…I was not treated well. My dad was a drunk, and my mom was never there.… (*Continues.*)

Trauma-centered psychotherapists will be dispassionate but clear. They will speak about the trauma and tell the client that together they will revisit the pain in order to get it out and that the client will feel better as a result. The therapist will be optimistic but direct.

The principle of immediacy also states that the therapist should address the client's distressing memories whenever they emerge. Commonly, when clients begin to talk about a traumatic event, they are reminded of other aspects of the event or of other events, and then show their distress nonverbally. These signs of distress are signals to the therapist to inquire immediately about this distress rather than to wait until the narrative of the other event is completed. This principle can be very helpful in handling clinical emergencies when clients become agitated and upset.

> A clinician with trauma expertise was called to the psychiatric emergency room to help with an urgent situation in which a newly admitted veteran was becoming increasingly out of control, threatening violence, and becoming incoherent. The clinician had never met the patient before. The actual reason he was being called was that the emergency room staff hoped that he might accept the patient into his inpatient unit. However, they framed the request as one of needing his expertise. The patient was ominous looking and pacing furiously up and down the hallway. When the clinician came onto the unit, the patient called out, "Get the f—k away from me!" The clinician did not know the man's psychiatric or medication history. The staff also had little background information on him, considering him to have paranoid schizophrenia. The clinician looked directly at the patient and then went into a small conference room, leaving the door open. The patient came in shortly and stood. The clinician said, "You wouldn't be acting this upset without a very good reason." He sat down. The clinician went to the door and shut it slowly and then sat down. The patient was obviously expecting a psychiatric examination. The clinician looked him straight in the eyes and said, "Something really bad happened to you." The patient teared up, and his face immediately softened. The clinician said, "Got it. Must have been really bad. I'm sorry." The patient then burst into tears and told the clinician that he had just been discharged from the navy and that 3 months earlier he had been anally raped by three servicemen on board his ship, where he had been humiliated and called "their woman." A male staff member on the unit had said something that reminded him of his rape, and the patient had exploded. That discussion took about 2 minutes. He was then completely calmed down. The clinician said, "God, I'm really sorry. It makes a whole lot of sense. Would you like to get some help with this?" The patient nodded, and they shook hands. They came out onto the unit, where the staff had collected a code team to grab the patient. This was obviously no longer necessary, and the staff members were a bit perplexed because the clinician had been in the room with the patient for no more than 3 minutes.

The clinician had been asked to do the obvious: to calm the man down. However, attempting to calm him down by asking him to calm down would likely have escalated him, because without an understanding between them that he had been anally raped and humiliated, there was no reason for him to calm down. In this case, the clinician's immediate focus on asking what had happened to the man and listening to him led to a change in the man's behavior.

The principle of immediacy also requires the therapist to begin each session with a question regarding some aspect of the client's traumatic experience. It may not matter what the question is as much as that the therapist is there to work on what the therapist and client say they are there to work on.

A trauma-informed supervising clinician was called to the waiting room by the receptionist because a 10-year-old girl was extremely upset and had barricaded herself in the small area between the outside door and the glass door to the waiting room. Her therapist, a trainee, was trying to calm her down by talking to her through the glass door, and the foster mother was sitting somewhat frightened on a couch. The supervisor knew that this child had been abandoned by her birth mother many times as a young child, that the foster placement was relatively new because she had just disrupted her previous foster home, and that this was the second or third session at the clinic. The therapist was trying to get her to open the door, and the child was pressed up against the door and appeared nearly out of control, possibly contemplating hitting her head against the door.

> SUPERVISOR: What is upsetting you, Ellie?
> ELLIE (*shouting*): Nothing! I'm not moving! You can't get in here!
> SUPERVISOR: Something got you upset that reminded you of bad things. (*To therapist.*) What happened in the session?
> THERAPIST: She got upset out of the blue when it was time to end. She ran out of the room and down here.
> SUPERVISOR: Ellie, are you remembering when your birth mother left you alone?
> ELLIE: (*Silent.*)
> SUPERVISOR: It was bad when your birth mother left you all alone.
> ELLIE: Yeah.
> SUPERVISOR: It must have been scary to be left alone.
> ELLIE: Yeah. (*Looks down and releases the pressure on the door a bit, but therapists do not try to open it.*)
> SUPERVISOR: We want to know all about it. We are not going to leave you all alone. Your foster mother is going to take you home, and you are coming back here to talk more about your birth mother and what she did to you.
> ELLIE: I hate her.
> SUPERVISOR: It is sad.
> ELLIE: (*Bursts into tears and stands away from the door. The therapist opens the door and gestures the foster mother to come forward, as Ellie runs to her and embraces her.*)

The therapist made a mistake by trying to get the girl to open the door rather than immediately addressing the traumatic event, which was the cause of her distress. As soon as the client realized someone was interested in what upset her, she began to calm down. Even then, the therapists did not move to open the door, because the child was barricading herself into the space so as not to be removed or left alone—a fear that the end of the session apparently had evoked in her. Only after a fuller explication of her fears and memories had been accomplished, and she released her hold on the door, could the door be opened and her relationship with the therapist and foster mother be recovered. Note that in each of the previous two examples, the clinician had never met the client before, so no therapeutic alliance had been established. The effectiveness of each intervention was entirely due to the content of the clinician's approach, which focused on the patient's trauma schemas and memories.

ENGAGEMENT

The principle of engagement concerns the psychological location of the therapist in relation to the traumatic experience of the client. Because the experience of a traumatic event often causes the individual to feel completely alone, cut off from others, and unable to communicate what happened, the traumatized individual may assume that another person has little interest in his or her trauma. Therefore, the usual warm but neutral stance of the therapist in general psychotherapy may be experienced by the client as that of a disinterested bystander. In addition, a neutral, receptive stance places the therapist outside of the traumatic event, as if the primary means by which what happened can be communicated to the therapist is through the words of the client.

The principle of engagement states that the therapist, from the beginning, demonstrates psychological involvement with the traumatic event, by placing himself or herself in close psychological proximity to it and asking experience-near questions (described later in this section). Instead of the usual receptive look, the therapist should show engagement through forward posture and animated gaze. The difference might best be characterized by the difference between how one looks at someone in a job interview and how one looks at a child when checking for ticks. Again, examples from general medical practice are cogent: One wants one's doctor to have his or her full attention on the physical examination of the body, regardless of the discomfort.

If the therapist places himself or herself psychologically too far away from the traumatic event, it will be harder to elicit details of the trauma, and the client is more likely to criticize the therapist for asking too many questions. Unfortunately, when this criticism comes, most therapists back off further, and the process deteriorates more. When the client criticizes the therapist for questioning too much about the trauma, the therapist should first consider whether he or she has been too distant.

The clinician demonstrates engagement in four ways: through gaze, posture, experience-near questioning, and affective response. The first way is through *gaze*. The therapist's gaze should be animated, alive, and active. The client should feel examined. In training, beginning therapists in actual sessions often appear neutral, receptive, and blank and fail to notice that the client is becoming more and more upset. Trauma is such an alienating experience for clients that an essential component of therapist behavior is to be natural, human, alive, and present. The emphasis is not necessarily on being *warm* but rather on being *interested*.

The second way the therapist shows engagement is through *posture*. Many therapists sit back in their chairs and then sit back farther as the client gets into the details of the trauma. This behavior goes against the principle of engagement, which suggests that during trauma inquiry, therapists should sit up in their chairs and, as the client begins to provide details of their traumatic experience, should sit forward just a bit more and sometimes even lean forward. Although this advice seems perhaps too specific, it is generally good practice. Even minute backward movement by the therapist may be perceived by the client as abandonment, whereas forward movement may be perceived as an indication of the therapist's involvement.

Third, the therapist shows engagement through *experience-near questioning*. This type of questioning communicates to the client that the therapist is actively imagining being in the scene with the client, looking around, and asking questions about what is happening, unlike the usual form of questioning, in which the therapist relies completely on the client to provide the details. For example, the following inquiry communicates that the therapist is outside the event, like a reporter.

> CLIENT: Then he got on top of me.
> THERAPIST: What happened next?
> CLIENT: I guess he raped me.
> THERAPIST: Tell me more about that.
> CLIENT: Well, he held me down and, uh, raped me, hard.
> THERAPIST: Did he say anything?
> CLIENT: No, oh, yes, he told me to shut up.
> THERAPIST: What happened after he raped you?

In contrast, the following demonstrates experience-near questioning.

> CLIENT: Then he got on top of me.
> THERAPIST: How heavy was he?

CLIENT: I can't remember. Heavy.
THERAPIST: Did he press down on you?
CLIENT: Yes.
THERAPIST: Where?
CLIENT: On my neck (*rubs her neck*).
THERAPIST: Where were your arms?
CLIENT (*beginning to get upset*): My arms…I grabbed his hands, I was chok-
   ing.
THERAPIST: Sweat?
CLIENT (*crying*): Yes, I couldn't get a hold. That's when he told me to shut
   up.
THERAPIST: Was there a pillow?
CLIENT: (*Bursts into tears.*)
THERAPIST: What about the pillow?
CLIENT (*choking*): It was to my left side (*gestures*). I saw him look at it. I
   thought he was going to suffocate me with it.
THERAPIST: That's terrifying.

The therapist communicates that he or she is imaginally present in the event, wondering about the weight, the touch, the pillow, the sweat, and so on. In this case, these questions led very quickly to important details about the client's fears.

Sometimes, however, the therapist's questions are not on the mark, but errors and missed guesses still tell the client that the therapist is present, trying to see what the client experienced. Errors may bring forward other details.

THERAPIST: Was there a pillow?
CLIENT (*becoming aroused*): No.
THERAPIST: There was something else. What?
CLIENT (*upset*): My scarf.
THERAPIST: What about the scarf?
CLIENT: I saw him look at it and I thought, oh my God, he is going to
   strangle me with it.
THERAPIST: Was it close enough for him to reach it with his hand?
CLIENT (*very upset*): Yes!

The therapist's job is to imaginally enter the scene as described by the client and, using knowledge of similar situations as well as imagination, to "look around" and ask questions about the environment, objects, actions, or other sensory aspects of the experience that the client has not yet mentioned. This experience-near questioning is more important than simply progressing chronologically through the main actions of the event. The therapist should demonstrate interest in the client's narrative by delving into the particulars of each statement rather than being concerned about getting through the timeline of the event. The devil is in the details, and the axioms of avoidance and incompleteness (see Chapter 2, "Axioms of Trauma-Centered Psychotherapy") suggest that the client is not going to offer up the details immediately. What the therapist questions are sensory details of the scene, not potential acts of the perpetrator, which might become leading questions. The therapist does not usually ask questions such as, "Then did he hit you?" or "Were you worried that he was going to kill you?"

The fourth way the therapist demonstrates engagement is through *affective response*. The therapist needs to be able to conduct the trauma inquiry dispassionately, without showing anxiety or fear. However, this statement should not be interpreted to mean that the clinician should not show affect. The therapist should maintain a warm, compassionate tone throughout the session; however, when the client begins to describe truly horrible aspects of his or her traumatic experience, the therapist should not remain unaffected. It is useful for the therapist to demonstrate some of the affect that reflects having heard something horrible by making statements such as these: "That was terrible," "That must have been scary," "I am sorry that happened to you," "Whoa," "Oh my God," "I can't believe that," and "That is so intense."

Many therapists hesitate to say things like this because of fear that the client may feel worried about them or because of concern about stealing the affect from the client. In general psychotherapy, these concerns have merit. However, trauma-centered psychotherapy is different terrain: truly horrible events are being described, and for the therapist not to become engaged with the material or the client at this time would constitute a major deviation from the frame. Therapeutic neutrality is to be judged in context. Therapists planning to do trauma-centered work need to be prepared to engage fully with clients' experiences. If a therapist does not fully engage, the client may resist, quit, or act out (discussed in Chapter 9, "The Gap: When the Trauma Schema Emerges in the Therapeutic Relationship").

EMOTIONALITY

The principle of emotionality states that in doing trauma-centered work, the therapist should expect the client to become emotionally upset. Traumatized clients are very upset. The experiences they have had are intolerable, overwhelming, and terrifying. In the past, as noted in Chapter 1, "The Developing Cultural Context of Trauma-Centered Psychotherapy," having the client experience a catharsis, or become flooded, was seen as an essential element in the treatment. In recent years, particularly in Western societies, greater concern has been expressed about emotionality. Increasingly, in both public and professional discussions about trauma treatment, becoming emotional has been reframed as "being retraumatized," "overstimulated," "flooded," and "ungrounded" (Craemer et al. 2004). The range of acceptable emotional expressions seems to have been greatly reduced. It is important, from a trauma-centered perspective, to differentiate crying from being retraumatized and to distinguish between shouting in pain and dissociating. Doing trauma-centered work, which brings the client and therapist in proximity to the minute details of the terror, will unleash powerfully felt emotions of sadness, anger, fear, guilt, and shame. Trauma-centered psychotherapy is not predicated on these emotional expressions, and the intent of the work is not to induce them; rather, they will happen as a natural course of the treatment if it proceeds successfully. It is important for the therapist to feel comfortable with high levels of emotional expression and not to attempt to dampen, suppress, avoid, or control them. This means that on occasion clients will burst into loud crying, or shouting, or uncontrollable sobbing. Such expressions will not go on forever and will not harm the client. The most harm that will be done may be to the equanimity of the people in neighboring offices.

Concerns over safety need to be differentiated from the natural expression of intense emotions that result from trauma-centered work. When the work reaches one of these points at which emotionality runs high, it can shake the therapist's calm to the bone, for what is being expressed is so deeply upsetting. The following is an example, and it is an upsetting example, so be forewarned.

> A 30-year-old man lived in a rural area in the western United States. He was a gentle man, a musician and a carpenter. He was separated from his wife, who suffered from depression. They had twin boys, age 5. One day, when he arrived at her home to pick up his boys, he found no one home. Then he heard the car idling in the garage. He opened the garage door to find his wife and two boys in the car, with a hose from the exhaust pipe leading into one window. They were all unconscious. He immediately pulled all three out of the car and laid them on the ground and called 911. The ambulance came within minutes, and they told him that his wife was dead. The two boys were still barely alive. They arrived at the hospital shortly, and both boys were intubated and attended to by a team of doctors and nurses. Within an hour, the doctor told him that one boy was failing fast and was about to die. At the client's request, they removed the child from the equipment, and the man picked up his little boy and held him tight, whispering in his son's ear as he passed away. Shortly after the doctors removed his son from the room, they told the client that his other son was also not going to make it, and then he too was removed from the equipment, and the client held his second son in his arms as he too passed away. The client remembers how his boys felt against his

chest. He remembers how he felt that he was falling into a bottomless pit, from which he has never returned. He feels like he has been submerged in an ocean ever since.

There is no boundary to the emotionality of this experience, for the client for sure, and to some degree for the therapist. In this case, the therapist, who had his own son, felt deeply upset and saddened when he heard the details of this event, and his eyes teared up in the session. He said to the client, "I am so sorry" and "That is overwhelming." When the emotion comes, as it did many times during the therapy, there is no point in getting in its way. Teaching the client affect regulation skills would not likely modulate the experience of grief over this incident. What this client required was a therapist who could tolerate the depth of emotion that such an event entails. In this case, the therapist actively imagined being in a similar situation with his own son, which allowed him to become aware of numerous aspects of the situation that served as the basis of further questions for the client.

CONCLUSION

In trauma-centered psychotherapy, the therapist will begin the process of reviewing the traumatic incident immediately, will psychologically engage with the incident, and will expect and tolerate the strong emotions that arise. All three of these principles—immediacy, engagement, and emotionality— derive from the fundamental premise of trauma-centered psychotherapy, which is for the therapist to achieve proximity to the traumatic event and the client's traumatic experience, and to not give in to the natural protective instincts to avoid or distance oneself from the horror.

STUDY QUESTIONS

4.1   What are the three main principles of trauma-centered psychotherapy?

4.2   Does the principle of immediacy conflict with establishing safety in the therapeutic encounter? If not, why?

4.3   How can a neutral stance by the therapist make the trauma client feel uncomfortable?

4.4   What are the main elements of the therapist's engagement?

4.5   Why is it important that trauma-centered clinicians feel comfortable with expressions of strong emotion from their clients?

4.6   Does the trauma-centered approach discourage teaching clients affect regulation skills before engaging in the trauma inquiry? Explain your answer.

CHAPTER 5

The Four Main Techniques

The axioms and principles of trauma-centered psychotherapy (see Chapters 2 and 4, respectively) provide a firm basis for every session during which this work is conducted. Once the trauma-centered frame is established with the client (see Chapter 3), the therapist can begin to implement the four main techniques that are used to impact the client's trauma schemas. These four techniques are described in this chapter (Table 5-1). Other techniques used for specific situations or clients are described in later chapters.

GETTING THE DETAILS

The first main technique of trauma-centered psychotherapy is to inquire into the details of the client's traumatic memories, which is to begin during the initial taking of the trauma history. The devil is in the details, but the details are typically glossed over or avoided in the client's initial descriptions of the event. The last detail of the event to be shared is often the worst. As long as details remain unshared, they continue to be sources of pain for the client and ultimately become symptoms in that they continue to support the trauma schemas. Just as in having a splinter, the pain continues until the very last piece is removed, which requires more and more digging. As anyone knows who has removed a splinter from a child's finger, the child struggles between the pain of the splinter and the pain of the treatment (i.e., the needle), and the situation is no different in trauma-centered psychotherapy. In Chapter 7, "Continuing the Trauma History," we demonstrate how the

59

TABLE 5–1.   Four main techniques of trauma-centered
                      psychotherapy

Getting the details
   The therapist takes time to inquire about minute details of the traumatic event.
Decoding current behavior
   The impact of trauma schemas are identified in descriptions of current issues.
Introducing discrepancy
   Trauma schemas are challenged by introducing discrepant information to the
   client.
Disclosing the perpetrator
   The name and identity of the perpetrator are mentioned frequently.

---

therapist proceeds with getting the details from a client, but it is sufficient
to note here that one should assume there are always more details. Whenever the therapist has the thought that "more details are not necessary now,"
it is almost always a sign that he or she has just missed something.

As the trauma inquiry is proceeding, the client is always one step ahead
of the narrative: because the client speaks after having had a thought, while
the client is speaking about item A, he or she is simultaneously thinking
about item B. Thus, if the therapist notices a quiver or sign of arousal as the
client speaks about item A, the visible reaction is more likely to be about
item B, which has yet to be uttered. It is therefore usually a mistake for the
therapist to think that the upset is about item A, and the therapist is encouraged to halt the inquiry and go back and inquire for more details, which
should reveal item B. The therapist seeks more details about one moment
rather than resuming the chronological narrative. This type of questioning
is vertical rather than horizontal, nonlinear rather than progressive. The
following examples demonstrate the two types of inquiry.

Chronological (Horizontal) Narrative

I knocked on the door to my mom's bedroom and I heard a moan. I entered
and said, "Good night, Mom." She was lying in the bed looking at the ceiling. I saw her face. I walked over and kissed her on the forehead, and she
said, "'Good night, love," in a whisper. I left the room and closed the door.

Detailed (Vertical) Narrative Inquiry

> CLIENT: I knocked on the door to my mom's bedroom and I heard
>   a moan.
> THERAPIST: [Possible questions:] Where is your mom's bedroom
>   in relation to yours? What kind of door is it? How loudly did

you have to knock? What kind of moan? Was it different than you have heard before?

CLIENT: I entered and said, "Good night, Mom." She was lying in the bed looking at the ceiling. I saw her face.

THERAPIST: [Possible questions:] How did you enter? How did you say, 'Good night'? What did you see? Was there a smell? Was she still or moving in her bed? What color were the sheets? Were her eyes open? Describe her face. What was her skin like?

CLIENT: I walked over and kissed her on the forehead, and she said, "Good night, love," in a whisper. I left the room and closed the door.

THERAPIST: [Possible questions:] What kind of kiss? How did her forehead feel? What did you see when you got close? How did she say "good night" to you? What kind of whisper? Did she look at you? How long did you stay there? Was there a smell? How did you close the door? What did you do immediately after closing the door?

Each of these questions will elicit more information, which in turn should be subject to further detailed questions. In this actual clinical case, what was revealed was that the client, age 9, was aware that her mother had been incontinent and bloodied from her own self-mutilation over the past week, but in order to survive, the client had to psychically blind herself to the situation by describing only her and her mother's physical actions.

The therapeutic effect of getting the details is essentially exposure: by revealing these bits of experience, the client is exposed to the upsetting material, and over time his or her fear conditioning will diminish.

If in the course of a trauma inquiry the client suddenly becomes distressed after a question from the therapist, this usually means that the therapist has just moved on and missed a detail that the client was thinking about. It is important for the therapist to say immediately, "I can see I just missed something. You must have been having a thought about something, and I moved on. What was it?" Not infrequently, the client is not fully aware of what he or she was thinking either, so the therapist should back up and ask a more detailed question about the item just mentioned.

CLIENT: I knocked on the door to my mom's bedroom and I heard a moan. I entered and said, "Good night, Mom." She was lying in the bed looking at the ceiling. I saw her face. I walked over and kissed her on the forehead, and she said, "Good night, love," in a whisper.

THERAPIST: Tell me more about what she looked like.

CLIENT: She was quiet, staring at the ceiling.... I think her eyes were closed.

THERAPIST: Then what happened.

CLIENT: (*Upset.*) I don't know why I have to go through this. I already told my case worker all about it. It's stupid.

THERAPIST: I can see I just missed something. You must have been having a thought about something and I moved on. What was it?

CLIENT: I don't know.

THERAPIST: Was it something about how your mom looked? How were the sheets? What did the rest of her body look like?

CLIENT: They were red.

THERAPIST: Red?

CLIENT: From blood, I think.

THERAPIST: The sheets were red, from blood.... How did that happen?

CLIENT: I think she was cutting herself.

THERAPIST: That's terrible. Could you tell when you looked at her?

CLIENT: I didn't want to look at her.

THERAPIST: Understandable.

In this case, the therapist would have made an error by addressing the "I already told my caseworker all about it" issue.

In addition to learning more details through this inquiry, the therapist learns about the client's major trauma schemas—that is, those core ideas that are formed as a result of the trauma that continue to operate as the basis of current behaviors in the present. Understanding these structures becomes the work of the next technique: decoding.

DECODING CURRENT BEHAVIOR

The second major technique, decoding current behavior, is used after the initial phase of treatment, once the client's basic trauma schemas have been discovered and the sessions turn to discussions of current events. Trauma-centered psychotherapists will be listening for signs of the client's trauma schemas in his or her narratives of current events and particularly for problematic issues that the client raises. Identifying the overlap between present behaviors and trauma schemas can be called *decoding*.

Decoding derives its benefits by providing insight to the client about the impact of his or her past traumatic experience on the present. Clients are often amazed by how much of current behavior has been infiltrated with memories of the past and patterns of thought that distort current perceptions. Decoding proceeds by the therapist 1) noticing a change in affect or energy when the client speaks a certain phrase or word or 2) remembering an important sensory item from the traumatic event and noticing it being repeated in a different context. Usually, the therapist at that point merely repeats the word or phrase while looking at the client. For example, the therapist might say, "Yellow umbrella…Hmm. Does that call up anything about your father's beatings?" or "Broken pliers…Hmm. Did you ever have a bad experience with broken pliers?" The following is a more detailed example.

THERAPIST: Tell me more about that.

CLIENT: My boss called me into her office, and I knew from the start that she was going to harass me again. There she sat, in her *big* chair, looking all smug, ready to tell I was a lazy worker again. I was trying to stay composed, but then the bitch picked up that *pencil* of hers and pointed it at me, and I lost it. I turned and slammed the door and walked out of the building!

THERAPIST: The pencil?

CLIENT: Yeah, that f—king pencil! Pointed right at me.

THERAPIST: I'm wondering if this is in any way similar to the way your mother mistreated you when you were little. Did she ever use a pencil?

CLIENT: (*Laughs.*) Why, yes she did! She was a schoolteacher, remember, and she just sat all day correcting papers in her big fat chair in the living room, and when she'd lecture me, she'd point her pencil at me.

THERAPIST: She had a big chair too?

CLIENT: What do you mean?

THERAPIST: You said your boss was sitting in her big chair.

CLIENT: Yeah.

THERAPIST: Did your mom ever accuse you of being lazy?

CLIENT: All the time.

THERAPIST: Seems like your boss' big chair and pencil were triggers of your memories of your mother, and set you off.

CLIENT: That's weird. Was I just filling in?

THERAPIST: Could be. You were making an assumption that the boss was going to tell you that you were lazy, but I think that may not necessarily be the case.

CLIENT: You think I should check this out?

THERAPIST: Yes. You developed this idea that female authorities are bloated and abusive from your experience with your mother, but not all of them are. And not all of them are going to accuse you of being lazy.

An important consequence of effective decoding is demonstrating to the client the presence and impact of the trauma. This is especially effective when done with children in front of their parents or foster parents, who often view the children's bad behavior as having nothing to do with the past. Once the link is demonstrated to the client or family, adherence to trauma-centered therapy and enthusiasm for examining the traumatic events will be much more consolidated.

INTRODUCING DISCREPANCY

The third major technique is introducing discrepancy into the therapeutic dialogue. This technique is generally used after the details of the traumatic events have been obtained and the person's trauma schemas have been iden-tified and are being decoded. Decoding examines the *similarities* between the present and the past, whereas introducing discrepancy examines the *dif-ferences* between the present and the past. The therapeutic mechanism of this technique is the correction of distorted cognitions (a major element of cog-nitive-behavioral therapy). The general error made by the trauma schema is that because there is only similarity between then and now, the two are the same. In this way, the distortions by the trauma schema are an active source of distress, symptomatology, and dysfunction. The goal of treatment is to challenge and alter these schemas when the client applies them to his or her current thoughts and perceptions of self and others.

The therapist introduces discrepancy immediately following a decoding and then works with the client by going back and forth in a repetitive man-ner, pointing out both the similarities and the differences between the past and the present. This technique is demonstrated in the following dialogue, which varies only slightly from the previous example.

> THERAPIST: Seems like your boss' big chair and pencil were triggers of your memories of your mother and set you off.
> CLIENT: That's weird. Was I just filling in?
> THERAPIST: Could be. You were making an assumption that the boss was going to tell you that you were lazy, *but I think that may not necessarily be the case.*
> CLIENT: You think I was wrong?
> THERAPIST: Perhaps. You developed this idea that female authorities are bloated and abusive from your experience with your mother, *but not all of them are. And not all of them are going to accuse you of being lazy.* You might want to check this out.

The two italicized sentences illustrate the beginning of introducing dis-crepancy by the therapist with this client.

The therapist usually begins with the concept that not all of a certain class of people will do what the perpetrator did. The therapist in the exam-ple stresses this natural logic until the client appears to give in to the idea, at which point the two can attempt to address the important question: Al-though every female in authority may not accuse the client of being lazy, does *his boss* think he is lazy? Whereas a therapist may be able to stand his or her ground as an expert on people in general, a client is at an advantage around the specific question if the person in question is known only to the client. In group therapy, a therapist can have the client directly ask the other group members how they perceive the client, but in individual therapy, the op-tions are much more limited. First, the therapist can ask the client to check it out directly with the party and then report back in the next session. Second, the therapist can make a statement that the current situation is different from that of the past, to which the client may disagree, holding to his or her point of view as determined by the trauma schema. The therapist then should state that he or she disagrees with the client in a calm but firm manner. It is helpful for the therapist not to communicate being upset that there is a disagreement. This is difficult for many therapists who are more familiar with a client-centered or psychodynamic approach to therapy, in which empathy and unconditional positive regard are central. Holding calmly to a disagreement is very difficult, because having a disagreement generally implies that one person is wrong, and this propels each participant into an active attempt to persuade the other person to agree with him or her or at least to back off from his or her assertion. However, a therapist's holding to a disagreement with the client without being controlling can have a positive effect in softening the client's trauma schemas.

> CLIENT: Well, it would be really hard for me to check this out directly with my boss. She was definitely planning to tell me something bad, that's for sure.
> THERAPIST: In hearing you describe this, I really don't think so. There may be some similarities between the interpersonal style of your mother and your boss, but the two situations are completely different, and unless I am way off here, I don't think your mother had a chance to phone your boss to fill her in on what to say!
> CLIENT: So you disagree with me?
> THERAPIST: I disagree with you on this one.
> CLIENT: But you have never met my boss. How would you know?
> THERAPIST: Because it is not possible for your boss to mean the same thing that your mother did.
> CLIENT: Unless I am lazy.
> THERAPIST: Are you lazy?
> CLIENT: No!
> THERAPIST: Then our disagreement stands.

In this dialogue, the therapist holds to the disagreement, despite never having met the client's boss or mother. The therapist's position, supported by the fact that past and present are not the same, continues to exert an influence on the client's trauma schemas by preventing closure.

An extremely important nuance is that trauma schemas divide up the world in a relatively rigid and overly generalized fashion, in order to lower the client's anxiety; therefore, the distortions in behavior are upsetting to other people but comforting to the client. Paradoxically, when other people act in ways consistent with the generalization proposed by the trauma schema (e.g., that all female bosses think I'm lazy), the client may feel slighted again, but at least the world is the way it is, and the client feels prepared for it. A trigger for upset is when the other person does not act in line with the trauma schema, because the client is thrown into a state of ambiguity and uncertainty about reality. For instance, for the client in the example, when a female boss acts nice or makes a compliment, which is discrepant from the schema, the client may feel off balance, and then worry that the boss is "setting me up," that "tomorrow I'll get the real deal," or that "clearly there is a conspiracy to humiliate me." The trauma schema tells the client that when other people are nice or intimate or interested, he or she is in greater potential danger and must make even more effort to self-protect, withdraw from the situation, or go on the attack. These behaviors usually make the other person feel less nice, intimate, or interested, resulting in the relationship settling back into one more consistent with that perceived by the trauma schema.

This dynamic may be at the heart of certain acting out behaviors among children and of disturbances in the relationship between client and therapist. These situations are discussed in more detail in Chapter 8, "Conducting Ongoing Treatment: Decoding the Trauma Schema in Current Behaviors," and Chapter 9, "The Gap: When the Trauma Schema Emerges in the Therapeutic Relationship."

DISCLOSING THE PERPETRATOR

The fourth main technique is bringing attention to the perpetrator. There is a tendency in trauma work to focus on the injury the victim sustained. For example, clinicians look for evidence of child abuse in the child. Because it is the victim who approaches professionals for treatment, it is the victim who receives the attention. Too often the perpetrator is not involved—he or she might be in jail, at an unknown location, or dead. The perpetrator often is protected by law against false accusation, whereas the victim struggles to heal and must seek out financial and other help on his or her own. The entire traumatic event becomes located within the victim. It is not uncommon for linguistic conventions to depersonalize the violent act: the discussion is about the rape, the physical abuse, the sodomy, or the accident and not about how the client's father raped her, his mother beat him, his uncle forced him to have anal sex, or the intoxicated truck driver ran over her 6-year-old brother. These more accurate descriptions are significantly more upsetting because they reveal the relationship between the perpetrator and the victim.

As a result, after some time, the memory of the trauma becomes embedded within the representation of the victim. Several linguistic examples demonstrate this concept among entire populations. The basis of Polish jokes worldwide is that the Poles were the victims of violence from both Germany and Russia, between which they are located. Their country disappeared for 125 years when Germany, Russia, and Austria divided it up. The Poles never won a battle and were perceived as poor fighters. This has now turned into the perception of them as foolish, weak, and incompetent. Other examples are the terms *Indian giver* and *Indian summer.* Both terms derive from the U.S. government's promising to give land to the Indians and then taking back their promise. *Indian giver* is used to refer to someone who gives to Indians, and *Indian summer* refers to a summer that comes in late fall but will soon be "taken back." The wording of both terms, with "Indian" first, transfers the character trait of untrustworthiness from the white man to the Indian. Another example is the term *black slavery*, which also eradicates the mention of the European white people who organized and implemented this horror. The proper term should be *European slave trade.* Similarly, instead of the *Jewish Holocaust,* the more appropriate term would be the *Nazi Holocaust.*

In a sense, the author of the traumatic event is the perpetrator. Using the fourth technique, disclosing the perpetrator, the therapist attempts to reallocate the responsibility for the injury to its proper place. The therapist needs to make this effort consistently and frequently, as the client raises strong resistance. This technique is also useful for cases involving natural disasters in which the client views the perpetrator as someone who let the client down (see discussion of axiom 4 in Chapter 2, "Axioms of Trauma-Centered Psychotherapy"), and for cases in which the client is the perpetrator, in which situation the therapist should address this fact and then allow for the emergence of the perpetrator behind the perpetrator, if one exists.

The lack of mention of the perpetrator is another form of avoidance on the part of the client, the therapist, and society. The victim's memory of the perpetrator lingers long and is burdensome. At the same time, the victim remains on alert for the resurgence or return of the perpetrator. Too often, the victim finds the perpetrator in interactions with others with whom he or she is intimate. Through the natural frustrations and arguments within relationships and families, the client's intimates will at times act in ways that remind him or her of the perpetrator, and the client will then apply his or her trauma schemas to these interactions, and soon the client's current relationships take on aspects similar to the original trauma. In the absence of the real perpetrator, new people are recruited. Disclosing the perpetrator helps the client to externalize the perpetrator, providing a basis for the client to differentiate the past from the present and the traumatic assaults of the perpetrator from the relatively minor aggressions of the people the client lives with now. This process will be accompanied by an increase in the affects of fear and shame, which are closely attached to the perpetrator.

The purpose of frequently disclosing and mentioning the perpetrator throughout trauma-centered psychotherapy is to help the client and his or her spouse or family to remember who in fact authored the injury and to allow the client to relate in a less-burdened manner with those who care for him or her. As described in Chapter 14, "Trauma-Centered Group Psychotherapy," and Chapter 15, "Trauma-Centered Couples and Family Psychotherapy," disclosing the perpetrator will be an important component of effective treatment, precisely because the dynamics of a hidden perpetrator can be very damaging to the client's social relationships.

Quite often when the perpetrator is not an intimate friend or family member, the victim more easily forgives the individual for being a bad person, and instead focuses anger at those who are on the victim's side but who did not help soon enough or fully enough. When the traumatized client is in family therapy, therefore, a great deal of anger can be expressed toward other family members but very little anger expressed to the perpetrator.

Another reason the perpetrator goes unmentioned is fear. The perpetrator is often a person of power, especially in the midst of the event. The perpetrator is known to be potentially violent, or crazy, or drunk, and most people prefer to keep their distance from such a person. The classic situation is when the therapist meets with a battered wife and boldly supports her attempt to leave her husband, seek a shelter, or press charges. Then the wife leaves the session and meets her husband, who drove her to the appointment, in the waiting room. In the next session, the wife explains that she threatened to press charges against her husband because the therapist advised her to, and her husband expressed a wish to harm the therapist. At this point, many therapists back off, out of fear for themselves.

The specific techniques for disclosing the perpetrator are *naming*, *reframing*, and *describing*. It is interesting that in many cases the perpetrator is not named. For example, although a victim may know her rapist's name, during the trauma narrative the client refers to him as "him" or "the man" or even eliminates the pronoun entirely, as in this statement:

> After I was hit, I tried to run out of the room, but I was grabbed hard and thrown to the ground…then I was raped over and over again…I saw the blood from my head dripping on my sleeve.

The perpetrator has been edited out, as if he were "he who cannot be mentioned." Therefore, the therapist first must establish the name of the perpetrator, both his or her formal name and any nickname or other name the client may have used to refer to the perpetrator. Second, the therapist needs to use this name when asking questions about the event. Third, the therapist needs to gently interrupt the client's narrative and insert the perpetrator's name to help the client practice using the name. Thus, the previous narrative is changed to the following:

> After I was hit *by John Wyeth*, I tried to run out of the room, but I was grabbed hard *by John* and thrown *by John* to the ground…then I was raped *by John Wyeth* over and over again…I saw the blood from my head *from the wound John had caused* dripping on my sleeve.

A therapist may find a client becoming uncomfortable with this procedure, because the fear in the victim's memory is attached to the perpetrator to a greater extent than are the injuries endured.

The second technique for disclosing the perpetrator is to reframe the narrative description of the event and its associated trauma schema to place the authorship and responsibility for the traumatic event onto the perpetrator. The client may represent the event as if he or she were harmed by some impersonal force, thereby sealing his or her view of self as helpless rather than describing the act as a conscious, intentional, harmful, or evil action on the part of another person. Not placing the responsibility and agency for the event onto the perpetrator subtly supports the view that the perpetrator did not mean to do it, or did it because he or she had previously been harmed, or was provoked to do it; these kinds of excuses subtly promote the idea that the victim shares the responsibility for the event. In the example discussed earlier, the client speaks only in terms of "I" as if she were the central actor in the event. Not only was the perpetrator not named, but each sentence was constructed to remove the perpetrator from a position of agency. The description could be reframed as follows:

> *John Wyeth hit me*, and then when I tried to run out of the room, *John grabbed me hard and threw me* to the ground, causing a cut on my head. Then *John got on top of me and raped me* over and over again. The blood *from the wound John caused* dripped down on my sleeve.

The purpose of this technique is to establish and reestablish that the traumatic event belongs to the perpetrator, not the victim, and to shift within the mind of the victim that the traumatic story is not only a story of survival, but a story of perpetration.

The third technique for disclosing the perpetrator is to help the client describe the perpetrator, in as much detail as possible, as experienced during the course of the traumatic event. It is natural for therapists to tend to ask clients to describe themselves and how they felt during events; indeed, discovering what mental processes were at work in a client during an event and how these became distorted trauma schemas is an obvious and relevant task. However, in addition to that work, the therapist should go over the client's narrative and develop it in terms of descriptions—intimate descriptions—of the perpetrator: the look, smell, and feel of his or her body, face, and actions. During the event itself, the victim is often almost entirely focused on the perpetrator, not on his or her own inner self. In an impending car accident, as one is slamming on the brakes and bracing for the collision, one is not attending to internal stimuli but instead is completely fixated on the onrushing rear end of the car ahead. Reexperiencing symptoms, such as intrusive memories or flashbacks, often consist of concentrated images of the perpetrator, such as his or her face or groin or body. Thus, during the trauma inquiry it is useful for the therapist to bring the client's attention to details of both the perpetrator and the client. In the earlier example, a filled-out version of the story may look like this:

> John Wyeth hit me *with his fist. I remember he was sweating, and his eyes were barely open because he was drunk. He held me by the arm with one hand, and I can remember the large blue school ring he wore on the hand he hit me with. Now I realize that it was that ring that cut my head.* Then when I tried to run out of the room, John grabbed me hard. *His hand dug into my elbow and he shouted, "You bitch!"* and threw me to the ground. *He looked down at me and grinned. His teeth were funny, crooked. I saw the bulge in his blue jeans. He rubbed his crotch and grinned again. I remember he spit on me.* Then he yelled, *"Open your legs, bitch." I guess I did because then he kicked me in the vagina with his shoe, no boot— yes he had cowboy boots on. I think I passed out because the next thing I knew* John Wyeth was on top of me, *his penis inside me. John's body pressed down on me and he rammed himself into me over and over again. John's breath was foul from drinking and not brushing his teeth. I remember thinking then, "He should have brushed his teeth, he'll get cavities." John had one tooth missing, and another was really sharp, like a vampire. Anyway, I don't remember feeling anything by that time except wanting him not to drool on my face, so I turned my head away and that's* when I saw the blood from the cut John had made on my face all over my upper sleeve. *John had his face resting on my neck, I felt his scratchy beard, and then I remember thinking he is a vampire and he wants my blood, and he is going to bite my neck and suck my blood or something, but that's when he pulled out and then hit me again on my head and I blacked out.*

Through the process of bringing the perpetrator forward as a central figure in the story, where the person is made responsible for his or her actions, which are intimately described, it is common for the listener to be filled with hate or disgust for the perpetrator. In stories that focus on the fears and injuries and survival of the victim, the listener tends to feel sad and helpless.

The effect of disclosing the perpetrator in the trauma narrative is to remove his or her presence from the self-image of the client, to redraw the boundaries of the traumatic event in their proper place, and to reveal and locate the cause of the injury outside the victim. This is accomplished by bringing the perpetrator's presence forward and confronting not only the client, but also the therapist and indeed society at large, with the problem of what to do about those who perpetrate. This is a hard, but necessary, thing to do.

STUDY QUESTIONS

5.1   What are the four main techniques of trauma-centered psychotherapy?

5.2   What is the difference between chronological/horizontal inquiry and detailed/vertical inquiry?

5.3   What is the most important reason to get the details of a traumatic experience?

5.4   Define the technique of decoding.

5.5   What are the most likely elements to be decoded in this short narrative by a client who had previously experienced a trauma:

> "My boss was really enraged with Bob, so much so that he grabbed him by his shirt, no collar, and yelled at him, so I came over and told him to release Bob's collar and calm down. It was crazy, like there was foam coming out of his mouth or something, and Bob just took it and sat down in his chair. My boss looked at him with contempt and then spit into Bob's wastebasket and stormed off. I was really upset. Bob just whimpered."

5.6   Introducing discrepancy means pointing out to the client the differences between which things?

5.7   Why is it common for people not to mention the perpetrator in trauma narratives?

5.8   What are the three main ways of disclosing the perpetrator?

5.9   Fill in the blanks:

> "Mr. Smith held Vivien down on the bed and raped her" is a _____ of "Vivien experienced a sexual assault by a Mr. Smith."

> "Tell me more about how Mr. Smith looked at that moment when he was on top of you" is using the technique of _____.

CHAPTER 6

The First Session

The aims of the first session are to establish the trauma-centered frame by employing the three basic principles of immediacy, engagement, and emotionality (see Chapter 4, "Principles of Trauma-Centered Psychotherapy") and to begin the trauma history. Many reasonable elements of the standard first session in psychotherapy may also be achieved but are not as critical. These include clarifying the presenting complaint, gathering important demographic and family history, and giving the client initial impressions of his or her diagnosis or treatment plan. The various aspects of the first session will be illustrated through the following transcript of a session.

> The client is a 34-year-old single white woman who mentioned on the initial phone call that she was depressed because she had just broken off a relationship with her boyfriend and that she has had trouble with relationships ever since she was raped at age 22. The therapist and client have never met. The client enters the therapist's office and sits down.

> THERAPIST: (*Looks at her for a moment.*) I understand you were raped when you were 22.
> CLIENT: (*Neutral.*) Yes.
> THERAPIST: Tell me about it.
> CLIENT: I was working as a secretary in an office, and a coworker had sex with me against my will one day after work.
> THERAPIST: I don't understand.
> CLIENT: I think it's why I've had problems ever since being intimate with my boyfriends. I just haven't felt comfortable getting close, you know.... I just broke up again, after 3 years (*looks sad*).

THERAPIST: The rape must have been upsetting.

CLIENT: (*Looks up at the therapist, who leans forward slightly.*) It was.

THERAPIST: I'm sorry you had to go through that. Was the co-worker someone you knew before the rape?

CLIENT: Yes,…he was a supervisor, not my supervisor, but anyway someone in the office in charge of another division. I knew him maybe for a year.

THERAPIST: What was his name?

CLIENT: Matt.

THERAPIST: Tell me what happened.

CLIENT: Well, for a couple of weeks I had the feeling he was watching me, looking over at me, you know, seemed interested, as a guy (*blushes*).

THERAPIST: You mean you assumed that he might be attracted to you?

CLIENT: Yeah, and he was fairly handsome and smart, so I guess I was flattered. He was always polite with me in the hall. We didn't work together and all, but one day he came by my desk and said that I looked nice in my dress. I wasn't prepared for what…(*slight pause*) happened the next day.

THERAPIST: (*Looks directly into her eyes and offers a warm smile.*)

CLIENT: (*Becomes tearful and then bursts into tears. After perhaps 20 seconds, takes a tissue out of purse and wipes face.*) I'm sorry.

THERAPIST: It must have been upsetting, but I'm afraid that's what people come here to do. Tell me what happened the next day.

CLIENT: I don't know if I can. It was terrible.

THERAPIST: Of course you don't have to tell me, but my guess is that you came here to tell me about the rape. This is what I do, and I believe I can help you.

CLIENT: It was at the end of the day. He came over to my desk and asked me if I could stay to help him file some papers because his secretary had already left. I said okay because we often did that for each other in the office; it wasn't a big office or anything.

THERAPIST: His office was near to yours?

CLIENT: Yes, just down a hall.

THERAPIST: He had his own office?

CLIENT: Yes.

THERAPIST: Was it the kind with a glass section so you could see into it when the door was closed?

CLIENT (*becoming upset again*): Yes, there was this glass panel alongside the door.

THERAPIST: I see. Show me how the glass was.

CLIENT: (*Motions with her hands in a vertical manner, but is now crying and breathing more loudly.*)

THERAPIST: What are you thinking about now? What are you seeing?

CLIENT (*crying while talking*): I, I see him (*points*), him.

THERAPIST: Who?

CLIENT: My supervisor, Tim.

THERAPIST: Where are you?

CLIENT: I'm on the floor, in the office.

THERAPIST: Matt is on top of you?

CLIENT: Yes, he is raping me.

THERAPIST: You are on the floor, and Matt is on top of you, raping you, and you look over through the glass and see your own supervisor? You're looking up at him?

CLIENT: Yes (*crying*).

THERAPIST: And he is looking at you.

CLIENT: No, he's smiling.

THERAPIST: Smiling at Matt?

CLIENT: (*Holds her hand in a thumbs-up position.*)

THERAPIST: Oh my God. That is terrible. You couldn't scream for help…

CLIENT: Because Matt was whispering to me to stay quiet.

THERAPIST: And because Tim thinks you are consenting, he walks out of the office (*client shows distress*). What happened before Tim left the office?

CLIENT: He turns off the main office lights.

THERAPIST: So you are alone with Matt in a darkened office.

CLIENT: And Matt continues to rape me for a long time.

THERAPIST: Where was your dress?

CLIENT: He had thrown it in the corner.

THERAPIST: I see. Now I am going to ask you a couple of direct questions regarding the rape itself. He penetrated you vaginally?

CLIENT: Yes.

THERAPIST: Anally?

CLIENT: Yes.

THERAPIST: Did he force you to masturbate him?

CLIENT: Yes.

THERAPIST: Oral?

CLIENT: Yes.

THERAPIST: Manually?

CLIENT: No.

THERAPIST: Going back a bit, when Matt first got you into his office, what did he do?

CLIENT: He looked around to see if anyone else was in the hallway and then closed the door. He said he had seen how I had looked at him, and he thought we just should get down to it. I said no, I didn't want to have sex with him, and then he got very angry and grabbed me.

THERAPIST: Where did he grab you?

CLIENT: By my belt (*becomes upset*).

THERAPIST: What did Matt do with your belt?

CLIENT: (*Starts crying again.*)

THERAPIST: It must have been bad.

CLIENT: (*Nods.*) He pulled it off me and wrapped it around my neck.

THERAPIST: That must have been frightening. What did he say?

CLIENT: "You are just a dog. But my dog. And you will do as I say. Take your dress off." I did, and then he unzipped his pants and pushed me down on the floor.

THERAPIST: On your stomach or back?

CLIENT: On my knees.

THERAPIST: He entered you anally first?

CLIENT: Yes (*coughs*).

THERAPIST: The belt was still around your throat?

CLIENT: Yes, I could barely breathe....It was so painful.

THERAPIST: Where was the pain?

CLIENT: My knees, he pressed down on my knees. It was a tile floor. Finally, he turned me over on my back and...and (*coughs*)...entered my vagina (*coughs*).

THERAPIST: Had Matt wiped off his penis before entering your vagina?

CLIENT: (*Looks up at therapist with horrified look on face.*) No, it was disgusting.

THERAPIST: I can't even imagine. Horrible. It was then that your own supervisor came by and looked in?

CLIENT: Yes, about then.

THERAPIST: And Tim gives Matt the thumbs up because he thought the two of you were consensually having sex and he was doing the guy-to-guy signal?

CLIENT: Yes.

THERAPIST: Was your belt still around your neck?

CLIENT: No, I had taken it off when he put me on my back.

THERAPIST: How long did this last after that?

CLIENT: About an hour.

THERAPIST: We will have a chance to talk more about this, because I know there is so much more that happened, but tell me, how did it end?

CLIENT: He told me that I was a great lay and that I had better not tell anybody, and that even if I did, he had Tim as a witness that I was going along with it, so no one would believe me. (*Looks up at therapist.*)

THERAPIST: He also said something else.

CLIENT: Yeah. He said that he was available anytime I wanted to be "taken" by him.

THERAPIST: And...

CLIENT: He said I looked good in a collar. (*Therapist grimaces.*) I got home that night and called in sick for 2 days and then quit the following Monday.

THERAPIST: That was terrible.

CLIENT: I've never told anyone about this, in this much detail.

THERAPIST: I can imagine. And I assume there is more.

CLIENT: Do you think this is why I am having trouble with guys now? It was a long time ago.

THERAPIST: I am sure that it is a major reason. Exactly how it has interfered we will figure out in future sessions. There are so many aspects that seem important. The fact that someone you knew came by and did not know to help you must have been devastating.

CLIENT: Yeah. You know, I always seem to break off a relationship when we are about to "go public" with it.

THERAPIST: That might relate to how you thought when Tim saw you and perhaps misunderstood.

CLIENT: Yeah.

THERAPIST: I appreciate your courage in describing so many details of your traumatic event with me today. How do you feel now?

CLIENT: Better. Terrible (*laughs*)!

THERAPIST: Yeah. That is what we will do here. Get into the details so we can help you feel less frightened of what happened to you and to discover what ideas you developed afterward that are now making intimate relationships difficult. Is this time a good one for next week?

CLIENT: Yes, this is a good time.

THERAPIST: Do you have any questions for me?

CLIENT: I should have talked about this a long time ago.

THERAPIST: I look forward to seeing you next week. In the meantime, feel free to call me if you have any questions.

CLIENT: Thank you.

Below, we repeat this session, pointing out essential elements of the therapist's technique and also explore variations of the therapist's interventions and client's responses.

THERAPIST: (*Looks at client for a moment.*) I understand you were raped when you were 22.

CLIENT: (*Neutral.*) Yes.

THERAPIST: Tell me about it. [The therapist begins immediately with the traumatic event. Immediacy.]

CLIENT: I was working as a secretary in an office, and a coworker had sex with me against my will one day after work.

THERAPIST: I don't understand. [Not understanding.]

CLIENT: I think it's why I've had problems ever since being intimate with my boyfriends. I just haven't felt comfortable getting close, you know…. I just broke up again, after 3 years (*looks sad*).

THERAPIST: The rape must have been upsetting. [The client attempts to move away from the event after briefly summarizing it and minimizing its horror. This is called a *jump*. The therapist moves back again to the rape. Avoidance. Immediacy.]

CLIENT: (*Looks up at the therapist, who leans forward slightly.*) It was.

THERAPIST: I'm sorry you had to go through that. Was the coworker someone you knew before the rape?

CLIENT: Yes,…he was a supervisor, not my supervisor, but anyway someone in the office in charge of another division. I knew him maybe for a year.

THERAPIST: What was his name?

CLIENT: Matt.

THERAPIST: Tell me what happened.

CLIENT: Well, for a couple of weeks I had the feeling he was watching me, looking over at me, you know, seemed interested, as a guy (*blushes*).

THERAPIST: You mean you assumed that he might be attracted to you? [This is probably a mistake, for the therapist should notice the blushing and assume it may relate to "watching me," "looking over," "as a guy," or a thought she had after that. This emotional lift in the narrative is called a *bump*. The therapist here assumes it is about attraction, when it is more likely related to "being watched," which comes up later in the trauma narrative. *Alternative response:* Therapist: Watching you, as a guy? Client: Yeah. I felt it was creepy.]

CLIENT: Yeah, and he was fairly handsome and smart, so I guess I was flattered. He was always polite with me in the hall. We didn't work together and all, but one day he came by my desk and said that I looked nice in my dress. I wasn't prepared for what…(*slight pause*) happened the next day.

THERAPIST: (*Looks directly into her eyes and offers a warm smile.*) [The therapist introduces a pause here to allow what she was thinking or feeling to be present rather than pushed to the side in the ongoing flow of the narrative.]

CLIENT: (*Becomes tearful and then bursts into tears. After perhaps 20 seconds, takes a tissue out of purse and wipes face.*) I'm sorry.

THERAPIST: It must have been upsetting, but I'm afraid that's what people come here to do. [The therapist underscores the principle of emotionality.] Tell me what happened the next day.

CLIENT: I don't know if I can. It was terrible.

THERAPIST: Of course you don't have to tell me, but my guess is that you came here to tell me about the rape. This is what I do, and I believe I can help you. [The therapist is establishing the trauma-centered frame.]

CLIENT: It was at the end of the day. He came over to my desk and asked me if I could stay to help him file some papers because his secretary had already left. I said okay because we often did that for each other in the office; it wasn't a big office or anything.

THERAPIST: His office was near to yours? [The therapist imagines being in the office and asks a question about the environment that underscores the principle of engagement.]

CLIENT: Yes, just down a hall.

THERAPIST: He had his own office?

CLIENT: Yes.

THERAPIST: Was it the kind with a glass section so you could see into it when the door was closed? [Again, a question that comes from imagining one is there. Engagement.]

CLIENT (*becoming upset again*): Yes, there was this glass panel alongside the door.

THERAPIST: I see. Show me how the glass was. [The therapist stays with the glass because client indicated by her upset that it held some importance.]

CLIENT: (*Motions with hands in a vertical manner, but is now crying and breathing more loudly.*)

THERAPIST: What are you thinking about now? What are you seeing? [This sensory element is an important piece of client's traumatic experience. The therapist does not mind disrupting the chronological telling of the event by zooming in on the details, because this will bring them closer to the traumatic moments. He also shifts into the present tense as a means of matching how the client seems to be processing the event.]

CLIENT (*crying while talking*): I, I see him (*points*), him.

THERAPIST: Who?

CLIENT: My supervisor, Tim.

THERAPIST: Where are you?

CLIENT: I'm on the floor, in the office.

THERAPIST: Matt is on top of you? [Again, imagining being there. Engagement.]

CLIENT: Yes, he is raping me.

THERAPIST: You are on the floor, and Matt is on top of you, raping you, and you look over through the glass and see your own supervisor? You're looking up at him?

CLIENT: Yes (*crying*).

THERAPIST: And he is looking at you.

CLIENT: No, he's smiling.

THERAPIST: Smiling, at Matt?

CLIENT: (*Holds her hand in a thumbs-up position.*)

THERAPIST: Oh my God. That is terrible. [Being emotionally engaged and responding accordingly.] You couldn't scream for help…

CLIENT: Because Matt was whispering to me to stay quiet.

THERAPIST: And because Tim thinks you are consenting, he walks out of the office (*client shows distress*). What happened before Tim left the office? [Seeing her upset, the therapist immediately asks again about leaving the office.]

CLIENT: He turns off the main office lights.

THERAPIST: So you are alone with Matt in a darkened office.

CLIENT: And Matt continues to rape me for a long time.

THERAPIST: Where was your dress? [Her comment is called a *bridge*, in that it goes over a whole period of time, so the therapist brings her back to the previous moment with a question about a sensory element.]

CLIENT: He had thrown it in the corner.

THERAPIST: I see. Now I am going to ask you a couple of direct questions regarding the rape itself. He penetrated you vaginally? [The therapist now asks some direct questions regarding the rape. The intent is in part to discover what happened, but more importantly to communicate to the client that the therapist is capable of hearing anything.]

CLIENT: Yes.

THERAPIST: Anally?

CLIENT: Yes.

THERAPIST: Did he force you to masturbate him?

CLIENT: Yes.

THERAPIST: Oral?

CLIENT: Yes.

THERAPIST: Manually?

CLIENT: No. [The therapist wants to quickly get a sense of what acts Matt did, prior to continuing with the narrative, even if that means not going into detail about them yet. The therapist notes that the client answers these questions without a significant shift in distress; had she shown that, he would have immediately inquired further.]

THERAPIST: Going back a bit, when Matt first got you into his office, what did he do? [The therapist abandons the chronological line and returns to an earlier point.]

CLIENT: He looked around to see if anyone else was in the hallway and then closed the door. He said he had seen how I had looked at him, and he thought we just should get down to it. I said no, I didn't want to have sex with him, and then he got very angry and grabbed me. [This more open narrative may indicate that the client did feel the therapist was able to hear more.]

THERAPIST: Where did he grab you?

CLIENT: By my belt (*becomes upset*).

THERAPIST: What did Matt do with your belt? [The therapist asks in more detail about the element that evokes an emotional response.]

CLIENT: (*Starts crying again.*)

THERAPIST: It must have been bad.

CLIENT: (*Nods.*) He pulled it off me and wrapped it around my neck.

THERAPIST: That must have been frightening. What did he say?

CLIENT: "You are just a dog. But my dog. And you will do as I say. Take your dress off." I did, and then he unzipped his pants and pushed me down on the floor.

THERAPIST: On your stomach or back? [Again, imagining being there. The therapist might have asked about the sensory element "dog," but the client does not show much arousal when mentioning it.]

CLIENT: On my knees.

THERAPIST: He entered you anally first? [Not hesitating to follow the obvious implications of her previous statement.]

CLIENT: Yes (*coughs*).

THERAPIST: The belt was still around your throat? [Noting the cough]

CLIENT: Yes, I could barely breathe....It was so painful.

THERAPIST: Where was the pain? [Not assuming the pain was in her rectum.]

CLIENT: My knees, he pressed down on my knees. It was a tile floor. Finally, he turned me over on my back and...and (*coughs*)...entered my vagina (*coughs*).

THERAPIST: Had Matt wiped off his penis before entering your vagina? [Imagining being there and noting the cough.]

CLIENT: (*Looks up at therapist with a horrified look on her face.*) No, it was disgusting.

THERAPIST: I can't even imagine. Horrible. It was then that your own supervisor came by and looked in?

CLIENT: Yes, about then.

THERAPIST: And Tim gives Matt the thumbs up because he thought the two of you were consensually having sex, and he was doing the guy-to-guy signal.... [The therapist misses an important detail here by not noting her partial agreement: "about then."]

CLIENT: Yes.

THERAPIST: Was your belt still around your neck?

CLIENT: No, I had taken it off when he put me on my back.

THERAPIST: How long did this last after that?

CLIENT: About an hour.

THERAPIST: We will have a chance to talk more about this, because I know there is so much more that happened, but tell me, how did it end? [This is said when the time for the session to end is approaching, despite the fact that much more needs to be told.]

CLIENT: He told me that I was a great lay and that I had better not tell anybody, and that even if I did, he had Tim as a witness that I was going along with it, so no one would believe me. (*Looks up at therapist.*)

THERAPIST: He also said something else. [Noting the look. Incompleteness.]

CLIENT: Yeah. He said that he was available anytime I wanted to be "taken" by him.

THERAPIST: And... [Incompleteness.]

CLIENT: He said I looked good in a collar. (*Therapist grimaces.*) I got home that night and called in sick for 2 days and then quit the following Monday.

THERAPIST: That was terrible.

CLIENT: I've never told anyone about this, in this much detail.

THERAPIST: I can imagine. And I assume there is more. [Incompleteness.]

CLIENT: Do you think this is why I am having trouble with guys now? It was a long time ago.

THERAPIST: I am sure that it is a major reason. Exactly how it has interfered we will figure out in future sessions. There are so many aspects that seem important. The fact that someone you knew came by and did not know to help you must have been devastating. [Providing an example of a trauma schema.]

CLIENT: Yeah. You know, I always seem to break off a relationship when we are about to "go public" with it. [She demonstrates she understands this and is capable of decoding her schemas.]

THERAPIST: That might relate to what you thought when Tim saw you and perhaps misunderstood. [Decoding.]

CLIENT: Yeah.

THERAPIST: I appreciate your courage in describing so many details of your traumatic event with me today. How do you feel now?

CLIENT: Better. Terrible (*laughs*)!

THERAPIST: Yeah. That is what we will do here. Get into the details so we can help you feel less frightened of what happened to you and to discover what ideas you developed afterward that are now making intimate relationships difficult. [Underscoring the trauma-centered frame.] Is this time a good one for next week?

CLIENT: Yes, this is a good time.

THERAPIST: Do you have any questions for me?

CLIENT: I should have talked about this a long time ago.

THERAPIST: I look forward to seeing you next week. In the meantime, feel free to call me if you have any questions.

CLIENT: Thank you.

This case is a not an atypical first session. The therapist engaged immediately in the revelation of the trauma story and was successful in reaching several particularly upsetting core moments that have burdened the client. Despite the lack of session time spent on collecting the usual general information about the client, by the end of the session the client has developed a good sense of what this type of therapy will entail and a certain degree of confidence in the therapist's competence in implementing it. The client is likely to feel that the therapist is interested in her experience and is not afraid to delve into the details, no matter how horrible. This client demonstrated a willingness to tell her story and, at the end, some capacity to understand how the past rape is still living in her interpersonal relationships today. The therapist established the trauma-centered frame and in large degree followed the principles of immediacy, engagement, and emotionality. He made two mistakes by missing references to particular details but overall was attentive to the client's attempts at avoidance in her use of jumps, bumps, and bridges (to be discussed in Chapter 7, "Continuing the Trauma History: Getting the Details and Formulating the Trauma Schema"). The event, originally labeled a rape, was pulled apart into important sensory elements, such as glass, belt, and knees, that contained her terror. Beyond the rape itself, the traumatic event included being dominated and humiliated, being abandoned by her supervisor, and being left alone in a darkened office with her perpetrator.

USING WRITTEN AIDS

Although the experienced trauma-centered clinician will begin each session in a manner similar to that in the previous example and conduct the trauma history spontaneously, beginning therapists can use certain written aids that help to guide the inquiry and help both client and therapist stay on track. When the inevitable avoidance occurs, it is somewhat easier to return to the inquiry if a paper form is involved.

Traumatic Events Checklist

The first type of written form is a *traumatic events checklist* that the client is asked to fill out in the waiting room. An example of such a checklist is provided in Appendix B. The form lists most types of abusive and traumatic events and allows the client to note whether he or she was upset by them at the time and/or is upset by them at present. Clients often list many more events than they might have revealed spontaneously. Also, if a client presents one traumatic event immediately that the therapist feels is important to follow through with, this form lets the therapist know that there are still other potentially traumatic events to discuss.

After a client completes the checklist, the process might go as follows:

> CLIENT: (*Enters the room and is greeted by the therapist.*)
> THERAPIST: May I see the checklist you filled out? (*Looks at it.*) Now I understand that you are here to talk about your father's sudden death, but I see on the form that you checked off "plane crash." What happened there?
> CLIENT: (*Explains.*)
> THERAPIST: [Therapist may decide to 1) start at the top of the form and go through each item, or 2) ask directly about the most upsetting items such as the father's death and save the rest of the list for the next session.] Just so I have some idea of what you have been through, let's go briefly through this list so I know what happened. Okay, so when was the hurricane? [If it turns out that one of these events appears to be of greater importance or upset for the client than the stated reason for coming in, the therapist is likely to begin the inquiry with that event, leaving the rest of the list for later.]

The list provides a flexible and concrete method by which the therapist can maintain control over what events the client is asked to describe and may help the beginning therapist stay on track in the first few sessions.

Structured Interview

Another type of written aid is the *structured interview*, which is a detailed clinical interview that covers many of the most important traumatic events (see example in Appendix C).[1] Typically, the structured interview is used after the first session, when the client has brought up a number of traumatic

---

[1]Note that this interview is intended to extract only information about traumatic events. Other instruments, such as the Clinician-Administered PTSD Scale for DSM-5 (Weathers et al. 2014), measure PTSD symptoms and can be used to diagnose PTSD.

events, and a more thorough history appears to be warranted. The therapist introduces the interview in the following manner:

> THERAPIST: Well, last week you let me know about a number of different events that have affected your life, and it seems important that I learn about each of them as well as others. I have a special interview that helps with this, and I would like to use that today.
>
> CLIENT: Okay.
>
> THERAPIST: (*Begins reading the Clinical Interview for Assessment of Trauma History [see Appendix C] verbatim:*) "Now I am going to ask you about personal experiences that for one reason or another have been bad, unfortunate, or frightening to you, such as losing someone close to you, being physically or sexually mistreated, or being seriously injured...."

The interview begins with a general screening question. If the client answers in the affirmative, the therapist follows up with more detailed questions before proceeding through the trauma categories. If the client answers in the negative, the therapist asks follow-up questions, as prompted in the interview. The reason for the additional questions after a negative response is that a person may say that he or she has not been sexually abused but may answer yes about being forced to masturbate his or her father. The interview assumes that a measure of avoidance is present at each step (axiom 2).

Usually, a client is cooperative with this approach, because the formal paper-based interview provides a kind of credibility to the inquiry: the client can see that the therapist is following a standardized procedure. The client's mistrust in the process is therefore calmed. Without the form, the intimacy of the trauma inquiry can raise concerns that the therapist is just making it up or is being intrusive or has other motives. The interview also helps the therapist to gather important details that are revealed by the follow-up questions. The process of going through the form therefore serves as a way of establishing the trauma-centered frame and beginning the initial phase of treatment.

WHEN THE CLIENT REFUSES TO CONTINUE THE TRAUMA INQUIRY

Sometimes a client will directly challenge the trauma-centered inquiry, either tactfully by trying to discuss another issue or directly by refusing to speak any more about the trauma and questioning its value. For instance, the client in the long example at the beginning of this chapter might have challenged this inquiry.

CLIENT: I don't think that was as important as my problem now with my boyfriend. I really want to get back together with him.

THERAPIST: I understand that is really important, but before we can work on that, I need to have a fairly good idea of what happened during the rape so I can help you figure out its impact on your relationships since then.

CLIENT: How will that help me with my relationships now?

THERAPIST: Because it is possible that you are carrying forward fears and anxieties that took place during the rape into situations that involve intimacy and that you may have become overly sensitive to aspects of your partner's behavior without knowing why.

CLIENT: Okay. What do you want to know?

The first response to challenges should be an accurate re-presentation of information about trauma and its effects, presented with confidence. The therapist may refer to the clinical or research literature, give case examples, or present aspects of trauma theory. If the therapist works in a specialty clinic and has laid the proper groundwork as discussed in Chapter 3, "Establishing the Trauma-Centered Frame," the client will already have heard this information but will just need reassurance. The therapist should generally not give the client a chance to withdraw by making comments such as "This type of an approach is not always for everyone," "The data on success are still unclear," or "Sometimes certain patients find the work overwhelming and may want to feel stronger before beginning it."

If an educational response is not enough to resume the trauma inquiry and the client appears defiant or frightened, the therapist needs to respond as in the following example.

CLIENT: I have done this before, and I just get really upset and can't sleep and barely can go to work. I don't see the benefit of hashing all this over again. I have already told you about the rape, and I don't want to talk about it anymore.

THERAPIST: You don't have to talk about it, and I will not insist or force you to do so.

CLIENT: (*Usually stays quiet, expecting the "so we can do…."*)

THERAPIST: (*Stays quiet, looks directly at the client, smiles warmly.*)

CLIENT: Well?

THERAPIST: What happened to you was horrible, and you have been carrying the pain from it around inside you ever since.

CLIENT: [The client will have difficulty saying that it was not horrible and that there was no pain. He or she might say:] Yes, it was horrible, but I am not in pain about it anymore.

THERAPIST: Then why when you talk about it do you become so upset? Barely be able to go to work?

CLIENT: (*No answer.*)

THERAPIST: Generally people who have been through what you have feel afraid of feeling the pain again, and that is understandable, and also they do not believe that the pain will ever be relieved.

CLIENT: Yes.

THERAPIST: But it can.

CLIENT: I don't think so.

THERAPIST: Yes it can and does go away, and that is what we are here to do; this is what we do.

CLIENT: You seem awfully confident.

THERAPIST: That's an accurate observation.

This reassurance is usually sufficient. The therapist gives no opening to discuss anything else, no opportunity to practice something before getting back to the inquiry, and no offer to have the client come back later or refer him or her elsewhere. A client usually acquiesces at this point. Occasionally, one does not:

CLIENT: Well, that is not good enough for me. I can see that you are set on this point. I don't think I will be able to work with you.

THERAPIST: I understand, and that is fine. This is what I do. We are always here if you reconsider in the future....Let me know if you need a referral to another therapist. [Only at the last moment should one offer to make a referral. Unless the client was entirely mistaken about the work that the therapist does, the client has come to do the work and is likely to be back.]

CONCLUSION

The purpose of the first session is to gain access to the client's traumatic experience, at least to the point of the expression of some pain, so that the client gains confidence that the therapist is competent to handle his or her story. If successful, the therapist establishes the trauma-centered frame, begins to access the outlines of the traumatic memory, and reassures the client that his or her emotionality will be tolerated and contained by the process.

STUDY QUESTIONS

6.1   What is the main goal of the first session?

6.2   What written aids are helpful in the first session?

6.3   Halfway through the first session, the client says, "I don't feel that comfortable talking in such detail about what happened to me.... It's a bit much for me now. Can we talk about other things going on in

my life and get back to the trauma next time?" Which is the best response from the therapist, from a trauma-centered perspective?

A. I can understand your concern, and we should go at your pace,
   so certainly we can get back to it next time.
B. As you are aware, this is a treatment for your trauma, so I'm afraid
   that we have to keep working on it.
C. What feelings just came up for you to make you feel like it is too
   much?
D. As we talked about before, this process is likely to bring up painful memories, and you don't have to continue, but no matter what
   we do, we will return to this point, and I'm ready to help you with
   it. (*Looks quietly at client.*)

CHAPTER 7

Continuing the Trauma History

Getting the Details and Formulating the Trauma Schema

The aim of early sessions is to continue to acquire a detailed narrative of the traumatic event and the client's traumatic experience. This exploration serves several purposes: it helps to support the trauma-centered frame, it helps in constructing and understanding the client's trauma schemas and triggers, and it begins the process of imaginal exposure which in itself has therapeutic benefits. Throughout these sessions, the therapist will feel a need to address numerous other apparently pressing issues, such as family problems, legal issues, medications and symptomatic upsurges, and various other emergencies that serve to express the profound distress of the client. Although attending to some of these issues is appropriate and unavoidable, the experienced trauma-centered clinician will attempt to forestall doing so and instead continue to explore the upsetting details of the trauma story.

CONDUCTING THE DETAILED INQUIRY

In this section we describe in some detail the nuances of conducting a trauma inquiry. Although a chronologically coherent narrative will eventually emerge, that is not the intent of the early sessions. The therapist should be completely attentive to uncovering the thoughts and images arising within the client in the moment as the conversation proceeds. These are not likely to be in chronological order. Traumatic memories are often highly fragmented. They lie like a jumbled collage within the client's mind and are evoked by highly specific elements of words, images, and associations that occur in the conversation. True to the axiom of avoidance, the client will naturally and automatically attempt to thwart their direct expression. The result will be several different types of avoidant maneuvers, which we have named *stops, jumps, bumps, labels,* and *bridges.* The therapist will use the techniques of *looking around, zooming in, slowing down, repeating, backing up, pausing,* and *using present tense* as means of deepening this inquiry. The therapist will also avoid *agreeing with* or *accepting closure* from the client and instead model *not understanding.* All of these techniques have been used by experienced trauma therapists; by giving them labels, we hope to direct the reader's attention to the specifics of the trauma inquiry.

Avoidant Maneuvers

The following are various ways in which clients may cloak important details in their narratives.

STOPS

Stops are sudden pauses in narratives that usually indicate that clients are upset and either do not want to or cannot continue. Clients often try to collect themselves; they might say, "Do I have to go on?" Sometimes they just appear frozen. The following is an example of a stop: "He took me over to the corner of the room. He pushed me down on the floor…." When expanded, the statement becomes, "He took me over to the corner of the room. He pushed me down on the floor *and raped me.*"

JUMPS

Jumps are smooth shifts from one time point to another in the narrative as if there is continuity, but upsetting details are being avoided. Tracking the time in the narrative allows the therapist to pick up on even small jumps where the client moves over an upsetting detail. In retelling stories, many people use jumps to move things along and to keep the pace of a story. In a normal jump, unimportant details are eliminated. In a jump within a trauma narrative, *important* details are eliminated. For example, a client might say, "He took me over to the corner of the room. He pushed me down on the floor and raped me." Without the jump, the narrative would be as follows: "He took me over to the corner of the room. He pushed me down on the floor, *rammed his finger into my rectum, and grabbed me around the neck,* and raped me."

BUMPS

Bumps are slight disturbances in the natural flow of a narrative that signal the presence of an underlying thought or image that spontaneously arises and cannot be integrated or expressed. Examples of bumps include clearing the throat, small gestures, slight hesitations, changes in cadence, repeating a word, glances to the side, shifts in posture, changes in breathing, or changes in skin color or voice tone. A bump may occur in the therapist, who suddenly feels a jolt of anxiety. A bump is added to the previous example: "He took me over to the corner of the room. He pushed me down on the floor, rammed his finger into my rectum, and grabbed me…around the neck and raped me." The slight pause after "grabbed me" hid the details presented in italics: "He took me over to the corner of the room. He pushed me down on the floor, rammed his finger into my rectum, and grabbed me *very hard around the neck, and I thought he might be cutting off my circulation*, and raped me."

LABELS

Labels appear to describe something with its generic name—for example, sexual abuse, rape, ambush, accident, or punishment—rather than the specific action that occurred. The use of labels is intended to avoid the distress related to the details of the act. The term *sexual abuse*, for example, means many things and tells the trauma therapist very little about the event. People are not traumatized by *sexual abuse:* They are traumatized by the fear over, for example, having to suck their stepfather's penis. In our expanding example, the client uses the label *rape:* "He took me over to the corner of the room. He pushed me down on the floor, rammed his finger into my rectum, and grabbed me very hard around the neck, and I thought he might be cutting off my circulation, and raped me." This description hides the details and distress, which are included (in italics) in the following expansion:

> He took me over to the corner of the room. He pushed me down on the floor, rammed his finger into my rectum, and grabbed me very hard around the neck, and I thought he might be cutting off my circulation, *and then pulled off my panties and tried to enter my vagina with his penis, which was not erect enough at first, so he yelled at me, grabbed me harder on the neck, and fingered my anus for several minutes. Finally, he hit me in the small of my back, and I cried out, which seemed to turn him on enough to be able to enter me. He's a macho kind of guy, and I remember him saying all the time how seeing women fight turned him on. Anyway, after about 15 minutes, he finally stopped.*

BRIDGES

A bridge is a run of apparently relevant information that goes up and over an upsetting detail while maintaining a semblance of continuity. A bridge is often in the form of a commentary or additional information about the perpetrator or event. Whereas jumps simply shift from one point to another, bridges provide distracting material. While someone is in the traumatic event, they are not thinking of interesting commentary but focused entirely on the immediate horror. In the previous example, the following statement is a bridge: "He's a macho kind of guy, and I remember him saying all the time how seeing women fight turned him on." This is obviously a thought that has crossed the client's mind after the event. The bridge appears to provide new information but really serves to avoid another upsetting detail.

After the stops, jumps, bumps, labels, and bridges have been removed, the original narrative fragment—"He took me over to the corner of the room. He pushed me down on the floor and raped me"—becomes this (with the bridged-over text underlined):

> He took me over to the corner of the room. He pushed me down on the floor, *rammed his finger into my rectum, and grabbed me very hard around the neck, and I thought he might be cutting off my circulation, and then pulled off my panties and tried to enter my vagina with his penis, which was not erect enough at first, so he yelled at me, grabbed me harder on the neck, and fingered my anus for several minutes. Finally, he hit me in the small of my back, and I cried out, which seemed to turn him on enough to be able to enter me.* As he thrust himself into me, every once in a while he hit me again, hard, on the back, and then on the head. I cried, and then he laughed. I got sick to my stomach and threw up, but he kept pounding away. It was horrible. I felt like a slab of meat. I kept thinking what he was going to do to me after he finished. How long would I be dead before anyone would find me? *Anyway, after about 15 minutes he finally stopped.* He put his clothes back on, spit on me, and left the apartment.

The goal of trauma-centered psychotherapy is to transform the initial, oft-repeated, surface narrative of the former short example into the rich, upsetting, more truthful narrative.

Specific Techniques Used During the Trauma Inquiry

The specific techniques discussed in this subsection are used to open the narrative line. The therapist should use these soon after the client begins therapy, as the principle of immediacy suggests, and not wait for the client to get too far into an abridged version of his or her traumatic event. As soon as the therapist notes an avoidant strategy, these techniques should be used.

Randomly asking for more details will be less effective, because the avoidant maneuvers cover the way in to the deeper levels of the traumatic experience.

These techniques share a common quality: they disrupt the continuity of the chronological flow in the client's verbal report. They slow things down and allow for time to focus more closely on the event, and then more details and more emotionality typically arise. The client's symptoms, distorted thinking, and disturbed behaviors are driven by fear and shame, and it is toward that fear and shame that the therapist should journey. The typical paths that the client has marked out in discussing his or her trauma carefully avoid the trenches and potholes of the bad road; it will be necessary to drive the vehicle down that road.

Clinicians are directed to spend extra time in working through the *hot spots* (Foa and Rothbaum 1998), which are moments in the trauma narrative when the client becomes upset. Going over these moments in the narrative several times is required to attain desensitization. What is being described here, however, is identifying moments of effective avoidance, which are hiding areas of distress; these could be called *cold spots*. By using the following techniques, the therapist can help the client locate these areas of avoidance and allow the covered distress to emerge, becoming temporarily hot spots. Once exposed to the light of day and processed, these moments will fairly rapidly diminish in intensity. Ironically, a focus on only hot spots may miss additional pockets of distress and thereby delay more complete resolution of the client's traumatic distress.

LOOKING AROUND

As the client describes the scene, the therapist attempts to imagine being there and "looks around" in his or her mind for examples of potential objects, people, or actions. When an avoidant response occurs, the therapist then asks a question about the surrounding environment.

> CLIENT: He was on top of me, and I remember his weight was hurting my back.
> THERAPIST: What else was in the room? Was there a nightstand?
> CLIENT: (*Looks upset.*) Yes.
> THERAPIST: What was on the nightstand?
> CLIENT: A screwdriver.

ZOOMING IN

The client might mention a particularly interesting, complex, or important detail. Like a photographer zooming in closer, the therapist asks a question about the situation from close up.

CLIENT: He was on top of me.
THERAPIST: Did you see his face?
CLIENT: Yes, his face was right there.
THERAPIST: What was the skin on his face like?
CLIENT: Pockmarked, sweaty.
THERAPIST: What was his smell?
CLIENT: Wine.
THERAPIST: What part of the face was closest to you?

SLOWING DOWN

The therapist helps the client to slow down the narrative by saying, "Slow down a bit for me," as well as by speaking more slowly and intervening with questions to slow the pace.

CLIENT: The truck was coming rapidly down the street.
THERAPIST: What kind of truck?
CLIENT: I don't know, I'm not sure…
THERAPIST: Think about it a minute…
CLIENT: It was red, like a moving truck.
THERAPIST: And how fast would you say it was going?
CLIENT: Oh, maybe 30 miles per hour.
THERAPIST: Let's see, how fast is that?

REPEATING

After noticing an avoidant maneuver, the therapist may choose to repeat the client's word or phrase that was involved.

CLIENT: The truck hit her on her right side, hard.
THERAPIST: Hard.
CLIENT (*becoming upset*): Like a smack. I heard the sound…[stop].
THERAPIST: You heard the sound. Smack?
CLIENT: It was like a thunder clap…(*bursts into tears*). Everything went all over the place: clothing, bike parts, her body.

Another repeating technique consists of asking the client to repeat what he or she said, as in the following:

THERAPIST: I did not get that.…Could you repeat the part about the phone call?

This is a second example:

CLIENT: I walked up the stairs. I heard them, both of them, anyway I thought so. He was hitting them again, and I went to the door, but it was locked, and I shouted real loud. I didn't want it to be too late. I always worried I would be too late. Thank God I wasn't...

THERAPIST: Wait a minute, say that again for me: you were walking up the stairs and you heard them?

CLIENT: Yeah, the stairs, there were sounds. First I thought it was the stairs creaking, but then I realized it was Carly squealing.

THERAPIST: Squealing?

CLIENT: Well, shrieking, it was so upsetting. I never should have left them home that day.

BACKING UP

Similar to repeating and slowing down, backing up is used by the therapist to stop the client and go back to a former detail, not to repeat it but to start over again with a new question.

CLIENT: Yeah, the stairs, there were sounds. First I thought it was the stairs creaking, but then I realized it was Carly squealing.

THERAPIST: I need to back up here a minute. I don't think you told me how the kids got there in the first place that day? When did they arrive?

PAUSING

Pausing is perhaps the most powerful of the techniques the therapist can use during trauma inquiry. This technique is useful when the client comes to a point in the narrative and pauses or is becoming emotional while remembering something. Although the client might have come to expect the therapist to respond with a nod or uh-huh at this point, the therapist instead stays quiet and looks intently into the client's eyes, perhaps with a warm smile, and holds his or her gaze. Sometimes, the client allows himself or herself to cry and then say what he or she is remembering; at other times, the client just breathes deeply or says "wow." With pause, the flow of the narrative comes to a stop, and time slows down and sometimes halts.

USING PRESENT TENSE

Another useful technique is for the therapist to shift into the present tense when asking the client a question. This is done when it is evident that the client's degree of emotional engagement in the memory is high, for the purpose of intensifying the vividness of his or her remembering.

CLIENT: He held up the knife, and I could see it gleam in the light from the bathroom.

THERAPIST: What is the expression on his face?

CLIENT: I can't describe it....It was awful...gray...angry.

THERAPIST: Now what does he do?

CLIENT: He is breathing harder and harder....I am thinking he is going to stab me.

In this example, the first time the therapist shifted into the present tense ("What is the expression on his face?"), the client stayed in the past tense ("It was awful"), but the client did shift after the therapist's next present-tense question.

We do not generally recommend that the therapist instruct (and definitely not demand) the client to shift into the present tense for several reasons. First, if the client is not ready, the energy required to accommodate to the therapist's request in remembering to speak in the present tense can actually pull the client away from his or her emotional engagement with the memory, having the opposite effect as that intended. It is generally important to allow the client to narrate naturally and not to bring attention to the manner in which the client is narrating. Second, asking questions in the present tense follows the second principle of *engagement*—communicating to the client that the therapist is psychologically near to him or her. In fact, the therapist and client may naturally shift into the present tense as they both become engaged in the trauma-centered inquiry.

EXAMPLE OF TECHNIQUE USE

The use of these techniques will be demonstrated with the rape example from earlier in the chapter. (The client's avoidant strategies and the therapist's techniques are in listed in brackets, with the techniques underlined.)

CLIENT: He took me over to the corner of the room. He pushed me down on the floor.... [stop]
THERAPIST: He pushed you down on the floor. [repeating]
CLIENT: Yeah, and then he raped me. [jump and label]
THERAPIST: Okay, now let's slow down just a bit: he pushed you down on the floor and then what did he do? [backing up]
CLIENT: He rammed his finger into my rectum and grabbed me...around the neck. [Bump]
THERAPIST: How did he grab you? [zooming in]
CLIENT: Hard, very hard around my neck, and I thought he might be cutting off my circulation.
THERAPIST: Were you able to breathe? [zooming in]
CLIENT: Barely. I thought I was going to die, but I didn't....He just raped me. [Label]
THERAPIST: Raped you. [repeating]
CLIENT: Yeah, raped me....
THERAPIST: (*Stays silent and looks at her.*) [pausing]
CLIENT (*emotional*): First, he pulled off my panties and tried to enter my vagina with his penis, which was not erect enough at first, so he yelled

at me, grabbed me harder on the neck, and fingered my anus for several minutes. Finally, he hit me in the small of my back, and I cried out, which seemed to turn him on enough to be able to enter me. He's a macho kind of guy, and I remember him saying all the time how seeing women fight turned him on. Anyway, after about 15 minutes, he finally stopped. [bridge]

THERAPIST: That is horrible.

CLIENT: It really was.

THERAPIST: But I don't think I got something. Can we back up a minute? He hit you in the small of the back, and then somehow he got an erection? [backing up]

CLIENT: I think it turned him on.

THERAPIST: And then what happened? Did he hit you again?

CLIENT: Yeah, as he thrust himself into me, every once in a while he hit me again, hard, on the back, and then on the head. I cried, and then he laughed.

THERAPIST: He laughed. [repeating]

CLIENT: I got sick to my stomach and threw up, but he kept pounding away. It was horrible. I felt like a slab of meat. I kept thinking what he was going to do to me after he finished. How long would I be dead before anyone would find me?

THERAPIST: (*Stays silent and looks at client intently.*) [pausing]

CLIENT: (*Eyes filling with tears, she looks directly into the therapist's eyes.*) I didn't die though. (*Smiles.*) He put his clothes back on, yeah, and left the apartment. [bridge]

THERAPIST: He just put his clothes back on, while you were on the floor, the vomit next to you.... Was he looking at you? [looking around]

CLIENT: Sort of. He did spit on me.

THERAPIST: Hmm, did it hit you? [zooming in]

CLIENT: (*Laughs.*) No, he missed! (*Client and therapist just grin at each other.*)

Opening Up the Narrative Line

From these examples, it should be clear how competent trauma-centered inquiry will *open up the narrative line* of the client's memory. Close listening to each of the client's statements will reveal many avoidant maneuvers, and when attended to, each will open up a new detail, a new thought, or a new fear, which together help in constructing a more complex understanding of the client's trauma schemas. This process is never finished: there is always more detail that can be extracted. The convoluted, wrinkled nature of the client's initial trauma narrative and the goal of opening up this narrative line are illustrated in Figure 7–1.

In addition to the techniques discussed in the previous section, three general approaches to the client's narrative are also helpful in constructing a more detailed narrative. With these approaches, however, the trauma-

The Convoluted Narrative Line of Traumatic Memories

Bridge   Jump   Label   Bump   Stop

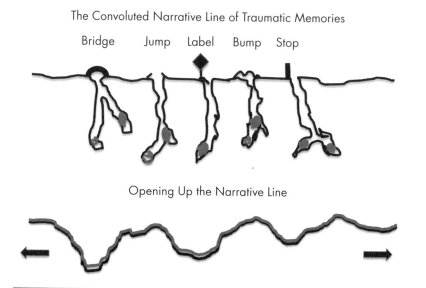

Opening Up the Narrative Line

FIGURE 7–1.   Comparison of initial trauma narrative and of narrative line after it has been opened up.

centered therapist will demonstrate a number of behaviors that deviate slightly from the norms of regular conversation, and therefore require some practice.

NOT UNDERSTANDING

It seems paradoxical that the prima facie essence of being a therapist—to understand—should be turned on its face with trauma clients; however, for them, not being understood is a fundamental aspect of their condition. The statement "No one can understand what happened" is both a truism, for the therapist was not there, and an accusation, for the therapist was not there. The typical methods used by a therapist to let clients know the therapist is with them—including the periodic nod, "uh-huh," "I understand," and "yes!"—not only do not challenge the avoidant strategies the clients are us- ing but also alienate these clients. Thus, when the therapist is inquiring about trauma, it is an excellent idea to let go of these habitual behaviors and instead periodically communicate that he or she did not quite understand: "I'm sorry, could you say more about that? I don't fully understand," or "I didn't quite get that: where was he when he said that?" or "Wait a minute, she screamed? Why did she scream?" These questions lead smoothly into asking the client to reveal more. They are often experienced by the client as demonstrating the therapist's curiosity, concern, and bafflement at the outrageous behavior of the perpetrator. Beginning therapists often express their anxiety about inquiring by becoming passive, occasionally softly saying "uh-huh" or nodding, and thereby losing the client. The technique of not understanding appears to be difficult for therapists to learn.

NOT AGREEING

Likewise, when the therapist appears to agree with a client's statement by nodding or saying "yes" or "uh-huh," he or she seems to be colluding with whatever avoidant strategy the client is using, even when the therapist does not know which one. In contrast, appearing slightly at odds with the client's statements suggests that there is something not right, incomplete, or a bit off with the narrative, and that is a far more accurate assessment of how the client feels. Because clients are constantly avoiding the truth, to some degree, they too feel that their statements are not quite right. Paradoxically, offering slight disagreement or a questioning stance will propel the client to provide more explanation and therefore more details of his or her experience. Because traumatic events are *unbelievable* (meaning overwhelming), it is a common experience for trauma victims to not be believed. Therefore, when the therapist moves slightly into this territory, and then appears to be won over by the client's narrative, more vivid details tend to emerge.

> CLIENT: Then he entered the room and literally jumped all the way over the bed on top of me.
> THERAPIST (*in a questioning tone*): What, he jumped all the way over the bed?
> CLIENT: (*Pauses.*) Well, anyway it felt like that.
> THERAPIST: Say more about how he jumped.
> CLIENT (*thinking*): He kinda gave a yell.
> THERAPIST: I don't know what you mean.
> CLIENT (*more energized*): Yes, now I remember. He came in, looked at me real hard, and then gave a deep…growl.
> THERAPIST (*again in a questioning tone*): He growled?
> CLIENT (*raising voice*): Yes, he growled like an animal. You should have seen the look on his face…(*becomes upset*). It was terrifying!
> THERAPIST: I can only imagine. Sounds terrifying.
> CLIENT: And then he leaped on top of me.

NOT ACCEPTING CLOSURE

People, when they speak and want to indicate they have come to the end of a thought or to the conclusion of their description, typically use tonal phrasing that may go up ("and that's how it ended!") or down ("and they never came back") to indicate closure. Such phrasings, as well as direct verbal content ("and that's the end of my story"), signal the other party to respond. Whenever a client uses these ways of indicating closure, the therapist should not use the typically expected verbal or nonverbal responses. Merely remaining quiet and looking at the client after he or she has appeared to conclude will disrupt this sense of closure and will often allow the diverted emotion or image to arise. Otherwise, the therapist should use one of the techniques described earlier in this chapter, such as backing up, repeating, or looking around, or should simply say, "Tell me more."

UNDERSTANDING WHY CLIENTS MAY GET UPSET AFTER THE SESSION

When a session ends only part way into this process, the client might go home and feel distressed and then might call the therapist the next day to say that he or she found the session really upsetting and may not want to return. The novice therapist will likely conclude that the reason for this lies in the information that the client provided in the session—that is, the incomplete narrative. Although this is possible, it is more likely that the client will be upset by the more upsetting details that have not yet been uttered. As the client is speaking to the therapist and using various jumps and bridges, he or she is usually aware of the more upsetting details that are being left out. Not infrequently, a client's distress after the session is due to the nearly but not quite expressed details. Therefore, it will be a mistake for the therapist to conclude that it was due to what was said and to retreat from the traumatic inquiry. Instead, the therapist is encouraged to comment that the client may have remembered a really upsetting detail that he or she did not have a chance to get out in the session and that the therapist may have missed this detail also. Quite often the client will agree with this and spurt out the detail on the phone and then feel some measure of relief and greater confidence in the therapist and the therapeutic process. The last detail is the worst, although one never gets to the last detail, for it is beyond words. One can only approach the edges of that abyss. Therefore, it is best said that the *next* detail is *worse* than the previous one, and thus it is usually good technique for the therapist to say at the end of a session that he or she assumes that there are more details yet to come.

FORMULATING THE TRAUMA SCHEMA

Trauma schemas are dynamic, relational structures that develop after a traumatic event and that serve to stabilize the person when he or she is disrupted by traumatic triggers in the present environment. Traumatic triggers are sensory or interpersonal stimuli that bear some resemblance to elements of the person's traumatic experience. Encountering them in the present sends the person into a state of ambiguity regarding the boundaries between past and present. Fearing an intrusion of the traumatic experience, the person employs the trauma schema in his or her interpersonal behavior to reestablish a firm distinction between the self and the danger situation and derivatives of the perpetrator. This often results in a misperception of the environment or others as dangerous or untrustworthy. Another way of saying this is that the person generalizes from his or her traumatic experience onto new experience that usually is not as dangerous to him or her.

Trauma schemas are organized in layers (Table 7–1; Figure 7–2). The first layer arises out of the extreme, pure experience of fear or shame, which prevents representation. The typical trauma schema arising from this layer is represented by this thought: "There are no words for my experience. No one can possibly understand me and what I went through, and I cannot explain it."

The second layer arises from the physical pain that the person experienced during the event. Toxic stress often expresses itself in actual physical pain, both at the time of the event and for years afterward (Schnurr and Green 2004). These pains are deep and enduring and are often continuously reexperienced in somatic and psychic forms. The following is an example of a trauma schema arising from this layer: "I am in a constant state of pain, and I cannot take it anymore. Nothing helps to reduce my pain."

The third layer arises from the specific sensory elements that were associated with the traumatic experience: colors, sounds, smells, objects, statements, and actions that were present or occurred at the time and that are indelibly etched in the person's mind. A specific example of a trauma schema related to this layer is the statement "I cannot be near churches ever. I must avoid churches at all times."

The fourth layer arises from the victim's thoughts about anticipated actions of the perpetrator that did not occur but might have. These arise within the victim during the event as he or she worries not so much about what is being done to him or her at the moment but about what might happen later that could be so much worse. The victim's memory of the traumatic experience usually includes these thoughts of what might have happened. The following is a trauma schema arising from this layer: "I am never safe. I am in imminent danger. Bad things are about to happen. The situation is hopeless."

The fifth layer of a traumatic experience arises from the lack of response by potential rescuers. The victim often thinks about why no one stopped or prevented what happened: "if only someone had come by," "if only some-

TABLE 7–1.   Layers of a trauma schema

1. Fear or shame

   The primary emotional state of the person in all its complexity during the
   traumatic event and immediately afterward.

2. Pain

   The primarily physical, bodily pain experienced during the event.

3. Sensory elements

   Any sensory stimuli experienced during the event, such as colors, sounds,
   smells, objects, and perceptions of the environment.

4. Anticipated actions

   Thoughts occurring during the event concerning what might happen next
   that evoked intense primary emotional arousal.

5. Lack of response

   Distressing thoughts about not being protected, saved, or responded to by
   others, that occurred during the event.

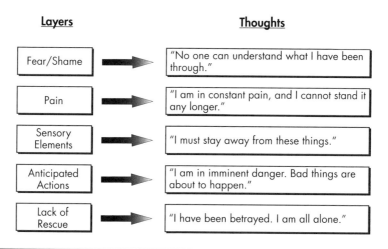

FIGURE 7–2.   Layers and thoughts within the trauma schema.

one had heard," "if only...." The trauma schema associated with this layer
reflects the victim's anger at being abandoned: "I have been betrayed. No
one is there for me. No one cares." This level is often called *homecoming
trauma* and is particularly damaging to current interpersonal relationships
(Johnson et al. 1997; Shay 2002).

   Using this model as a heuristic for understanding the trauma schemas
of clients will help therapists in their decoding work. Each phrase or ele-

TABLE 7–2. Analysis of clinical example in terms of layers of the trauma schemas

Layers	Items from the narrative	Potential trauma schemas	Potential current behaviors
Fear or shame	It was horrible.	I am terrified all the time.	Experience anxiety.
Pain	Rammed his finger into my rectum, grabbed me very hard around the neck. Grabbed me harder, fingered my anus, hit me in the small of my back; I cried out. He hit me again, hard, on the back, and then on the head; I cried, sick to my stomach and threw up.	I feel pain in my rectum, my neck, and the small of my back. I get sick to my stomach.	Go to gastrointestinal doctors, chiropractors.
Sensory elements	Corner of the room, pushed me down on the floor. Pulled off my panties; entered my vagina with his penis; not erect enough, he yelled at me. He thrust himself into me; he laughed, pounding away; I felt like a slab of meat; he spit on me.	I don't like corners of rooms, to sit on carpets, people yelling at me, laughter, raw meat, sex, spit.	Avoid corners, carpets, comedy, raw meat, sex. Get upset when people yell.
Anticipated actions	Might be cutting off my circulation. What was he going to do to me. How long would I be dead.	I worry about the circulation to my head. I worry that I am going to die.	Don't wear scarves; wear open-neck shirts. Feel claustrophobic, hard to breathe. Keep windows open.
Lack of response	Before anyone would find me.	No one will find me or know where I am.	Obsess about cell phone batteries dying. Won't go out alone.

ment in the narrative corresponds with at least one layer of the trauma schema, which includes fear or shame, pain, sensory elements, anticipated actions, and lack of response.

As Table 7–2 demonstrates, each element of the traumatic experience of the rape victim, as presented in the running example throughout this chapter, is associated with aspects of a trauma schema, which in turn underlies specific distorted behaviors in the present. As therapy proceeds, the combined inquiry into the client's experience, ways of viewing the world (schemas), and distorted behaviors will result in a comprehensive understanding of the nature and cause of the client's disorder. Many clinicians do not appreciate how specific these connections are and to what degree details in any one area (traumatic experience, schema, and behavior) can help identify details in the other areas.

CONCLUSION

Our intention in this chapter is to demonstrate the complexity, intricacy, and sophistication inherent in a competent trauma inquiry. Through guided and supervised practice, the clinician can learn how apply these techniques and intervene effectively. The client is likely to experience an integrated imaginal exposure and to identify his or her distorted cognitions arising from the trauma. This work provides a solid foundation for the therapeutic work ahead.

STUDY QUESTIONS

7.1　Match the items by placing the letters in the appropriate spaces.

　　A. Not agreeing　　　　___ "I'm not sure I get what you are saying here."

　　B. Not understanding　　___ "That is amazing, but tell me more about what happened in the boat."

　　C. Not accepting closure　___ "How could he have jumped that high?"

7.2　Match the items by placing the letters in the appropriate spaces.

　　A. Bumps　　　　　___ The client pauses because he or she is upset.

　　B. Jumps　　　　　___ The client uses the phrase "sexual assault."

      C. Stops   ___ The client clears his or her throat and becomes flushed while speaking.

      D. Bridges   ___ The client skips a few minutes of time in the narrative.

      E. Labels   ___ The client comments on an aspect of the city in which the event took place.

7.3   Name the seven techniques useful in getting the details of the traumatic memories.

7.4   What are the five layers of a trauma schema?

7.5   Name which layer is being represented in the following statements:

    A. "I know things will be worse in the future."
    B. "I don't believe it when people tell me they will help."
    C. "I can't stand the smell of boxwood."
    D. "I can get a headache at almost any time."
    E. "There's no way to describe it."

7.6   What is the major function of formulating the client's trauma schemas?

CHAPTER 8

Conducting Ongoing Treatment

Decoding the Trauma Schema in Current Behaviors

At some point, the initial phase of gaining a good understanding of the client's traumatic events and experiences will be achieved, although full understanding will never be reached. Additional information will be continuously revealed throughout the remainder of the treatment, sometimes even years later. Sessions will begin to transition so that a greater preponderance of time is spent on current situations and issues that arise in the client's life. Prior to making this transition, however, the therapist needs to have formulated the basic trauma schemas that the client developed in response to these events, as well as some of the triggers that may ignite these trauma schemas. These distorted forms of thinking, feeling, and relating are ultimately the targets of treatment, and identifying them within current circumstances will be the major activity of this phase of treatment.

Having a rich understanding of each of the layers within a trauma schema will be important in the process of decoding behaviors and linking them to schemas and thus to the original traumatic events. The trauma-centered therapist is encouraged to make an assumption that any aspect of current behavior may have a link to the client's traumas. When a particularly strong or obvious link emerges, the therapist will initiate a decoding inquiry, as demonstrated later in this chapter (see section "Examples of De-coding Process"). More experienced therapists can develop rather remark-able intuitive sensitivity to derivatives of the trauma schemas.

Therefore, although the content of the discussion between client and ther-apist begins to transform, the basic trauma-centered contract or frame for the work does not. The principles of immediacy, engagement, and emotionality should remain at play (see Chapter 4, "Principles of Trauma-Centered Psy-chotherapy"), because remnants of highly distressing memories can emerge at a moment's notice.

TECHNIQUE OF DECODING

The technique of *decoding* includes two of the basic therapeutic ingredients noted in the literature: repetitive imaginal exposure and cognitive restruc-turing. By frequently linking and then moving from current behavior to past traumatic memories, the client continues to be exposed to the under-lying fear or shame structures and thus continues to receive the benefits of desensitization that exposure provides. By untangling the current situation from the past situation, decoding provides a measure of differentiation be-tween present and past that helps the client reestablish stronger but more flexible boundaries and therefore restructure his or her current expectancies and behavioral impulses. The technique of *introducing discrepancy* into the client's experience is therefore at work here.

Additionally, the technique of *disclosing the perpetrator* is integrated into this phase of treatment. Of the many differences between the client's trau-matic past and present, the presence versus absence of the perpetrator is per-haps the most crucial. Because of the dynamics of trauma, many distorted trauma schemas, when employed, will cast the client's loved ones or close relationships in the role of the perpetrator, reflecting the confusion between past and present. Clients complain about being mistreated (again) by their families, employers, the government, and service people. They feel betrayed by friends, ignored by family, purposefully mistreated by supervisors, and ripped off by their attorneys, plumbers, and doctors. Being accused of these actions, the people in their lives withdraw from them, confirming to the cli-ents that they were against them from the beginning. One of the most im-portant elements in the phase of decoding and discrepancy is to raise the presence of the client's perpetrator within the discussion. In comparison to their perpetrators, their families, friends, attorneys, and bosses pale in evil. For clients, learning that they have been reviving and reliving their trau-matic experience by confusing those around them with their perpetrator can have a freeing and powerful effect. Thus, throughout each session, the therapist will frequently mention the name of the client's perpetrator(s) as part of the decoding procedure. The therapist, rather than asking about the client's "sexual abuse," "rape," or "accident," asks whether the client has been thinking about "your stepfather," "Ralph Jones," or "the truck driver" who hit his or her child. According to the fourth axiom, which states that trauma schemas are relational, people are hurt not by events but rather by evil people, incompetent professionals, or drunken drivers.

EXAMPLES OF DECODING PROCESS

The decoding process can be a powerful experience for a client. The following is a brief introductory example of the first of a two-session treatment of a 35-year-old single man who presented with panic disorder that had failed to respond to medication.

> THERAPIST: Hello. What happened?
> CLIENT: So I had a serious panic attack. I mean, I was working that day, February 3, and all of a sudden my heart started to jump out of my chest. I freaked out, had to stop. They sent me to the ER and checked me out, but everything was okay.
> THERAPIST: Tell me more about the panic attack.
> CLIENT: I was in this meeting and I was shaking. I don't know, it was a regular meeting. We were planning something I can't remember, but it didn't mean much to me, but I thought I was going to jump out of my skin or die! I was so embarrassed. When I got back to work, the guys really gave it to me. Then I had another attack that same day, and they sent me to a doctor who thought I was making the whole thing up to get out of work. Another doctor gave me some medication that made me sick. They think I'm crazy or something. So they sent me here. I'm not crazy, but I have no idea what happened here, February 4, no 3rd, yes, 3rd.
> THERAPIST: Has anything really upsetting or frightening ever happened to you on February 3rd?
> CLIENT: No, I don't know, no, let's see…February 3rd. Uh…
> THERAPIST: February 3rd.
> CLIENT: No, February 3rd? Wow. That was the day we invaded Iraq.
> THERAPIST: You were in the Persian Gulf?
> CLIENT: Yeah.
> THERAPIST: Did anything upsetting happen that day when you invaded Iraq?
> CLIENT: (*Becomes very upset.*)
> THERAPIST: (*Stays silent, looks intently at client.*)
> CLIENT: Oh, my God.
> THERAPIST: Bad.

CLIENT: Real bad.
THERAPIST: Tell me about it.

(*Client then tells of his experience, which included several terrifying brushes with enemy fire, and then a devastating attack on his unit, by mistake, by another U.S. combat unit, which killed several soldiers in his unit and nearly missed him. He had never told anyone about these incidents because they involved friendly fire.*)

CLIENT: So are you telling me that my memories of what happened that day are the cause for my panic attack?
THERAPIST: Seems likely. The day triggered your memories, and you re-experienced the fear that you had felt, but you didn't make the connection, so you felt you were going crazy. What do you think?
CLIENT: I can't believe it. So I don't have panic disorder?
THERAPIST: Probably not.
CLIENT: I'm not crazy?
THERAPIST: Nope. You had a terrifying experience in the Gulf. I can't imagine how frightening it was, but you got through it. Compared to that, this situation should be no problem for you.
CLIENT: Thank you. Lot to think about.

(*The client returned 2 weeks later for another session, in which he reviewed again his combat experiences. He had not had another panic attack. Treatment terminated, and a year later [in February] the therapist received a postcard from the client, who thanked the therapist and wrote that he had taken February 3rd off that year.*)

The general process of decoding follows a series of steps. First, the therapist (and sometimes the client) identifies an element in the client's narrative of a current event as a *trigger*. This is then used to explore *links* between the current situation and the past traumatic event. The *similarities* between the present and past situations are noted. Then the therapist highlights the *differences* between the past and present events, particularly regarding the original perpetrator and the current challenger (i.e., the person who is enrolled as the perpetrator in the current scenario). Once these connections and differences are fully discussed, the therapist may review the process, pointing out to the client in an educational manner how the trauma schema was evoked and played out.

In the following case example, a single, male client in his 50s is at a session after a year in treatment.

CLIENT: I had an important meeting last Thursday. The board was reviewing my proposal, and there was a lot of discussion and questions about it....I was recommending that they completely rehaul their infrastructure; an old factory building needed to be taken down and replaced—toxic waste, you know. I have a lot of support, but this was the meeting that I had to stand up for my views and take a few hits. I was really excited. Anyway, weird, I wake up Thursday morning early and find myself having completely tied myself up in the sheets from turning over and over in my sleep; my head is stuck in one of the pillows, like this, and it's nice and soft, and I have this funny thought: maybe I should show up at the meeting naked and wrapped up in these sheets, sort of like giving a speech as a Roman senator or something! Anyway, the meeting went fine, but I kept having that image in my mind all day.

THERAPIST: Interesting. So your dream seemed to be about your anticipation of this important meeting? [noting trigger]

CLIENT: Yes, definitely. I knew I was going to have to stand my ground, which is hard for me.

THERAPIST: Any thoughts about waking up like that, wrapped in sheets, head in your pillow?

CLIENT: Not really.

THERAPIST: When your mother abused you, was there a pillow involved? [linking with trauma]

CLIENT: (*Looks down.*) Yes.

THERAPIST: Say more about this.

CLIENT: She kept a pillow by my head in case I made a sound.... I remember how soft it felt compared to how rough she was.

THERAPIST: At times your mother restrained you with the sheets? [mentioning perpetrator]

CLIENT: That's right. And then used them to clean me up afterward. Amazing.

THERAPIST: Seems like a lot of parallels here. [pointing out similarities]

CLIENT: Yeah, the meeting was about cleaning up,...toxic waste (*laughs*).

THERAPIST: And standing up for yourself.

CLIENT: Making noise. Instead of not making any noise.

THERAPIST: After your mother cleaned you up, did you get up, stand up?

CLIENT (*tearful*): I couldn't....It hurt too much.

THERAPIST: But you stood up to the board. [introducing discrepancy]

CLIENT: I did stand up to them, and made noise.

THERAPIST: What do you say to your mother now?

CLIENT: Can't hold me down any more.

THERAPIST: Things are different now. [introducing discrepancy]

CLIENT: Yeah, I've rehauled my infrastructure.

In this example, the client's trigger appeared to be standing up for himself in front of the board, which conflicted with a thought from his trauma schema: "I feel too frightened and weak to be able to stand up (to my mother) (for myself)." This schema developed from his experience of being tied down in his bed when he was ages 3–6 by his mother, who then sexually abused him by masturbating him and penetrating his anus with her fingers. The schema included the sensory elements of the pillow's softness, the sheets holding him down, and being cleaned up afterward. The elements of anticipated actions were represented by fears of being punished if he made noise. There were few references in his dream to primary fears or to lack of rescue; in fact, his dream reveals a substantial overcoming of these fears in his desire to speak to the board as a Roman senator. The richness of the interweaving of past and present, in the overlapping nature of toxic waste, rehauling infrastructure, and making noise, is impressive.

The therapist first made a link through a question about the client's prior abuse. The parallels quickly emerged and were commented on. Then the therapist pointed out the difference between past and present in that the client was able now to stand up, highlighting the discrepancy, and then suggested how both similarities and discrepancies are present in the client's choice to repair the world through his work. Throughout, the therapist mentions the client's mother in person, disclosing the perpetrator. The fact that the client and therapist had had a detailed mutual understanding of the client's trauma helped to facilitate a rapid decoding of this current event.

In the following case example, a male client in his 40s is at a session 6 months after beginning treatment.

> CLIENT: I'm leaving on my trip to Georgia with Sherry tomorrow, but I'm feeling anxious about it.
> THERAPIST: Say more.
> CLIENT: We're driving and not flying, so that's not a problem. It's funny, because I can't think of any reason I should worry about this trip. I was looking forward to it. I mentioned to Sherry yesterday that I was anxious about it, and she got angry. She's upset when my anxieties "ruin" things. I said, "Fine. Go without me." She said, "No, we'll just get separate rooms." I said, "No need for that. I'll just sleep in the car!" That upset her. I worry too much. Anything I can do about this? The trip is tomorrow.
> THERAPIST: What are you worried about?
> CLIENT: That's just it. I don't know. I've never been to Georgia.
> THERAPIST: You're worried about Georgia?
> CLIENT: Yeah.
> THERAPIST: And you have never been there?
> CLIENT: Nope.
> THERAPIST: When you were a kid, your dad never drove the family to Georgia? [noting trigger]
> CLIENT: Nope....We did go to Florida once.
> THERAPIST: (*Looks at client. Client looks back.*)
> CLIENT: We must have gone through Georgia.
> THERAPIST: Seems likely.

CLIENT: (*Remembers.*) Oh my God. We did stop in Georgia. It was late, and we passed the state line from South Carolina to Georgia, and we were looking for a motel, and we finally found one—it was awful looking—and my parents got out and had a huge argument in the parking lot. My dad said she had ruined the whole trip. He was really yelling. He took us kids into the room and forced her to sleep in the car. We were terrified. [linking with trauma]

THERAPIST: Did your father hit you or your brother or sister? [mentioning perpetrator]

CLIENT: Of course. I wanted to go out to be with my mother, but it was too cold.

THERAPIST: Must have been horrible. Did you sleep?

CLIENT: Not one minute. We were worried about Mom in the car and maybe more worried about Dad.

THERAPIST: So no mystery why you are anxious about going to Georgia: the fight between your father and mother, her having to sleep separately in the car. [pointing out similarities]

CLIENT: I can't believe that.

THERAPIST: And with Sherry, you worried that you would "ruin" the trip.

CLIENT: And that I'd have to sleep in the car.

THERAPIST: Are you going to ruin the trip? [introducing discrepancy]

CLIENT: I don't think so.

THERAPIST: Are you going to sleep in the car?

CLIENT: No.

THERAPIST: Are you going to hit Sherry, or is she going to hit you?

CLIENT: No.

THERAPIST: Are you your father?

CLIENT: My God, no.

THERAPIST: Are you your mother, who has to sleep in the car?

CLIENT: Definitely not.

THERAPIST: Are you going to go to Georgia?

CLIENT: Definitely. Maybe I can find that old motel? (*Smiles.*)

THERAPIST: I'll bet it's long gone, like your father. [mentioning perpetrator]

CLIENT: I visit his grave regularly, just to make sure.

THERAPIST: (*Smiles.*) No need to bring him along.

CLIENT: Thanks.

This dialogue is a good example of a decoding process that is mutually conducted by client and therapist, each of whom is familiar with the process. The client suspects that something is operating in his anxiety about the trip and presents it to the therapist, who simply asks if he had ever been to Georgia. The memories and connections tumble out in short order, and the client and therapist quickly put the pieces together and reveal the process that the trauma schema has produced. The result is a resolution of the behavioral inhibition against going on the trip, a clarification of the interpersonal conflict with his current spouse, and an emergence of a sweetly ironic sense of humor about his parents.

In the following case example, a woman in her 40s and her 6-year-old foster child, Sam, are in a session early in treatment.

FOSTER MOTHER (FM): The weekend went very badly. Eric was terrible all weekend, weren't you, Eric?

ERIC: (*Ignores her.*)

FM: Tell the doctor what I found in your closet. Tell him!

ERIC: (*Sits down on the floor and picks out a plastic hamburger from a toy bin.*)

THERAPIST: What did you find in his closet?

FM: It was disgusting. I thought there would be the usual clothing all piled up, but when I picked it up, I found a whole bunch of food, old food, lying at the bottom of the closet, some in open containers....The smell was awful, bugs crawling over it, and then I saw mouse droppings, yuck! Right, Eric?

ERIC: (*Shrugs shoulders and continues to play with the toy.*)

THERAPIST: What happened when you found it?

FM: Well, that's just it. I confronted him with it and told him to clean it up, but he refused. So I began to clean it out, and he went wild, saying he needed it. I told him I was taking every last bit of it, right Eric? And then he kicked me. Didn't you? In the 6 months I've had him, he's never kicked me before. Doctor, I don't know if I can keep him like this. This is too much.

THERAPIST: My guess is that he hoarded food in his closet for a reason. [noting trigger]

FM: God knows what that could be. It must have been there for weeks.

THERAPIST: Eric, when you were with your birth parents, was there ever a time when you didn't have enough to eat? [linking with trauma]

ERIC: (*Nods.*)

THERAPIST: I understand your birth mom was often away for some time—a day?

ERIC: Three days.

THERAPIST: Who else was around?

ERIC: No one. Just me and my sister.

THERAPIST: Who fed her?

ERIC: Me.

THERAPIST: Did your birth mom ever punish you by refusing to serve you food.

ERIC: (*Nods.*) We have no food.

THERAPIST: You have no food.

FM: Eric, we have plenty of food now. Why do you hoard food when there is plenty? I feed him all the time; he eats like a horse.

THERAPIST: Underneath, because of his past experience, he believes that he may not have enough food because his mother would not give it to him. [identifying trauma schema, mentioning perpetrator]

ERIC: So I hide it.

THERAPIST: So he hides it. Not to eat. Because it calms him down. [pointing out similarities]

FM: I see.

THERAPIST: Would your birth mom come into your room and take your food from you?

ERIC: Yes. She'd find it, and I'd get a whooping.

THERAPIST: What would you do? Hide from her?

ERIC: No. Kick her.

THERAPIST: Eric was at times not fed, so he developed the idea that there is no food, and he deals with that by hoarding food in his closet, even now, and when you came in and, appropriately, cleaned it out, it made him feel anxious, and the two of you got into a fight a little like his birth mom and he did. [explaining the process]

ERIC: A lot like.

THERAPIST: And he even kicked you. But he wasn't kicking *you*; he was kicking his birth mom. (*To Eric.*) Eric, that must have been so sad and scary, what your birth mom did to you. [mentioning perpetrator]

ERIC: (*Nods.*)

THERAPIST: But your foster mom here is not your birth mom. She is not going to harm you like your birth mom did, right Mom? [introducing discrepancy]

FM (*gently*): Not at all, Eric.

ERIC: (*Looks at his foster mother, then stands up and goes over to her and lies across her lap.*)

FM: I'm sorry, honey. (*Strokes his hair.*)

In this example, the result of the decoding and then differentiating process is to free up the child to seek comfort from the foster mother, who has been released from the hold of the perpetrating mother. The interpenetration of two situations, carried by the child's trauma schemas of "I will not have enough food" and "she will punish me if I ask for food," is diminished by the therapist's directly addressing the original traumas still burdening the child. The therapist follows the basic sequence: identifying the trigger, linking with the original trauma, pointing out similarities, introducing discrepancy, and then reviewing the process. The client is reexposed to an upsetting memory, and his distorted schemas are revealed and corrected. The intimate others in the client's life are differentiated from the perpetrator, which allows them to stay in proximity to the client and not to withdraw from him.

Conclusion

The process of decoding, introducing discrepancy, and disclosing the perpetrator is the method used for the remainder of the treatment process, which need not be of great length. Once a client and his or her family learn how this process works, they become increasingly able to identify the rise of their trauma schemas in current behaviors and become less reactive in challenging situations. A rather substantial calming down of their sensitivities to stress occurs.

Study Questions

8.1   What are the two main components of this phase of treatment?

8.2   Fill in the blanks:

In decoding, one identifies the _____, then points out the _____ between that and an element of the traumatic experience, noting the _____ between the past event and the current situation, and then emphasizes the _____ between the past and the present and between the perpetrator and the challenger.

CHAPTER 9

The Gap

When the Trauma Schema Emerges in the Therapeutic Relationship

Trauma schemas are evoked in current behaviors outside the session as well as increasingly by behaviors inside the session. Trauma schemas are interpersonal, relational structures that serve to stabilize the client's inner feeling of uncertainty regarding the boundaries between the past and the present, and between danger and safety. When these trauma schemas are employed, they usually surface as means by which the client externalizes his or her fear or shame and experiences danger emanating from the environment, usually from another person. The other person (in this case the therapist) will feel misunderstood and unfairly blamed. The unfortunate paradox is that in the attempt to reduce ambiguity (and the possible reexperience of fear), the trauma schema re-creates the division between victim and perpetrator from the original event, imposing the past upon the present, again. When this occurs within the therapeutic interaction, it is called the *gap*.

The gap is a disturbing event for most therapists. Until this point in the therapeutic relationship, the client has been operating within his or her usual neurotic schemas regarding the therapist, one of which may be "I am so thankful to you for being here to listen to my story, which I have shared with no one else." This is a particularly gratifying schema for the therapist, and indeed empathy, understanding, and connection may be evident in the conversation between client and therapist, as in any psychotherapy. As long as the therapist and client remain within this territory, all goes well, because the problematic material is being avoided. As a rule of thumb, if the treatment is moving along smoothly and there is a good feeling of connection between therapist and client, trauma-centered psychotherapy has not fully begun. The rise of the gap brings forward into the relationship between therapist and client the proximity to the terror and the need to cut the bridge between self and other for protection. One moment the therapist appears to be doing well, and the next he or she is enrolled in one of several disturbing roles that are intrinsic to the trauma schema.

THE TRAUMA GRID: VICTIM, PERPETRATOR, BYSTANDER, AND COLLABORATOR

The four main roles in a trauma schema are the *perpetrator*, who committed the act; the *victim*, who was harmed by the act; the *bystander*, who is on the side of the victim but, because he or she is frightened, does not intervene to stop the act; and the *collaborator*, who is on the side of the perpetrator and who allows or aids the perpetrator but does not actually participate in the act (Johnson and Lubin 2000). Most trauma schemas rigidly define these roles despite the fact that in most cases the boundaries among them are quite ambiguous and overlapping. Thus, in the trauma schema, the victim is the *innocent victim*, for if the victim in any way evoked or allowed the perpetrator's behavior, he or she would also be a collaborator, as victims are often accused of being. In the trauma schema, perpetrators must be completely bad or evil, whereas often they too act out of schemas produced by prior victimizations, turning them into part-victims, which the defense attorneys point out in court. Collaborators, when confronted, claim to have been intimidated into helping, thus becoming bystanders. Victims are accused of making false claims and thus are turned into perpetrators. These ambiguities of real life are often hashed out in court; they remain deeply upsetting to the trauma victim, who seeks to cleanly compartmentalize these four roles of the trauma event.

Why is the role of the rescuer not included in the trauma grid? Unfortunately, although this role may emerge within the therapist or friends and family members, the rescuer is not a role in a trauma schema precisely because there would have been no trauma if the victim had been rescued. Trauma occurs when the fire trucks come too late to put out the fire, the cavalry took the wrong turn, the neighbors looked the other way, or no one called for help. Any therapist who attempts to enact the rescuer role within his or her relationship with a trauma client will soon learn of this folly: the client will reject

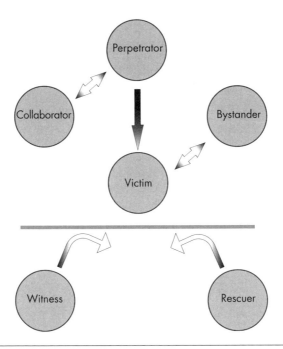

FIGURE 9–1.   The trauma grid.

The trauma grid includes the four main roles of perpetrator, victim, collaborator (on the side of the perpetrator), and bystander (on the side of the victim). The roles of witness and rescuer are rejected by the trauma schema.

him or her and express deep resentment of the therapist's wish to help when the tragedy has already concluded. "You are too late," the client will say.

What of the role of the witness? Therapists often say that they become witnesses to the testimonies of their clients or witnesses to their clients' stories. Indeed, many clients are seeking witnesses. The true witness was a person who was present at the traumatic event and who can testify to what happened but, unlike the bystander, was not in a position to intervene. At times in certain traumatic events, there are eyewitnesses, such as news media staff in war or natural disasters. There are at times people far from the event who videotaped it, as in the Rodney King event. However, in most traumatic events experienced by clients, such as sexual abuse occurring in the home, rape, combat, and domestic violence, there are no witnesses: all who were there can be placed in one of the four primary roles.

Thus, an essential reality of psychotherapy with trauma victims is that therapists are witnesses to their clients' traumatic stories or narratives, without being witnesses to their traumatic events. This discrepancy is the primary source of instability in the therapeutic relationship that evokes clients' trauma schemas.

When these trauma schemas occur, the therapist will be placed in one of the primary roles. The client may accuse the therapist of being a cold-hearted *bystander* who is voyeuristically listening to the horrors of the client and planning to write a paper about him or her; or of *collaborating* with or secretly agreeing with "those who do not believe me"; or of *perpetrating* various harms upon the client, such as being late, not returning phone calls, not caring, and retraumatizing the client just like the perpetrator did. Ironically, in these moments, the therapist will feel *victimized* by the client and feel offended that his or her efforts to help have been rebuffed. The therapist may begin to feel suspicious of the client and wonder if the client is exaggerating or lying about the trauma (collaborator role); may find himself or herself feeling helpless to change the situation for the client (bystander role); or may find himself or herself wishing to be rid of the client (perpetrator role). All of these situations arise when the level of intimacy between therapist and client rises to a point that triggers the trauma schema, whose function is to reset the boundaries between therapist and client. It is best for the therapist to consider such enactments as inevitable.

In fact, in addition to being inevitable, the rise of trauma schemas within the therapeutic relationship may be a sign that the therapist has done his or her job of evoking the trauma history and engaging in decoding the client's behaviors. That is, these moments can be viewed as opportunities for corrective intervention by the therapist. It is important for trauma-centered therapists to anticipate these moments, to not view them as mistakes, and to be prepared to deal with them effectively. The remainder of this chapter is devoted to presenting methods to deal with these moments.

These gaps—disruptions in the continuities in the therapeutic relationship—occur regularly with traumatized clients, because at the moment of a traumatic event, the client had to break the connection to the perpetrator out of overwhelming fear or shame, damaging their capacity for empathy and emotional experience. In topics outside the influence of a trauma schema, the client may be able to maintain a normal empathic relationship with the therapist. However, whenever the topics turn toward the trauma and the accompanying trauma schemas are evoked, sudden eruptions of gaps in the relationship will occur. Because the job of the therapist is to bring the client into proximity to these topics, the emergence of gaps is expected.

In moments when the influence of trauma schemas in the client's everyday behavior can be decoded for him or her, the client learns to identify and then differentiate the past from the present. This work is done in the session, which remains at a distance from these situations at home or work. Although this work is important, it is not occurring in the heat of the moment, as working in the gap is. Thus, clinically, these are not challenging moments to be managed but rather inevitable appearances of traumatic damage that provide opportunities for healing.

The trauma-centered therapist might be conceptualized as a *failed witness*, in that the therapist does attempt to listen to and hear and be witness to the client's experience. The client responds naturally with great hope and appreciation for someone, finally, to be interested in and capable of being present in his or her story. However, as this witnessing takes place, the realization occurs to both parties that no amount of empathy and no amount of witnessing will have any impact on the traumatic act, which has already occurred and will remain in the client's memory. No amount of sympathy brings back the murdered wife or the amputated leg or the innocence of the child. It is at this moment, when good intentions break upon immutable loss, that the gap arises. The actual relationship in the present moment, that of a witness to a teller's story, collapses into a relationship within the trauma schema between two of the four primary roles.

For the client, this moment is familiar and disturbing, for again hope has been raised and dashed. The client reaches out for help in this moment to the person who has appeared to cause the break: the therapist. The situation escalates as the therapist alternates between approach and retreat, both now triggering further distress. The therapist, too, feels disrupted and disoriented, misunderstood and helpless. Relying on his or her ability to create and maintain continuous attachment through empathy and reasoning, the therapist now finds these methods to be useless and, even worse, to be the cause of the problem. As the therapist reaches out to help the struggling client, the therapist's fear of being pulled in or cut out also rises. Whatever the therapist says now appears to be the wrong thing. Indeed, it is this collapse in connection, in empathy, that leads to what has been called both *compassion fatigue* and *vicarious traumatization* (Figley 1995; Pearlman and Saakvitne 1995). Knowing the limits to one's role as witness and anticipating the gap will help the therapist to prevent these outcomes.

RESPONDING TO THE GAP

In this section, we describe the five steps the therapist can take in responding to the gap (Table 9–1). Although more serious gaps tend to arise once the therapy has commenced, it is not unusual for some gaplike moments to arise even in the first session. Handled properly, these challenges can greatly improve the likelihood that the client will continue in the therapeutic relationship.

TABLE 9–1. Responding to the gap: the five steps
1. Restating the problem   Using the client's words, the therapist restates the observation or complaint without any additional interpretation.
2. Linking to the trauma   The therapist immediately continues to state that he or she can understand the client's distress about the current situation because of what the client has been through before, mentioning the client's traumatic experiences.
3. Acknowledging harm   The therapist continues immediately by acknowledging that those events caused the client severe or enduring harm and then waits for a response from the client.
4. Pointing out the discrepancy   The therapist points out that even though there are similarities between the current situation and the past traumatic event, there are also differences, including intent, degree of harm, and ramifications.
5. Recognizing the failure to prevent the traumatic experience   The therapist continues by acknowledging that he or she was not available to have prevented or curtailed the client's injury in the past and is indeed sorry that the client had to go through the horrible experience.

Step 1: Restating the Problem

The therapist begins by immediately restating the problem or complaint using the client's words. This indicates to the client that the therapist has heard the client, and the client will find it difficult to disagree. Using the client's exact wording is important, because he or she will be excruciatingly sensitive to any interpretive twists the therapist gives, assuming that the therapist will attempt to squirm his or her way out of blame. Immediately following the restatement, the therapist should continue into step 2.

Step 2: Linking to the Trauma

The therapist should state his or her understanding that the client is particularly sensitive to what the therapist has done because of what the client lived through in his or her traumatic experience. At this step, having knowledge about the client's traumatic experience and, more importantly, the client's major trauma schemas will pay off. The therapist has only the amount of time during this restatement to make the connection between the behavior that upset the client and the client's past. If the therapist's restatement is fairly accurate, he or she will know because the client will pause; if the therapist is too far off the mark, the client will resume his or her attack, and the therapist should immediately rephrase his or her restatement and understanding of its link to the client's trauma.

Step 3: Acknowledging Harm

The therapist then points out that the traumatic event had caused the client tremendous harm. This statement is often most effective when said after the client pauses to process what the therapist said in step 2. This acknowledgment of harm brings an emotional as well as an intellectual dimension to the therapist's response. In this step, the therapist should draw on his or her own sense of traumatic injury and suffering, putting aside for the moment any irritation at the client's seemingly overreactive, unjustified criticism of the therapist's behavior. If effective, this statement should provoke some agreement from the client and sometimes more information about how he or she had been injured.

Step 4: Pointing Out the Discrepancy

The therapist points out that he or she had no intention of harming the client, which makes the current situation different from the traumatic event. The therapist should emphasize lack of intention and not that the therapist did not harm the client. In fact, sometimes the therapist has to say that he or she did harm the client but clarify that this harm is different from the past harm. At this point, the therapist should mention the client's perpetrator by name and deed, so that the client is presented with images of both the therapist and the perpetrator simultaneously. This will facilitate the client's process of differentiation. If effective, the client should become a bit calmer and more introspective.

Step 5: Recognizing the Failure to Prevent the Traumatic Experience

The therapist then states his or her wish that he or she had been present to prevent the client's injury or that it had never occurred and then acknowledges that the therapist was not present. This statement should be made in the spirit of sadness and mourning (e.g., "If only I had been there to help, but I wasn't") rather than bravado (e.g., "If I had been there, I would have taken care of it"). Sometimes it may be effective to say, "And even if I had been there, I would have been too terrified to intervene, just like everyone else." The aim of this step is to create a shared feeling of the failure to undo or rectify the traumatic reality.

EXAMPLES OF RESPONDING TO THE GAP

The following is a brief example that illustrates an effective response to the gap in the therapeutic relationship. The client is a 55-year-old combat veteran.

> CLIENT (*enraged*): You're late, 10 minutes late.
> THERAPIST: You are upset that I was 10 minutes late [restatement of problem], and I can understand why that is important because of the time you called for air support and it came late. [linking to trauma]
> CLIENT: And my unit was overrun.
> THERAPIST: And your unit was overrun, meaning over 15 of your buddies were killed, needlessly, causing you great harm. [acknowledgment of harm]
> CLIENT: Yes.
> THERAPIST: And I wasn't here for you at the start of this appointment, but I can tell you that unlike in the situation back then, I had no intention of causing you any harm and that nothing like what happened then will happen here with me. [pointing out discrepancy]
> CLIENT: It just brings it all back.
> THERAPIST: I only wish I could have been there to ensure that you had the air support you needed, but I wasn't. It was a terrible loss. [acknowledging failure to prevent] I can see you are sad.
> CLIENT: It was horrible.
> THERAPIST: What are you seeing now in your mind about it? (*Trauma inquiry continues.*)

In contrast, the following is an example in which the therapist does not utilize the steps. The client is a 30-year-old woman.

> CLIENT (*enraged*): You keep looking at the clock. Are you listening to me at all, or are you thinking of your next client? You know, I really resent the fact that you do not seem to care about what I've been—
> THERAPIST: I was just checking the time. I'm sorry, but—
> CLIENT: You're not sorry, and not only that, we have just had to spend time dealing with this instead of getting to what really counts, so I need a couple more minutes.
> THERAPIST: You are being unreasonable, I think we can—
> CLIENT: Unreasonable! You arrogant son of a bitch.
> THERAPIST: There is no point getting so upset.
> CLIENT: That's it! I can't stay here! (*Leaves the room and slams the door.*)

The following example begins as the previous one did, but the therapist's response to the gap is more effective.

CLIENT (*enraged*): You keep looking at the clock. Are you listening to me at all, or are you thinking of your next client? You know, I really resent the fact that you do not seem to care about what I've been—

THERAPIST: You are upset that I was looking at the clock, very upset [restatement of problem], and for good reason, because I can understand why this is such a sensitive issue for you given what your dad did every time he visited, looking at the clock and seeming not to care about you. [linking to trauma]

CLIENT: Yeah.

THERAPIST: When you were being abused by your stepfather and hoping that your dad would figure it out… [linking to trauma]

CLIENT: He never did.

THERAPIST: And he never did, and that caused you incredible harm and made you feel hopeless. [acknowledgment of harm]

CLIENT: I used to run out of those visits early.

THERAPIST: Really. I can imagine. But even though I looked at the clock just like he did, it isn't because I don't care for you, and it doesn't mean you will be harmed like that because I am interested in what you have to tell me. [pointing out discrepancy]

CLIENT: Sometimes I'm not sure of that.

THERAPIST: I only wish I could have been there to tell your father or somebody that you were being abused so it could have been stopped, but I wasn't and no one was. [acknowledging failure to prevent]

CLIENT: (*Cries.*) If only he had figured it out.

THERAPIST: It would have been good. I'm so sorry he didn't. Is there something that I haven't figured out? That you need to tell me before you go?

CLIENT: No, you know just about everything.

THERAPIST: But not everything.

CLIENT: (*Smiles.*) No, not everything.

THERAPIST: What were you thinking? (*Trauma inquiry continues.*)

As these brief examples illustrate, once the gap has arisen, the therapist should respond immediately in a nondefensive manner, directly acknowledging his or her behavior in the terms used by the client, or else an escalation will ensue. Generally, the therapist should not apologize but instead, as rapidly as possible, frame the client's outburst or criticism as justified in relation to the past traumas. Obviously, it is much easier to do this if the therapist knows what the traumatic events, experiences, and schemas are, which is why it is very important to have gained that knowledge as soon as possible in the early sessions, prior to these gaps occurring.

Sometimes the gap appears in the first session.

THERAPIST: Good morning.

CLIENT (*upset*): I did not fill out these forms; they are worded incorrectly, and I will not just give away my privacy to any so-called professionals based on their reputation.

THERAPIST: I see that your privacy is very important to you, no doubt for very good reasons. Have you been harmed by some so-called professional who misused your personal information?

CLIENT: Why, yes I have.

THERAPIST: That must have caused you a great deal of—

CLIENT: Agony. It was agony.

THERAPIST: And obviously that would be the last thing you would want to experience again with me.

CLIENT: Absolutely.

THERAPIST: It must have been bad. What happened?

CLIENT: (*Begins to explain events.*)

Becoming caught in these gaps with clients is the greatest source of strain for the therapist, even greater than listening to the details of horrific events. A therapist's *raison d'être* is to establish a caring, empathic alliance with the client, to be helpful, and in the gap the client rejects these possibilities and cuts himself or herself off from the therapist, sometimes brutally, leaving the therapist confused and sometimes resentful.

Gaps that arise in the beginning of therapy are means by which clients communicate quickly that they have been harmed and are opportunities to begin the trauma work. Gaps that arise later in treatment are more intimate and not only reflect new details that the client is having difficulty expressing, but more importantly are opportunities for healing of the profound isolation created by the trauma. Gaps that are poorly managed can lead to termination of treatment, greatly increased acting-out behaviors, and sometimes even litigation against the therapist. These gaps can be quite dramatic and intense, as in the following example.

CLIENT (*on the phone with the therapist*): I quit! Actually, I'm firing you. I am getting nothing at all from the therapy, you don't understand me, nothing has changed.

THERAPIST: What happened?

CLIENT: You are clueless. There's no point in even having this conversation.

THERAPIST: You feel I haven't helped you at all.

CLIENT: That's right!

THERAPIST: I haven't helped you at all, and I can understand why that is so important to you given the fact that your mother gave you up almost immediately because she felt she couldn't take care of you, and that led you to be moved from one caretaker to another for years...

CLIENT: My mother...

THERAPIST: ...causing you great harm, and if you sense that I don't care for you enough or at all, it brings back all that stuff about your mother which hurt you so much.

CLIENT: No one likes me.

THERAPIST: And something made you sense that I am like your mother and all the other therapists you have seen and left or been dropped from, and you are saying to yourself, "Here it goes again."

CLIENT: That's right.

THERAPIST: And so you are not going to believe me when I say that what is happening between you and me is not what happened between you and your mother. How I screwed up is not the same as how she screwed up.

CLIENT: (*Laughs.*) You screwed up all right.

THERAPIST: Someone should have been there to help your mother out to care for you. Someone should be there for you now to help you deal with things, and as much as I would like to have been there, or be there for you, we both know that I wasn't, and that I can't be, and that makes me sad.

CLIENT: So I'm quitting.

THERAPIST: And so you are quitting.

CLIENT: So?

THERAPIST: You are quitting. I am not quitting. You can come in if you want to our session on Monday. Up to you.

CLIENT: No way. Give it to someone else.

THERAPIST: I hope to see you then.

CLIENT: Goodbye. (*The client skipped the next session but came in the following week and resumed treatment.*)

Although this client remained upset and did not reestablish connection to the therapist during this interchange, the therapist was able to maintain the trauma-centered frame and his commitment to the treatment, preventing the client from escalating further.

The following is another challenging example.

A 19-year-old female client was sitting in her therapist's waiting room even though her appointment was not for several days. The receptionist, who knew the client, asked her if she knew that the appointment was not until later in the week, and the client nodded but did not leave. The receptionist then called and reported the situation to the therapist, who decided not to intervene. After 2 hours, the client left. She then did not show for her appointment 2 days later. The therapist called the client and left a message noting that she had missed the session and that she would be expected the following week. On the day of the session, the client appeared in the waiting room 5 hours before the session. The receptionist informed the therapist, who again decided not to intervene. The receptionist informed the business manager, who went out to the waiting room and in a somewhat pointed manner asked the client why she was there so early. The client refused to answer.

At the time of the session, the client came into the therapist's office and began to speak about some events of the week.

THERAPIST: You were sitting in the waiting room all day today.

CLIENT: What's it to you? What, did they let you know? I have my rights.

THERAPIST: Were you expecting me to come down and ask you to leave?

CLIENT: You probably don't care one way or another. I have no place to go. I wasn't causing a problem to anyone.

THERAPIST: You did not do this without a good reason. Given how many times you have been thrown out of agencies, and before that removed from foster home placements, and before that abandoned by your birth parents, something triggered your memories of being kicked out.

CLIENT: Nope.

THERAPIST: And given how much pain and suffering all that caused you, this is not a small deal. It's a big deal.

CLIENT: No, it's nothing. I was just sitting in your damn waiting room.

THERAPIST: So you must be thinking that I am going to kick you out of our treatment, and I assume that that worry would likely come up if you felt we were developing a good relationship, because then if we broke it off you would be hurt again, and our last few sessions have been very productive, I think. But unlike all your other relationships, I am not going to kick you out of treatment. This relationship is different from those, especially different from that with your birth parents.

CLIENT: I don't know what you are talking about. Can we get on with the session?

THERAPIST: You know, maybe you were thinking that my staff would try to kick you out and that I would come down and stop them, and that connects for me with a thought, a wish, that I've had that I had been around when you were with your birth parents or some of those foster homes, and I could have stopped them all from giving you up or kicking you out. But I wasn't there then, and I couldn't have stopped them even if I was.

CLIENT: (*Looks sad.*) Everybody throws me out eventually.

THERAPIST: You have had an amazing journey, with a lot of losses, but you have made it here to today, and I'm interested in working with you on everything.

CLIENT: I guess so. I have nowhere to go.

THERAPIST: I understand that you had nowhere to go, and that it must have been scary for you. I would have liked to have helped you then.

CLIENT: Okay. Can we get back to the session? I've got some things to talk about.

THERAPIST: Let's do it.

In this example, the therapist was able to navigate through the client's distress and return the client to the ongoing therapeutic work.

MOVING INTO MOURNING

The traumatic event in its core is inexpressible and unforgivable and cannot be adequately shared; in contrast, the trauma as a wound and record of a loss and the source of humility and spiritual strength is expressible, forgivable, and capable of being shared. This sharing occurs in the moments that the client and therapist acknowledge the loss and their failure to prevent it, and they can then proceed with the natural healing process of mourning that the traumatic reaction and schemas have prevented. These moments of failure bind one to another rather than keeping them apart. As treatment progresses, more and more of these gaps are resolved softly, in a jointly held sadness, in quiet reflection, and in dreams of repair. Chapter 10, "Long-Term Process in Treatment," discusses methods of reparation. Reparation follows mourning, which follows desensitization and imaginal exposure.

The reason mourning is forestalled in trauma is that the normal process of identification is disturbed. In normal mourning, one holds onto the lost person or object through identification. Eventually, one seeks the object or person again in new people and activities through reparation and rebuilding. In traumatic states, the person is drawn into identification with the aggressor or perpetrator, out of the fear, and until that identification can be loosened through desensitization, mourning cannot commence.

As treatment proceeds, and indeed following successful work with each gap in the therapeutic relationship, an approach to the process of mourning occurs. Mourning is the human being's natural method of healing from severe loss, and it is interfered with by trauma schemas. In mourning one moves back and forth across the boundary of time, feeling one moment the pain of loss, and then the next the fact that one has moved on. Trauma schemas do not allow this boundary permeability and instead rigidify these boundaries. As treatment proceeds, there should be an increase in a palpable sense of sadness and thoughtfulness within the sessions. What allows the traumatized client to move forward is the increasing sense that what has been lost (e.g., virginity, innocence, a loved one, a career, physical capacity) still lives on inside one, not as a reality, but as a desire. Thus, in working with the gap, it is the expression of the therapist's desire to have been there to help or to rescue (the present reality), coupled with the knowledge that that did not occur (the past reality), that may help the client to accept that wish. Indeed, the client will use that wish to motivate recovery, to apply to future actions and relationships, and to find in new activities and relationships that which was lost in the past.

STUDY QUESTIONS

9.1   Define the gap.

9.2   T/F   The rise of the gap in the therapeutic relationship indicates that the therapist has made a mistake in the trauma inquiry.

9.3   What are the four roles in the usual trauma schema?

9.4   Why is the role of the rescuer not present in a trauma schema?

9.5   Why is the experience of the gap so stressful for the therapist?

9.6   What are the five steps of a response to the gap?

9.7   T/F   When responding to the gap, it is important not to imply that the current complaint by the client is baseless because it is a displacement from a past trauma.

9.8   How does trauma interfere with the process of normal mourning?

CHAPTER 10

Long-Term Process in Treatment

Trauma-centered psychotherapy may be employed by therapists of any theoretical persuasion and at any time during the course of treatment. Generally, the work of conducting a thorough trauma history, identifying the trauma schemas, decoding current behaviors in terms of these schemas, and then differentiating the past from the present can be accomplished within a 4- to 6-month time frame, but often more quickly. The therapist may then decide to resume other methods that he or she believes are appropriate based on the entire set of needs presented by the client. After a course of trauma-centered psychotherapy, the therapist can continue to work on deepening the client's personal insight, providing encouragement and advice, extending the client's social capacities, and helping the client deal with current stressors and life decisions. When and if the client's trauma schemas emerge again forcefully, the therapist can apply the techniques described in this chapter. Trauma-centered psychotherapy is not a comprehensive treatment method for all problems; it is designed to facilitate the loosening of the traumatic event's grip on the person's functioning. Although many derivative problems may lessen or even disappear during this therapy, many others less connected to the trauma schemas do not.

In this chapter, we describe aspects of long-term treatment within a trauma-centered model, well after the initial phases have been completed. The focus is largely on basic principles of the work, because the variations

131

among clients in long-term treatment are vast. The decision to conduct long-term trauma-centered work is completely optional, and therapists may choose to return to their regular form of treatment with the client. For therapists interested in pursuing trauma-centered therapy throughout the duration of the treatment, this chapter will be of particular use.

The most important principle is to maintain the trauma-centered frame, which consists of the four main axioms and the three principles of treatment (see Chapters 2–4). The therapist continues to demonstrate interest in and curiosity about the original traumatic events, no matter how many times they have been discussed. The therapist remains steadfast in remembering the horrors of those times and reflects back to the client the thrill and wonder of each new advance in his or her functioning.

Despite the urge for closure and completion felt by both client and therapist, the therapist needs to remain open to hearing more details or hearing the same details in new ways throughout the treatment process. It is amazing how often clients in long-term treatment reveal new details, sometimes years after the initial trauma work has been done. These details are rarely offered by the client directly but rather almost always emerge in small disruptions in the flow of the discussion or in the therapeutic relationship. These disruptions are often so subtle and so easily brushed aside that therapists might at times have to interrupt the client to ask for details (e.g., "So what are you saying? That seems to relate to the moment you arrived at the hospital. Is there something else that you haven't told me about that moment?"). Sometimes the client will be discussing some well-reviewed issue and say something with a different tone, leading the therapist to pursue more details.

THERAPIST: What? What now?

CLIENT: What do you mean, "what"?

THERAPIST: What are you thinking about right now? Did a thought about your molestation just cross your mind?

CLIENT: I don't think so....What was I saying?

THERAPIST: You said, "I *hate* yellow."

CLIENT: Hmm. Yes, I did have the thought that the tile on the bathroom floor was a dirty yellow. So what?

THERAPIST: I don't think you ever told me that. Presumably, it is connected to something upsetting.

CLIENT: It does. Didn't I tell you that after he raped me and I was lying on the tile floor in the bathroom, he urinated on me. I remember thinking at the time that his urine matched the color of the tile.... (*Becomes tearful.*)

THERAPIST: He urinated on you....That is awful. I am so sorry. Had you told me that before?

CLIENT: I'm not sure.

THERAPIST: Neither am I.
CLIENT: Yeah. Thanks.

Remaining attentive for more details over time is to follow the principle of incompleteness with tenacity, for the monotonies of long-term treatment can dull a therapist's antenna.

Trauma-centered psychotherapy becomes effective when clients themselves learn to perform the basic techniques of identifying details, decoding their own behavior in terms of their trauma schemas, and differentiating the past from the present. Throughout long-term treatment, these skills are taught, practiced, and discussed by the therapist. Much of the therapist's work is to listen for the footprint of the client's trauma schemas in the current issues being discussed. The mutual awareness between client and therapist of the client's trauma schemas and their impact on current behaviors serves as a framework for the therapeutic relationship. A time comes when new problems or issues do not have strong links to the prior traumas. One client exclaimed, "I finally have a problem that's not connected to my trauma!"

Long-term treatment within a trauma-centered framework provides continued, repetitive exposure to the trauma narrative. A general principle is that the traumatic event should be mentioned in every session at least once. Thoughts and feelings associated with the traumatic event tend to build up slowly over time, even after successful exposure treatment. Having multiple reexposures, however brief, helps to provide ongoing desensitization to the client. These reexposures can be threaded into the therapeutic discussion at any time.

CLIENT: The dog was barking so loud, it was driving me crazy.
THERAPIST: And you couldn't tell your friend to do something about it because…
CLIENT: I didn't want to upset him. He loves his dog, blindly!
THERAPIST: You were able to tell your teacher about your father's porn habit, even though that upset everybody.
CLIENT: True, but I waited a year to do it.
THERAPIST: Oh, so if the dog had been barking…
CLIENT (*laughing*): For a year, I definitely would have told my friend to deal with it!
THERAPIST (*ironically*): Your patience has always been impressive.
CLIENT: Well, now it's patience; back then it was helplessness.
THERAPIST: Good to know that things have changed for the better.

Repetitive exposure is a central principle in the long-term treatment of trauma survivors. An important element within this reexposure is the mention of the perpetrator (or in the case of a natural disaster or accident, mention of the person[s] who let the client down), in addition to the client's injury. The client's injury is the result of the frightening event and therefore in some ways represents the end of the tragic story. The perpetrator is the author of the story, and it is the perpetrator's free will that is the source of the problem. Anxieties that are experienced later in life may be linked to some degree to the fears generated by the presence or absence of the perpetrator. In the perpetrator's absence, the client may experience the trace of the perpetrator in intimate relationships, thereby burdening the client's current situation with the shadow of the past. This dynamic is further examined in the presentation of group and couples/family therapy in Chapters 14 and 15, respectively. Nevertheless, reexposing the client in long-term therapy to the perpetrator by mentioning him or her is a recommended practice, preferably in every session.

As the desensitization effects of trauma-centered psychotherapy take hold, more and more of the client's available energy is freed up to attend to the tasks of his or her current life. Throughout this process, a certain amount of mourning usually occurs, as past and present become more differentiated, and the defenses against fear and shame give way to the awareness of the losses occasioned by the traumatic event. As noted before, this process of mourning is a natural way that humans process trauma, which posttraumatic stress disorder inhibits. In long-term treatment, mourning continues but is soon mixed in with the question "What next?" Given the fact of the traumatic event, how can a client live on? Various strategies—forgetting about it, just moving on, being thankful one has survived, and not using the event as an excuse for failure—have strong adherents, and if these strategies work for a client, they need not be questioned.

Within the trauma-centered framework, however, the intent is not for the psychotherapy sessions to allow endless revisitations to the horror or dwelling on one's injuries. As the therapy proceeds, an attempt is made to connect a client's newfound interests and pursuits with one's previous experiences. This process is conceived as making reparation, or repair. After a hurricane, people rebuild; after a fence has fallen, people repair it. In the act of reparation, the client is encouraged to find representations of what was lost in what is new. For example, in the choice of friends and spouse, in career and hobbies, and in political engagement or charitable giving, the traumatized client helps to repair the world in the name of what was lost, and in spite of the deeds of the perpetrator. Thus, many interactions between therapist and client are shaped by pointing out this reparative dimension in the client's current life. Although emphasizing the individual's strengths and finding ways of increasing his or her resiliency through engagement in healthy activities are good practices, it is also important for the person to make a conscious link between these positive interests and his or her traumatic losses. Having a foundation of meaning helps to sustain new activities and interests, for then each action a person takes is an act of healing.

An African American client entered treatment at age 32 after three inpatient hospitalizations for depression, which occurred shortly after his mother, with whom he had lived his entire life, had died. He had been brutally sexually molested as a child by men in the neighborhood, which he had not told anyone. They had drawn him into a corner shop with a promise for candy on his way home from school and taken him into a back room. He eventually dropped out of high school and lived with his mother, unemployed. After 6 months of trauma-centered work focusing on the sexual abuse, he began to feel better and applied for Social Security benefits. His siblings insisted that he babysit their children because he had nothing else to do, and he lived in the same apartment project they lived in. He resented this initially and was told by his siblings that this was the least he could do (being otherwise worthless). He was not paid. However, he was able to care for the children well enough that over time other families in the complex also sent their children to him. He ran his informal daycare well but still felt badly about himself. When during treatment, a connection was made that by keeping an eye on these children, he was protecting them from being abused, he became more engaged. With the support of the therapist, he developed the idea, or dream, that he would be able to repair some of the damage done to him by caring for children. On his own, he then volunteered to be a school crossing guard, a job he took extremely seriously. He was very tall and big, so when he went into the intersection to stop traffic, it stopped. A year later, he was honored by the town as the year's best crossing guard. His family and neighbors in the apartment complex likewise shifted their attitudes toward him and honored his excellent care of their children by paying him. Within 3 years of his hospitalizations, he had achieved a completely new adaptation in the world. He frequently reminded his therapist, "From the time the children are in my sight—as I go into the intersection to stop traffic, and as they cross the street and then go on to the school—they are safe. Completely safe. Not in danger like I was as a kid." It is the double entendre of being safe from traffic and safe from sexual molestation that makes this adaptive behavior so reparative. His intersection was but a few blocks away from that original corner store where 20 years before no one had kept an eye on him, a fact from which he and the therapist drew pleasure in every session.

It is important that the therapist keep a focus on the relationship between clients' positive behaviors and achievements, and their recovery from their traumatic experiences. A large part of this process is to reframe their recovery in terms of the increased risks that they are willing to take, rather than celebrating general improvements in mood or symptomatology. Trauma schemas attempt to reduce risk by clarifying and simplifying the boundaries between safety and danger. Transforming the statement "All men are bad" to "Some men are bad and some are good, and I will be able to tell the difference and protect myself if I need to," entails not feeling safer but tolerating greater risk, for indeed, some men are bad. Standing up for oneself may lead to being criticized, becoming intimate with another may lead to painful rejection, and getting back to driving on the highway may increase the chance of an accident; however, all of these involve increased participation in life, engagement with other people, and feeling emotions more strongly. Traumatized individuals, perhaps more than any other people, can understand the boldness, the courage, and the sacrifice it takes to be fully in the world. Understanding the link between their past experiences and their current functioning is a contribution that long-term trauma-centered psychotherapy can make to their recovery.

Sometimes clients will work on a frequent and regular basis for a period of time and then terminate treatment, but more often clients continue in long-term treatment, with the frequency of visits being gradually reduced, perhaps from once a week, to once every 2 weeks, to once a month, and then to once every 3 months. A model for this type of treatment pattern is the periodic checkup. For patients with enduring problems, periodic checkups with their doctors are useful. During these checkups, the doctor does not waste too much time chatting about a person's everyday life, but looks again at the bloodwork, checks for new moles, or pokes again at the tender spot in the abdomen to see if the condition has reared itself again. Likewise, in trauma-centered work, during these periodic visits, the purpose is not so much for the therapist to catch up with the client about his or her life, but for the therapist to inquire directly about the client's memories of the trauma and to name and discuss the perpetrator, in the context of reexposing the client to the traumatic material. If the client goes "ouch," it may mean that the trauma schemas have reasserted themselves to some extent and may require some attention. From a trauma-centered point of view, the therapist is not doing his or her job if he or she avoids bringing up the client's original traumas, out of concern for upsetting him or her during these infrequent visits.

Long-term trauma-centered psychotherapy is more of a continuation of a basic agreement between client and therapist to maintain their vigilance on the potential influence of the client's trauma schemas than a specific method of treatment. It is perhaps more of an attitude, a sentiment, and a commitment that respects the significance and power of the traumatic event in the client's life.

STUDY QUESTIONS

10.1 T/F In long-term work, new details of the past traumas are rarely disclosed.

10.2 T/F In long-term work, the traumatic events are mentioned in every session.

10.3 T/F In long-term work, clients learn how to employ the techniques of trauma-centered treatment themselves.

10.4 T/F In long-term work, the therapist generally discourages the client from finding ways of repairing his or her losses, because this would support denial that the trauma occurred.

10.5 T/F In treatment checkups, it is not necessary to ask the client again about his or her traumas.

10.6 T/F The process of reparation involves engaging the client not only in positive activities but also in activities that are meaningfully linked to the suffering and experiences the client has had.

CHAPTER 11

Handling the Edges

Engaging in trauma-centered psychotherapy brings the therapist into close proximity to extreme states of terror, helplessness, and isolation. Although most clients will experience the therapeutic hour and space as a safe haven from the bustle of the world about them, occasionally clients' abilities to maintain their composure will be overcome by the confrontation with their past experiences, giving rise to very challenging situations for the therapist. The trauma-centered therapist should be trained to expect such moments and be able to handle them. The most common challenging experiences include dissociative reactions, violent reactions, disruptive behaviors outside of the session, substance abuse, and having no memories of the abuse, which are discussed in this chapter.

DISSOCIATIVE REACTIONS

In the course of working with traumatized individuals, the therapist may encounter in clients sudden, severe dissociative reactions such as fainting, pseudoseizures, blanking out and being nonresponsive, gagging, head-banging, curling up in a corner, singsong noises, and other forms of sudden collapse. These issues are to be differentiated from working with clients who have dissociative identity disorder, which is discussed in Chapter 12, "Working With Clients With Dissociative Identity Disorder."

These dissociative reactions are most likely to occur when clients are transitioning into and out of the therapist's office, when they are in public areas such as waiting rooms or bathrooms, and when other people are near. They may also occur within the session when exploring trauma material. Although these reactions are common psychological defenses and behaviors, they are often dramatic and disturbing, causing an undue amount of anxiety among office staff or other people. Witnesses somehow feel that these clients are in danger and that efforts should be made immediately to bring them out of the dissociated state, such as by calling 911, using smelling salts, hugging or rubbing them, or whispering in their ear.

Fortunately, these reactions do not last for long periods of time and are rarely dangerous to the client. The therapist should remember that as psychological defenses, these reactions are employed to lower the client's anxiety. Because these reactions indicate dissociation, the client is on some level fully aware of what is going on, even if afterward he or she is not able to remember the experience.

It is helpful for the therapist to understand that these reactions occur with some frequency, that they are not a sign of something gone terribly wrong, and that one can manage them in a safe and reliable way. In most cases, the client will return when he or she has calmed down or needs to. When one goes to an oncology treatment center, one sees people who have lost their hair. When one goes to a trauma clinic, one occasionally sees people who are dissociating.

The following is an example of the successful management of a severe dissociative reaction that occurred in the first session.

> A man came with his wife for his first session with a new therapist. He had been in treatment for 10 years for diagnoses of depression, bipolar disorder, borderline personality disorder, and factitious disorder. He had been hospitalized numerous times, medically, for seizures and diagnosed with seizure disorder and had been taking antiseizure medications for 5 years. He had undergone numerous computed tomography and magnetic resonance imaging scans, neuropsychological tests, and cardiac workups to assess the cause of his seizures. Finally, his primary doctor began to suspect a psychological cause and referred him to the therapist. No one in over 10 years of intensive medical and psychological treatments had documented or inquired as to whether the man had a trauma history.
>
> The couple described the client's history and their difficulties in getting him the right treatment. Fifteen minutes into the session, when he was asked about his relationship with his mother, the man's eyes rolled back in his head and he pitched forward head first onto the floor, where he shook and gagged as if having a seizure. It was quite dramatic and convincing. His wife sat next to him and placed her hand under his head, whereupon he began banging his head onto the floor, now cushioned by his wife's hands. The therapist remained in his chair and calmly asked the wife how often the client did this. She replied, "Whenever anyone asks him about his mother." The therapist

told her that it appeared that he had had experiences early in his life, probably involving his mother, that he had a hard time facing and that he had developed this means of dealing with it, or more accurately avoiding it. She said that he was usually out for 10–15 minutes and that he would not remember anything. The therapist continued to talk with her about the client's history, and the client slowly stopped moving and then, reorienting himself, came back, sat up in the chair, and continued the session. He said that he had only a dim memory of what had happened.

The therapist explained to the client that he had come to the right place, because obviously something had happened with his mother that upset him. The client nodded calmly and provided a few details of his mother's emotional and verbal abuse. Near the end of the session, his wife said, "You know, you are the first doctor who did not freak out when he did this. Doctors usually call for an ambulance, order tests, and then do not want to see him again. He has been kicked out of two group programs for doing this." The couple continued in treatment for a year, during which time he had three more seizures, each of lessening intensity, and then were transitioned to a regular provider near their home. The client was able to discuss his childhood in much more detail, including possible sexual abuse by his mother at an early age. Two years later, the therapist learned that the client had continued to do well.

In cases of chronic or frequent dissociative reactions, it is often helpful to have a family member either in the session or nearby, in the waiting room, so that the therapist can educate him or her about the behavior and continue to talk with someone while the client is in a dissociative state. Helping the family and others in the client's support network, including providers, understand the nature of the dissociative behavior can significantly decrease the level of distress, panicked efforts, and interpersonal conflict that such reactions typically engender.

Having a family member present is helpful also because it allows the therapist to carry on the trauma-centered conversation while the client is dissociating. However, even when there is no one else in the room, the therapist should consider continuing to speak about the traumatic events. The therapist should assume that the client or some part of the client is listening and taking in the information. Continuing the discussion about the traumatic roots of the behavior while the client is dissociating therefore may serve a purpose and not be a waste of time.

In the following case example, the client is an 18-year-old female.

THERAPIST: So then what did he do?
CLIENT: He said that his penis was a long stick and that it would go through me up to my neck and maybe even out my throat, it was so big.
THERAPIST: You were 7 when your uncle said this?
CLIENT: About. It was part of his game.

THERAPIST: Game?

CLIENT: He asked me to indicate on my stomach where I thought his penis had reached. (*She stares.*)

THERAPIST: That is terrible. Did this game have a name like the others?

CLIENT: (*Continues to stare, unresponsive.*)

THERAPIST: Emily, I assume you are dissociating now because a memory came up that upset you—something that you remembered as we were talking about your uncle's talk about how big and long his penis was, and the game he made you play.

CLIENT: (*Continues to stare.*)

THERAPIST: You were talking just before you dissociated about having to indicate on your stomach how far you thought his penis reached, so it seems possible that you had a memory about that or perhaps of being in pain (she flinches)—yes in pain, some kind of body pain as he was having sex with you, penetrating you I believe you said from behind....

CLIENT: (*Looks uncomfortable, squirms.*)

THERAPIST: Did he cause some pain as he did this? (*She winces, begins to breathe harder.*)

THERAPIST: Seems likely, and when you come back here, we can talk about it because it must have been very distressing to you what he did.

CLIENT: He pulled my head back.

THERAPIST: He pulled your head back. Hard?

CLIENT: (*Tearful.*) Yes, very hard....Hurt my neck. (*Brings hand up to rub her neck.*)

THERAPIST: He did what we call very sadistic acts.

CLIENT: Yes. (*Looks at therapist.*)

THERAPIST: Welcome back. We were talking about your uncle having you play a game.

CLIENT: I don't remember.

THERAPIST: You were telling me that he had you point on your stomach where you thought his penis reached, when you dissociated a little, because you remembered him pulling your head back hard, which hurt a great deal.

CLIENT: I had forgotten that. (*The session continues.*)

In this session, the therapist is not derailed by the client's dissociative departure and gently continues to think aloud about what the client had said, offer ideas as to what had upset her, and provide some educative information about what the therapist was thinking, assuming that the client could hear everything. The therapist does not abandon the trauma-centered work to address the dissociation as the problem but instead maintains a commitment to exploring the event, which the client eventually returns to, rejoining the therapist in this effort.

VIOLENCE AND PROPERTY DAMAGE

On occasion, traumatized clients, either children or adults, will become so highly charged or angry in sessions—at themselves, the therapist, or family members—that they will lose control and exit the room, slamming the door; throw or break objects; scream; or cut themselves. Although these unfortunate events are sometimes due to the intensity and horror of their memories alone, these events may mean that the therapist did not intervene correctly.

Violence is a complex and not well-understood behavior, despite its significance in human misery. For traumatized persons, becoming violent is usually due to feeling cornered, with no room to move. Violent acts also communicate to others that the client has not felt understood, that something from the traumatic event is reoccurring, and that by becoming violent the others around the client will be forced to take the role of either victim or perpetrator (depending on whether they decide to withdraw from or restrain the client). Violent acts are also stabilizing acts, for they bring closure to ambiguous processes such as talking about feelings or about the trauma, and they create definitive boundaries between the client and others near him or her. In the following two cases, therapists managed to intervene effectively when patients became violent. The first case occurred in a hospital setting.

> A trauma-centered clinician was called to the emergency room of a psychiatric department. An emergency code had been issued because a 35-year-old man had become suddenly violent. He was standing in the hall of the unit with a pool stick, which he held in a threatening manner. The code team and hospital police were crowded at the other end, not sure what to do. The man was screaming, "Get the f—k away from me!" although no one was around him. Every few seconds, he smashed the pool stick against the wall near him. The clinician, who had never met the man, was told that the patient was diagnosed with paranoid schizophrenia and was currently psychotic. The clinician was given the authority to approach him while the code team waited behind him. When the clinician stepped forward, still 10 feet away, the patient shouted again, "Get the f—k away from me!"

> CLINICIAN: What happened? You would not be so upset unless something happened.
> PATIENT (*shouting*): You wouldn't understand.
> CLINICIAN: You are not doing this for no reason. There is a good reason for this. Tell me. Did someone try to attack you?
> PATIENT (*enraged and shouting*): What the f—k do I have to do to get it across to you people?
> CLINICIAN: Okay. Who tried to attack you?
> PATIENT: (*Pointed down the hall to the common room where other patients were sitting.*) That white motherf—ker called me a n——r!

> CLINICIAN: That's really upsetting. I'm sorry about that. No won-
> der you are upset, especially because that has probably hap-
> pened before. What happened before?
> PATIENT: (*Looking at clinician intently and softening grip on pool stick.*)
> When I got almost beat to death in school by a bunch of white
> boys.
> CLINICIAN: How old were you?
> PATIENT: Ten.
> CLINICIAN: That was terrible. No wonder.

Then the patient burst into tears and dropped the pool stick. When the clinician approached him, the patient lay his head on the clinician's shoulder, before being quietly escorted to the safe room.

The following case occurred in an outpatient child guidance clinic.

A 10-year-old girl in her second therapy session, with her foster mother present, became upset and rushed out of the room, through the waiting room, and into the small foyer. The two therapists and the girl's foster mother followed her into the foyer. The foster mother moved toward her, whereupon the girl pulled a doorstop out of the wall and threatened to stab the woman with the nail end of the doorstop. A discussion ensued as the girl took the doorstop and jammed it into the wall of the foyer, damaging the wall, and then periodically jabbed her skin with it and scratched herself, a little deeper each time. The outside door had a single-pane glass panel that she could easily have broken. Previously in the session, she had been talking about her childhood abuse by her birth parents, which consisted of severe neglect and physical beatings. At the time she ran out, the topic had shifted to mundane aspects of her school life and activities at home. In the foyer, the therapist started talking.

> THERAPIST: You are doing this for a reason. Something came up
> in the session that you weren't able to tell us. We missed
> something.
> CLIENT: (*Jabs the wall harder.*)
> THERAPIST: What did we miss?
> FOSTER MOTHER (FM): Honey, stop doing that!
> CLIENT: (*Shouts, jabs the nail along her arm.*)
> THERAPIST: You don't need to try to stop her. She is trying to tell
> us something that we missed in the session. Something about
> what happened to her with her birth mother.
> CLIENT: No.
> THERAPIST: Birth father.
> CLIENT: (*Calms down.*)
> THERAPIST: Her birth father. What did he do to you?
> CLIENT: (*She begins to scratch hard near the lower part of her forearm.*)
> THERAPIST: Are you trying to get out, cutting off the…
> CLIENT: Ropes.

THERAPIST: The ropes?

CLIENT: He tied me to the chair when he had to leave to do drugs.

THERAPIST: So he left you alone, tied you up with ropes, and you tried to get out of them? Makes a whole lot of sense. (*To foster mother.*) Did you know about this?

FM: No, I didn't.…It's horrible.

THERAPIST: So you are remembering the time you wanted to get out of the ropes.

CLIENT (*in a soft, childlike voice*): I'm scared.… (*She drops the doorstop and runs over to her foster mother to receive a hug.*)

FM: I'm here, honey. I had no idea.

THERAPIST: Thank you for telling us. (*She is now completely calmed down.*)

In both of these examples, had the therapist attempted to control or eliminate the violent behavior, the individuals would have escalated quickly into even greater violence. In both examples, the violent behaviors were triggered by stimuli in the present situation that overlapped with the individuals' traumatic experiences but that remained unexpressed. The therapists or hospital staff had previously missed or not asked about the traumatic experience.

Therefore, when a client becomes extremely angry or upset and initiates a violent sequence of behaviors, it is likely that the therapist has missed an element of the client's traumatic experience. The therapist then should directly inquire into it, framing the client's behavior as "making sense" or "having a reason," even when the therapist does not know the reason. The assumption is made that the client became upset about a not-yet-expressed memory (axiom of incompleteness), that he or she is afraid (axiom of fear), and that the behavior is intended to avoid the direct expression of the memory (axiom of avoidance). Obviously, the sooner a corrective intervention is made in the escalating behavior, the better. However, in both of the preceding cases, the client had already initiated actual violence (e.g., smashing the pool stick against the wall; jabbing herself with the nail). It was still preferable to focus on the possible trauma-related aspects of the behavior prior to attempts to restrain the client. Even if the therapist is incorrect about details of the client's experience, the fact that someone is trying to approach this experience is often sufficient to begin to calm the client down.

BEHAVIORS OUTSIDE OF THE SESSION: ARRESTS, SELF-HARM, AND HOSPITALIZATIONS

Not uncommonly, clients may become involved in disturbing situations outside and between therapy sessions. The therapist discovers that the client has been arrested and is in jail, is or was hospitalized, was injured in an accident and hospitalized on the medical unit, or was sexually or physically assaulted. The therapist may learn of these behaviors by receiving a phone call, usually panicked, from the client who is in the middle of the event; or from the client or another professional or family member who calls the therapist well after the event; or from the client at his or her next session. In all of these cases, the therapist has little control over what happens. Frequently, the therapist is not consulted by the police or the hospital. The client may not tell the other professionals about being in treatment with the therapist, or the client may tell them that the therapist is to blame for the disturbed behavior (sometimes because of talking too much about the trauma). At times, the harmfulness of the events is greatly exaggerated by the client in the heat of the moment, and at other times, the client's report to the therapist may be completely accurate.

Therapists should know how to manage these events as professionals (e.g., direct the client to the emergency room, have easy access to basic information about potentially acting-out clients, be able to summarize useful clinical information quickly to police or hospital staff, regularly assess the client's acting-out potential and offer hospitalization if necessary). However, it is also important to know how to manage these behaviors in ways that further the trauma-centered treatment. Acting-out behaviors by the client can be used to hinder or stop the exploration of the trauma or, indeed, to constrain or even end the trauma-centered work itself. Unfortunately, other professionals may attribute the behavioral problem to the trauma work and even recommend that the treatment be switched to another provider or altered in ways that support avoidance.

> After having been seen three times by a new trainee at a trauma clinic, a client stole alcohol from her parents' cabinet, became intoxicated, drove their car, and crashed it into a tree. She was hospitalized at a local psychiatric hospital, and the staff quickly concluded that it was the trauma treatment that had triggered this event. In actuality, the trainee was highly avoidant and had not even begun to discuss the client's trauma (being abducted). In a staff meeting 2 days prior to the acting-out behavior, this trainee's supervisor had instructed him to begin the trauma inquiry "before she reenacts her abduction."
>
> Her parents withdrew her from treatment on the recommendation of the hospital, whereupon she continued to act out frequently over the next 6 months while being treated with supportive psychotherapy. That therapist finally recommended that she return to the trauma clinic. In the following sessions, which did address her trauma, she revealed details of her abduction, which included all the elements of intoxication, a cabinet, a car, and a tree.

The basic principle is that when the therapist learns of an untoward event outside of a session, he or she should first and foremost (after attending to the immediate safety of the client if necessary) consider the action to be the client's attempt at communicating some new detail about his or her traumatic experience.

A 22-year-old client with a long history of borderline personality disorder–like symptoms caused by years of sexual abuse (incest) and emotional neglect called the therapist late at night in a panic. The phone call sounded as if she was outside on a street in the middle of people screaming and/or fighting. She was mostly unintelligible. The therapist was able to call her back the next day. The client answered calmly. She described going to a bar with a male friend who became solicitous of her and had taken her into the bathroom and attempted to have sex with her, possibly initially with her consent. She changed her mind and told him to stop, and he did not; a fight ensued, causing a commotion in the bar. The staff called the police and pulled her and the man outside, whereupon she accused her friend of trying to rape her. She was hysterical, and the police officer did not believe her. He sent the man away and had her sit in his car to try to calm down. At one point, he must have reached over to pat her on the shoulder, which she took as his attempt to abduct and rape her. She began hitting him, and he defended himself and threatened to arrest her. When another police officer arrived on the scene, she accused the first one of rape, and it was in the middle of this discussion that they let her make the call to the therapist's office.

The following is the remainder of the phone call between the therapist and the client the next day.

CLIENT: I'm going to press charges.
THERAPIST: What an upsetting event.
CLIENT: Why do you care? You were no help.
THERAPIST: You tried to go out and have a good time with your friend, and it turns into him trying to use you, like so many times before in your life.
CLIENT: Yeah.
THERAPIST: And it possibly reminds you of when your brother came into your room, and you thought he was going to talk with you and instead he tried to have sex with you, because "that's all that you're worth."
CLIENT: But it was the cop who tried to rape me.
THERAPIST: And then you went in to tell your mother or father what your brother did, and they wouldn't believe you, or they'd slap you, or…
CLIENT: They'd touch me too.
THERAPIST: Or your dad would touch you too, and then you'd tell your mother and she'd say, "Get out of my house," and blame you for all the trouble, and you'd end up alone, like last night.
CLIENT: (*Cries.*) No one cares for me.
THERAPIST: I'll even bet that the second police officer who came last night was a female.

CLIENT: Yes.

THERAPIST: Just like your mom, and what did that officer tell you?

CLIENT: To get the hell out of there.

THERAPIST: And she let you go, just like your mother did.

CLIENT: Yup, just like my mother did.

THERAPIST: We're going to work on this. It's a big problem.

CLIENT: It's a big problem.

THERAPIST: See you tomorrow for our session?

CLIENT: Okay.

A 14-year-old boy was removed from his biological mother because of his out-of-control behaviors and her emotional neglect. He had been physically and sexually abused during visits with his father at age 8 after his parents divorced. On one occasion, when the visit with his dad lasted over a month, the father arranged for a child pornographic ring to film several men having sex with his son. The boy was terrified and felt trapped, hoping each day for his mother to come back to take him. After he was placed at age 14 in a residential treatment setting, the staff arranged to have a trauma-centered clinician come to the facility to provide therapy twice a week. In each of these sessions, the client discussed many details of his frightening and humiliating experience. After 2 or 3 months, he ran away from the facility and with some friends drank and took drugs. He was arrested early in the morning and returned to the facility. A large staff meeting was called to discuss this incident. The leadership of the facility had raised concerns about the trauma work as potentially too upsetting to the client, even though he had been reasonably well behaved for several months prior to the event.

STAFF: So Mark, do you have any thoughts about why you ran away last weekend?

CLIENT: Nope. Felt like it.

STAFF: Something must have been going on?

CLIENT: F—k you!

STAFF: Have you been working on your coping skills in the group?

CLIENT: (*Shrugs shoulders.*)

STAFF: He has participated well in group activities in general.

STAFF: He has been on independent status for over a week now.

CLIENT: Go f—k yourself!

THERAPIST: In the past, Mark has run away when he has felt trapped. When he was with his father, all he could think of was that he wanted to get out of there, and he constantly wondered when his mother was going to come and get him. (*Mark calms down.*) Was there any activity regarding his mother last week?

STAFF: Well, yes. She contacted the unit and wanted to visit him.

THERAPIST: Was Mark told that his mother might come to visit him?

STAFF: Yes, I did, over a week ago, but I told him we weren't sure when she would come. I think I told him maybe Friday.

THERAPIST: So Mark, is it possible that when you heard about this, you were reminded of having to wait for your mother when you were at your father's house, and then when she didn't come on Friday, that's why you ran away on Saturday?

CLIENT: She never came.

STAFF: She wasn't supposed to come.

THERAPIST: No, I think he means back when he was 8. She never came.

CLIENT: She never came for me. She hates me.

THERAPIST: I believe that the reason Mark ran away on Saturday is that he felt that what had happened to him before was happening again, and that made him feel trapped, and he had to get out of here, even though "here" is really "there."

STAFF: What do you think about that, Mark?

CLIENT (*to therapist*): When is our next session?

In this case, the persistent application of the trauma-centered approach resulted in new and useful information about Mark's past and present behavior and was associated with a lessening of his activation in this meeting, as well as improved management by the residential staff. For young clients with a trauma history, anxiety and traumatic reaction are often being triggered by memories of their abuse, resulting in a tremendous variety of acting-out behaviors. Effective trauma treatment will largely reduce these acting-out behaviors, although along the way they will still occur. It is important that their occurrence should not be reactively attributed to trauma-centered work.

SUBSTANCE ABUSE TREATMENT

Helping the family and others in the client's support network, including providers, understand the nature of the dissociative behavior can significantly decrease the level of distress, panicked efforts, and interpersonal conflict that such reactions typically engender.

The use of substances is widespread in most societies, and these substances interact in complex ways with mental health conditions. Among traumatized individuals, substance abuse is common, being one of the most frequent comorbidities of posttraumatic stress disorder (PTSD) (Foa et al. 2009; Kessler et al. 1995). Clients presenting for trauma work, therefore, may be social drinkers, may have periodic episodes of abuse, or may have significant substance use disorders. Many clients will have been prescribed benzodiazepines for anxiety, or narcotics for sleep or pain, and some will have developed dependency on these medications. Clients may use drugs or alcohol as a means of treating the anxiety and hyperarousal of their

PTSD, as another means of avoidance, or as part of an independent substance use disorder.

Within the mental health field generally, it is widely held that trauma treatment, and even any exploratory psychotherapy, may threaten the sobriety of a client with substance abuse and therefore should be delayed until well after the client has established sobriety and has demonstrated the capability of regulating intense affect (Foa et al. 2009). This view, of course, presents challenges to conducting trauma-centered psychotherapy, especially because so many traumatized clients have substance abuse issues (Briere and Scott 2006).

First, if the client is intoxicated during their session, psychological work cannot be effectively conducted and the therapist must inform the client that he or she cannot attend sessions while under the influence.

Second, for those clients who do not have a substance use disorder but who report having an episode of abuse, the therapist should treat this behavior as a form of avoidance on the part of the client, usually indicating distress over a detail he or she did not discuss in the previous session. It is critical that the therapist's commitment to the trauma inquiry is not derailed by the episode of substance use. Nevertheless, it may be important to inquire about the details of the episode, because often the client's use of substances may be a way of communicating to the therapist that substances were involved in the traumatic event.

A female client in her early 40s began trauma-centered psychotherapy to deal with a severe incident of sexual abuse. At the age of about 22, she had been gang raped while attending a party in a private home. The first several sessions went extremely smoothly, and the client was able to offer many details of the horrific event and reported feeling significant relief. She failed to show up for the fourth session, however, and the therapist assumed that he had missed something in the previous session. The therapist called her, but she did not respond. She arrived at the fifth session and informed the therapist with great embarrassment and anxiety that she missed the previous session because "I stole a bunch of Xanax from my daughter and slept through the session. My husband was really alarmed, and he is worried that trauma work may be too much for me." Rather than attend to this issue, the therapist immediately asked her if there had been any drug use during the gang rape. The client looked shocked and replied, "Oh, yes! It was a couple of hours into the rape; you know, I was locked up in one of the bedrooms, and I was crying and resisting, and one of the guys gave me a bunch of pills, benzos I think, and I fell asleep until the morning." He apparently found the pills in the medicine cabinet in his sister's bathroom, which the client realized immediately linked to her stealing the pills from her daughter's medicine cabinet. The therapist asked her what this man's action meant to her, and she said, "I felt thankful that he gave me those pills, like he was concerned about me, even though he was one of the guys who raped me." This led to a very productive discussion about her confusion about the incident and her perpetrators, which revealed that a year after the rape she briefly dated the man who had given her the pills. She continued in trauma treatment for 6 months and progressed rapidly. In this case an incident of substance abuse was linked to undisclosed details of the client's traumatic experience.

Third, for those clients who do have a substance use disorder, it is recommended that they engage or continue to engage in a substance abuse program during the course of trauma-centered psychotherapy. In such cases, collaboration with the provider of the substance abuse is very useful, so that if episodes of substance use occur, both providers will support the continuation of the trauma work. For clients with an independent substance use disorder, improvement in their functioning and the stability of their sobriety can nevertheless still be gained, even though their substance use disorder will remain after trauma treatment.

Despite the fact that trauma treatment lowers clients' arousal and reactivity, decreases their anxiety, and desensitizes them to traumatic triggers, the idea persists that clients with substance use disorders cannot handle talking about their traumatic experiences. These clients do in fact have difficulty maintaining their sobriety, but for a plethora of reasons. It is therefore recommended that each client be considered individually, on the basis of their interest in doing trauma work as well as the degree to which their providers feel that their traumas are interfering with their functioning. In many cases, attending to the traumatic experiences in an organized and detailed way will lead to dramatic improvement in the client's substance abuse.

Roger, a 35-year-old male with a history of severe physical and sexual abuse by a neighbor from the ages of 6 to 12, was referred for trauma treatment. His parents had asked a neighbor, Mr. Morgan, to babysit because they trusted this middle-aged man. Morgan immediately began to intimidate and threaten Roger, inducing tremendous fear to the point where Roger felt that the man was all-powerful and could kill his parents if he said anything. Once Roger was under his control, Morgan sexually molested and physically beat him several times a week. Roger sometimes slept over at his house and went on short trips with him to a vacation house where he was molested.

Roger did poorly in school, dropping out of high school and never being employed. He revealed his trauma at the age of 18 after his perpetrator died. He lived with his parents, who took him to doctors and therapists over a period of 15 years, with no effect. In his late 20s, Roger developed a dependency on the narcotic OxyContin, increasing his daily use to high levels. He demanded that his parents drive him into dangerous neighborhoods to purchase the drug. He was hospitalized on numerous occasions on detox, substance abuse, and psychiatric units, and participated in intensive outpatient treatment programs. He made many suicide gestures and one serious attempt, in which he had nearly died. He was open about his early childhood abuse, but his providers unanimously believed that he should not do trauma work, and several believed that it was the trauma work that he had done in his early 20s that migh have caused his turn to OxyContin. Nevertheless, he was referred to a trauma therapist when staff at his outpatient program felt they had run out of options.

The therapist was initially reluctant to accept this client, given his substance dependence and the lack of support from his other providers, who knew him well. However, Roger was insistent that his memories were haunting him and that he wanted to talk about them. Given the severity of the situation and the enmeshment within the family, the therapist insisted on having the parents join the sessions, which Roger initially rejected. The therapist was finally able to convince him, and treatment began. After the third session, however, Roger overdosed on his OxyContin and had to be taken to the emergency department. Treatment continued and appeared to be productive. After the tenth session, Roger professed feeling suicidal and was hospitalized for 1 week, then participated for 3 weeks in the hospital's intensive outpatient treatment program. Against the recommendations of hospital staff, the family and Roger returned to trauma treatment.

However, by this point in the treatment, the therapist had been able to access Roger's childhood fears, during the abuse, that his parents would be killed by Mr. Morgan. These fears were nearly of psychotic proportion: Roger worried that they might be in danger even now from "things Morgan put in place" 25 years before. When these details were revealed and explored, some of Roger's current behavior regarding his parents could be decoded and then differentiated from the past. For example, his taking his parents into dangerous areas to purchase drugs was a reenactment of their being in danger from Morgan. As Roger experienced the reduction in his fear for his parent's safety—in the present—he showed huge relief. Within 3 weeks of this work, he had reduced his OxyContin usage significantly, and by 5 weeks, he stopped taking the pills. When his parents asked him why, he said, "I'm surprised. I don't feel like I need them anymore."

Roger has not been hospitalized, had a suicide gesture, or used pills of any kind, even after a knee surgery. Six months after initiation of trauma treatment, he took his GED and enrolled in a local community college. Several months after this he began a part-time job as a landscaper. He moved into his own apartment close to his parents, with whom he maintained frequent contact. Four years later he graduated with a bachelor's degree and entered a physical therapy master's program. Treatment—which included the parents—continued for 6 years, with sessions reduced to twice a month during the last 3 years. Ten years after treatment began, Roger continues to be stable and successful.

In this case, what appeared to be a primary and independent substance use disorder was in fact a coping mechanism used by the client to manage his PTSD. When the substance abuse is so directly linked to the trauma, trauma-centered psychotherapy can have rapid and significant effects. Unfortunately, it is not possible to determine the degree of linkage without conducting a trauma inquiry.

Each client with co-occurring trauma-related and substance use disorders should be evaluated as an individual, taking into account the relationship between his or her trauma schemas and use of substances, interest in and motivation to engage in trauma work, the level of support from substance abuse providers, and the severity of the consequences of any possible loss of sobriety. This evaluation should be an ongoing collaborative effort among client, therapist, and other providers as the trauma treatment proceeds. The therapist should not conclude that trauma-centered psychotherapy is contraindicated on the basis of an increase in symptomatology at the beginning of treatment. As in the initiation of any medical treatment, premature cessation may prevent the client from receiving the main effects of the intervention.

No Memories of Abuse

Occasionally, a client will be referred who believes that he or she might have been abused despite having no memories of abuse. In some cases, a previous therapist has suspected early childhood abuse and encourages the client to meet with a specialist. In other cases, a client may have seen a program on television or read a book about posttraumatic stress disorder and feel that he or she has all the symptoms.

Unfortunately, one cannot employ a trauma-centered psychotherapy method if there is no trauma or if there is no memory of a trauma. The clinician should determine whether the client is sincere and credible and whether it is worth attempting to help him or her remember what happened. We generally do not recommend launching into an intensive memory recovery process, because it may unnecessarily force an otherwise natural process of emergence. It is best simply to tell the client that if the abuse occurred, then the memories are likely to emerge when they need to. When that happens, the process can begin.

Clients with this type of presentation often have dissociative symptoms or even dissociative identity disorder. In the latter case, the host personality may not remember but senses the presence of other personalities that do remember. In this situation, the therapist should proceed to engage with the dissociated parts and conduct a trauma inquiry as described in Chapter 12, "Working With Clients With Dissociative Identity Disorder." A careful evaluation of dissociative symptoms at intake is therefore highly recommended.

STUDY QUESTIONS

11.1 T/F Dissociative reactions in treatment are not generally harmful, and the best strategy is to wait them out.

11.2 T/F When a client is threatening violence, the therapist should not attempt to control or eliminate the behavior at first, but rather should try to connect the behavior to a past traumatic experience.

11.3 T/F Clients' disruptive behaviors outside of the session are often a way of communicating a new detail of their traumatic experience.

11.4 T/F Trauma-centered psychotherapy is possible even when the client has no direct memories of abuse.

CHAPTER 12

Working With Clients With Dissociative Identity Disorder

The treatment of clients with dissociative identity disorder (DID), or multiple personality disorder, is a specialized area requiring a great deal of experience (Putnam 1989). The complexity of these clients' presentations, the chaotic alterations in their behavior and interactions with others, and the bizarre nature of their symptoms justify referring these clients to clinicians who specialize in treatment of DID. Unfortunately, traumatized clients often do not come to therapists with a sign that identifies them as having DID. They often are unaware of the disorder. Thus, it is common for DID symptoms to present well into treatment, when referral to another clinician may be too disruptive for a client. Therefore, clinicians using a trauma-centered approach should be sure to make a thorough evaluation of dissociative symptoms as part of their initial assessment but also need to know how to handle and treat clients with DID that emerges during the course of trauma-centered psychotherapy.

DISSOCIATION AND PRIMARY PERSONALITIES

The main challenge in working with clients with DID is that their primary defense in the face of anxiety or threat is to dissociate, which interferes with their ability to integrate and remember their trauma narrative. As a result, clients who dissociate may be among the most difficult to treat with exposure therapy. Because the trauma inquiry will inevitably approach these areas of threat, the client with DID will likely dissociate instead of becoming aroused or angry. Thus, the client may avoid the gap (see Chapter 9, "The Gap: When the Trauma Schema Emerges in the Therapeutic Relationship"), a situation that prevents the clinician from working on the client's distorted trauma schemas.

From a trauma-centered psychotherapy perspective, a useful assumption to make is that all of the primary personalities were present at the original traumatic event. It was during this highly traumatic moment that the child used dissociative defenses to split his or her developing self-representations into pieces. Continuing to keep these personalities separate is another way in which the client avoids remembering the traumatic event. Thus, a trauma inquiry is likely to evoke these defenses. Dissociation has both structural dimensions, in that the original act of dissociation resulted in relatively enduring alterations in personality structure, and process dimensions, in that dissociative defenses are used when needed on a temporary basis. Thus, in response to a trauma inquiry, the client may use the same form of avoidance by forming secondary personalities as a means of protecting himself or herself from reexperiencing the anxiety of remembering the event. This may explain why some clients with DID develop additional personalities as a result of being in treatment.

In trauma-centered psychotherapy, however, the central interest is in uncovering and processing the traumatic event and the client's experience. Therefore, the primary personalities, all of whom were present at the event and hold a piece of that experience, are to be privileged over the secondary personalities that emerge as a result of the therapeutic inquiry. The therapist should show less interest in these secondary personalities.

The therapist should demonstrate a neutral or even indifferent attitude toward the drama of the client with DID. Despite the usually bizarre or interesting names and qualities of the personalities, the therapist should maintain interest and focus on what happened to the person-as-a-whole and communicate that interest directly to the client. Therefore, it is best not to inquire too much into the various qualities of each personality other than name and age and not to become interested in their relationships with each other. We do not recommend making charts, diagrams, or lists of personalities. All of these acts serve to continue the client's avoidance of remembering the whole event and may produce additional and more dramatic personalities.

There are many types of primary personalities. In clinical practice, however, four or five basic types are common. The first is often an *innocent child* who is preserved without the memory of the trauma and who is protected from remembering by the other personalities. The personality may speak in a childlike voice or be speechless. Second, there may be a *witness figure* who saw what happened from a distance. This figure is often cold and rational and is occasionally cynical or critical. Third, there may be an *angry, protective figure* who identifies with the power of the perpetrator, but in order to protect the other figures from intrusion by an outsider. This primary figure may be differentiated from secondary protective figures in that he or she has a retaliatory dimension as a result of having been present at the perpetration. Fourth, there may be an *acting-out figure* who identifies with the perpetrator's view of the victim; this figure is risk taking, sexual, wild, or aggressive and is often responsible for the client's becoming revictimized. Finally, there is the *host personality*, who may serve as one of the above or may be a separate figure, who is the public face of the person. Generally, there are rarely more than three or four primary personalities.

Interestingly, there is usually not a figure who is frightened, because the dissociation was employed to prevent such a feeling. When a personality does show signs of fear or emotional arousal regarding the traumatic event, this may be a sign that progress toward integration of the story is taking place.

Throughout the therapeutic work, the therapist will treat the client as one person with the host's formal identity. In inquiring about what each identity knows about the traumatic event, the therapist will ask, "What did you see happen to Carol [the client's name]?" The therapist will also tell the client directly about the assumption that all the personalities were present at the time of the trauma and were split up to prevent remembering. An example of this intervention is provided later in this chapter (see Lindsay's case in "Case Examples").

TREATMENT APPROACH

In a trauma-centered approach to clients with DID, the therapist will be interested in the integration of the trauma story, not the integration of the personalities (which may be the subject of a treatment for DID). During reconstruction of the trauma narrative, the intensity of the splitting among the personalities diminishes, sometimes to the point of personality integration.

The therapist conducts the session in the standard trauma-centered psychotherapy manner, following the principles (immediacy, engagement, and emotionality) and techniques (getting the details, decoding current behaviors, introducing discrepancy, and disclosing the perpetrator) discussed in Chapter 4 ("Principles of Trauma-Centered Psychotherapy") and Chapter 5 ("The Four Main Techniques"), respectively. As this work proceeds, the client will evidence sudden shifts in personalities as a means of avoiding the rising affect associated with the remembering. The therapist can make a choice either to continue the inquiry with the new personality or to point out the avoidance and ask to speak to the first personality again.

As in standard forms of therapy with clients with DID, the therapist can talk directly to each personality (e.g., asking "Who is there?" to obtain name and age or "How do you know [the client]?" or "Where were you when [client] was molested by her uncle?"). The therapist may choose to *talk through* the host by having the host report what the other personalities are saying. Grounding techniques such as deep breathing, holding hands, or orienting to time or place may also be used when the client is highly dissociated, as long as implementing these techniques does not lead the inquiry astray.

It is important that the therapist not be surprised, overly interested, or upset when the client dissociates. If clients with DID do not dissociate, this may mean that the therapist is actively avoiding the relevant material. The therapist is encouraged to remind himself or herself that dissociation is a defense, which means that while dissociating the client probably feels more comfortable than previously and that it will not last long. Generally, the more action taken by the therapist to get the client back, the longer it will take. Examples of the recommended process are presented later in this chapter (see "Case Examples"). Once the client returns, the therapist may simply say, "Welcome back."

As the discussion proceeds, if any of the personalities appear to apply their trauma schemas onto current issues, the therapist, or relationships among the personalities, the standard method of handling these displacements is used: decoding their link to the original trauma and then providing a sense of discrepancy between the trauma and the present. If a personality attacks the therapist or treatment process, the standard method of working through the gap—acknowledging the problem, linking it to the original trauma, noting the harm, and then providing discrepancy—should be applied. Through these methods, the client learns that dissociating will not stop or divert the therapist from continuing to discuss and inquire about the original trauma. The foundational purpose of dissociation is therefore defeated. When secondary protective figures arise, the therapist should ask whether they were present at the original trauma and then tell them that the therapist does not wish to talk to them because the purpose is to find out what happened.

In milder forms of DID, in which the client has not differentiated into distinct personalities but rather has partially organized personality states with slightly different voices, postures, or demeanors, it is usually possible to conduct the sessions in the standard trauma-centered manner. Again, as long as the process of discovering the details of the traumatic event and the client's schemas is occurring, there is no need to find out more about the interesting aspects of these part-selves.

CASE EXAMPLES

In the following case, the client is a 30-year-old single woman.

> THERAPIST: Lindsay, after he got on top of you, what happened?
>
> CLIENT: (*Looks away, silent, shudders.*)
>
> THERAPIST: I can imagine that it was very frightening. He was on top of you. Did he feel heavy?
>
> CLIENT: (*Curls up in chair, shakes head.*)
>
> THERAPIST: I see. To whom am I speaking?
>
> CLIENT (*in a childlike voice*): Maarry.
>
> THERAPIST: Hello, Mary. And how old are you?
>
> CLIENT: Four.
>
> THERAPIST: That's very young. So you were there when Uncle Henry molested Lindsay?
>
> CLIENT: I don't know.
>
> THERAPIST: Well, Uncle Henry molested Lindsay when she was about 4. He got on top of her.
>
> CLIENT: He was heavy. Smelled bad.
>
> THERAPIST: Thank you. I am interested in finding out what happened to Lindsay back then. Where were you when Uncle Henry was on top of Lindsay?
>
> CLIENT: I was hiding in the closet.
>
> THERAPIST: Did you hear any sounds from Lindsay when she was being molested?
>
> CLIENT: (*Looks away, straightens up, yawns, then glares at therapist.*) Huh?
>
> THERAPIST: To whom am I speaking?
>
> CLIENT (*in a loud, harsh tone*): Why is it your business?
>
> THERAPIST: Because Lindsay and I are trying to remember what happened to her when she was 4 and her Uncle Henry molested her. He got on top of her and hurt her. He was heavy. That's what I know so far. Were you there?
>
> CLIENT: Yup. But you're not going to get a thing out of me.
>
> THERAPIST: I understand you are here to protect her, and I can understand why, given how harmed she was. It must have been horrible. Do you have a name?
>
> CLIENT: Some call me Jo.
>
> THERAPIST: Hello, Jo. Are you a male or female?
>
> CLIENT (*derisively*): Can't you tell? Female.
>
> THERAPIST: And what did you see? It was in the basement, and Uncle Henry was on top of Lindsay.
>
> CLIENT: The asshole nailed her.

THERAPIST: He penetrated Lindsay with his penis?

CLIENT: Yeah. What more do you want?

THERAPIST: Well, when the event happened, it so overwhelmed Lindsay that she divided herself into a couple of parts: you, Jo, who seem like a strong protector; Mary, who is innocent and 4 and hid in the closet...

CLIENT: We kept her away from him.

THERAPIST: And who else kept away from him. Are there others who were present?

CLIENT: (*Stares, looks down, nods.*)

THERAPIST: What's your name?

CLIENT: (*Looks up at the therapist, staring.*)

THERAPIST: Well, hello, I have met Mary and Jo, both of whom were present when Uncle Henry sexually molested Lindsay by raping her. I'm interested in what you know about what happened?

CLIENT: (*Stares.*)

THERAPIST: I'm sorry this happened to you. Lindsay, do you know who this person is?

CLIENT: (*Shudders, looks away and then back.*) I call her Little Miss Stupid.

THERAPIST: Was she present at the rape?

CLIENT: Yeah.

THERAPIST: What was she saying to you when I was asking her questions?

CLIENT: She was saying she wanted this to be over.

THERAPIST: I can understand that. But we are trying to put together what each of you remembers about Uncle Henry and what he did to you. What did Little Miss Stupid see?

CLIENT: She says she was floating overhead, looking down on Uncle Henry's back.

THERAPIST: Did he still have his clothes on?

CLIENT: (*Moves suddenly, with energy.*) Of course not, how else was he going to rape her!

THERAPIST: This must be Jo again. Do you understand why I am asking these questions? I want to know what Little Miss experienced during the rape and what she knows about it. This will be helpful in Lindsay's recovery.

CLIENT: Little Miss doesn't want to talk.

THERAPIST: Okay, but it seems that Uncle Henry was naked?

CLIENT: (*Nods.*)

THERAPIST: Had Henry ordered Lindsay to take off her clothes also?

CLIENT: Yes, except for her shoes.

THERAPIST: Shoes?

CLIENT: Uncle Henry insisted she keep her shoes on.

As illustrated in this example, the therapist attempts to continue to conduct the trauma inquiry despite the complexity of the different personalities.

He also makes explicit his rationale for inquiring and his basic assumptions about the cause of the divided self. He shows no particular excitement about the appearance of any of the personalities and does not try to get to know them in depth outside of their knowledge of the traumatic event.

The following is an example of the appearance of a secondary personality well into treatment.

> THERAPIST: And tell me more about what your wife said.
>
> CLIENT: She was being a bitch, nagging at me over and over again, like always.
>
> THERAPIST: What was she saying?
>
> CLIENT: Clean up, clean up! Over and over again.
>
> THERAPIST: I can understand why that was so upsetting to you, given how your grandfather had yelled at you to clean yourself up after he sodomized you, over and over again.
>
> CLIENT: (*Stares out window, says something unintelligible, mutters, then begins scratching at his forearm, hard, apparently trying to draw blood.*)
>
> THERAPIST: Who is here now?
>
> CLIENT: (*Speaks in a strange accent.*) Apoche.
>
> THERAPIST: Hello, Apoche. You are scratching yourself.
>
> CLIENT: (*Scratches harder.*) Tattoo.
>
> THERAPIST: We have not met before. Bill and I have been trying to put together what his grandfather did to him when he was 10 years old. We know his grandfather sodomized him on many occasions in his backyard shed. Were you present for that?
>
> CLIENT: You cannot speak about that.
>
> THERAPIST: I understand that you do not want Bill to get upset by this conversation. You may be trying to protect Bill. But since I am trying to help Bill with what happened to him, I am not interested in talking with figures who were not there. Do you understand me?
>
> CLIENT: Yes. I don't remember if I was there.
>
> THERAPIST: Okay. If you do remember something, please tell me. For now, I want to talk to Bill some more. Bill, I was saying that your wife's nagging you may have reminded you of your grandfather's abuse.
>
> CLIENT (*after a pause*): Yeah. I can see that.
>
> THERAPIST: How did you clean up after yourself, being in the shed?
>
> CLIENT: My grandfather had old rags in a corner barrel. I'd throw them into the manure pile outside the shed as I went back into the house.
>
> THERAPIST: I can't imagine how that must have felt.
>
> CLIENT: Just a whole bunch of shit, through and through (*smiles*).
>
> THERAPIST: You can say that for sure!

Clients with DID are accused of purposefully manipulating and performing, essentially because of their repeated use of dissociation as a means of handling stressful emotional situations. It is important that the therapist not be distracted by this sometimes disturbing, sometimes histrionic drama, and keep focused on the trauma-centered work. The truth and credible experience that lies underneath these strange symptoms and behaviors can be revealed by an active process of inquiry about the traumatic events. Once reached, the client's need for his or her dissociative defenses greatly diminishes.

STUDY QUESTIONS

12.1   What is the difference between primary and secondary personalities?

12.2   T/F   It is possible for new personalities to emerge in treatment in response to the trauma inquiry.

12.3   What are the common primary personalities?

12.4   T/F   The therapist should at all times maintain a neutral, slightly disinterested stance toward any dramatic presentations of the personalities.

12.5   T/F   In trauma-centered work with clients with dissociative identity disorder, the therapist works to integrate the client's dissociated identities.

12.6   What is the major challenge to trauma-centered psychotherapy in working with clients with dissociative identity disorder?

CHAPTER 13

Working With Clients With Borderline Personality Disorder

In this chapter, the process of conducting a trauma inquiry with clients who have borderline personality disorder (BPD) will be addressed. This process should not be confused with a method of treatment for BPD itself, which has been the subject of long-standing interest in the field of psychotherapy (Bateman and Fonagy 2006; Kernberg 1984; Linehan 1993; Masterson 1981). Like clients with dissociative identity disorder (discussed in Chapter 12, "Working With Clients With Dissociative Identity Disorder"), clients with BPD present unique challenges to the therapist in conducting a trauma inquiry. In work with clients with BPD, potential issues include their rapid shifts in affect; frequent threats to act out or harm self; tremendous need for reassurance and out-of-session contact; aggressive and critical attacks on the therapist based on intrusive but accurate collecting of personal information from the Internet and other sources; and engagement with other providers, agencies, and community authorities.

ROLE OF TRAUMA IN THE CAUSATION OF BORDERLINE PERSONALITY DISORDER

A vast majority of clients with BPD report having been abused, usually but not exclusively sexually abused, during childhood. The perpetrators are often family members or trusted adults who hold out a promise of love but betray a child by using the child sexually and then rejecting or abandoning him or her. Many authorities have proposed that BPD is a form of trauma-related disorder, in that clients demonstrate affect dysregulation, distortions in self-concept and interpersonal relations, and anxiety and depressive symptomatology (Bloom 1997; Courtois and Ford 2013; Herman 1992; van der Kolk et al. 1994). The clients' acting-out and self-harming behaviors may be actions triggered by memories of the traumatic abuse.

Others, including Paris (1996), have proposed that because not all clients with BPD report childhood traumatic events, BPD cannot be caused by trauma, which is simply a co-occurring condition. Paris notes that the relationship between BPD and childhood trauma is only correlational and statistical, even though in his own research, he found that 70% of clients with BPD reported childhood abuse.

The leading form of treatment for clients with BPD is *dialectical behavior therapy* (Linehan 1993). Although Linehan (1993) acknowledges the close relationship between trauma and the disorder, she recommends that the trauma inquiry be delayed until the client has learned to manage his or her affective behaviors and acting-out behaviors.

CLINICAL CHALLENGES

After deciding that the client with BPD is ready for a trauma inquiry, the clinician may face any of a variety of impressive challenges:

- Clients may resist having their problems explained by their traumatic experiences.
- Clients may be reluctant to provide details of their traumatic experiences.
- Clients are likely to experience the therapist as being inadequate, being harmful, and/or betraying them early and throughout the treatment.
- Clients may act out or report acting out after sessions in which the traumas are discussed and blame this discussion on the reason for their acting out.
- Clients may complain about the treatment to other agencies and providers, who will tend to agree that the trauma inquiry should be terminated or delayed.
- Clients may quit the treatment or fire the therapist and then insist on starting again with the agreement not to talk about the trauma.

Whereas the client with dissociative identity disorder, when triggered, will dissociate, the client with BPD will engage in much more problematic and challenging behaviors that will demand management from the therapist, leading to much stronger countertransference reactions from the therapist, usually of the type that desire the client to go away, confirming for the client his or her abandonment schemas and permeating the treatment relationship with the traumatic relationship with the abandoning parent. No matter how the therapist responds, it will not be sufficient for the client, who will escalate or threaten to escalate. The therapist's attempts to be nice to the injured child within the client will be experienced as a reenactment of the original seduction and lead to acting out, whereas being able to argue and disagree with clients without tension is likely to be experienced as a sign that the therapist is not afraid of them and result in diminished acting out. Handling these moments is part and parcel of treating clients with BPD and requires a steady and calm acceptance of failure coupled with the understanding that the real failure occurred long ago. The goal is to maintain an emphasis on feelings and inner states rather than engage in action language of what the therapist will do in response to what the client plans to do.

Therapists should use whatever strategies have been effective for them with clients who have BPD, whether these involve availability for phone contact, conjoint group therapy, or psychoeducational materials, as long as these methods do not interfere with the primary purpose of the trauma inquiry within a trauma-centered frame.

ESTABLISHING THE TRAUMA-CENTERED FRAME

We advise that the therapist establish the trauma-centered frame with the client in the first session and preferably in the first few minutes of the first session. Establishing and holding this frame is essential to the success of the trauma inquiry. The therapist should show no wobbling or compromise and should make it clear that in working with this therapist, the client has no option other than to address the impact of the childhood abuse on the client's self-image and current interpersonal problems. It may be useful for the client with BPD to simultaneously see another provider who will attend to his or her other needs; preferably, the other provider is linked with the trauma provider so that when the client with BPD complains to the other provider about the trauma treatment, that provider will remain neutral.

Clients with BPD may break off and resume the trauma treatment many times. This should be predicted to them, and they should be reassured that the therapist will tolerate this and will be available to resume the treatment whenever they are ready. It is not recommended that the therapist cease the trauma work temporarily to do other types of therapeutic work, for this will break the trauma frame, and it will be nearly impossible to resume the trauma-centered frame.

COLLECTING THE TRAUMA HISTORY

It is also important for the therapist to gather the trauma history in as much detail as possible immediately from the client and/or from previous providers and their reports. Very soon after beginning, the client with BPD may refuse to provide more details of his or her trauma as part of a challenge to the therapist who has proven to the client that he or she does not care about the client. The therapist may have several sessions in which the client is cooperative and can report what happened, and the therapist should take every opportunity to gather this information as accurately as possible.

On the basis of this early information, the therapist should construct, preferably with the collaboration of the client (although often this is not possible), the basic narrative that explains how the traumatic abuse by the perpetrator altered the client's internal and interpersonal world, producing enduring affective and cognitive schemas that are now operating in the client's current life, leading to frequent distortions and misinterpretations of other people's motives and actions. This narrative will be revised and filled in as treatment progresses, but having an initial basic narrative is useful in handling the gap work that will begin shortly. The story should be able to explain sufficiently the most problematic acting-out behaviors in which the client engages (e.g., suicidality, cutting, putting self in dangerous situations, disappearing, refusing to leave the office).

ENGAGING IN GAP WORK

Many clients with BPD seem to be living in the gap their entire waking day. They are constantly feeling cut off from or harmed or dismissed by people who come close to them. They initially draw people close to them with ingratiating or pleasant or idealizing attitudes, only to be deeply disappointed by minor fluctuations in the other's attention or care. The psychotherapeutic environment is the perfect fit for this gap to appear, given the role of the therapist to care for them and the need to examine difficult subjects that evoke deep feelings of betrayal and abandonment. These clients assume that eventually the therapist will turn on them and abandon them after having lured or seduced them into the promise of a caring relationship. To prove their expectation, they mistreat and attack the therapist and wait for him or her to withdraw, and if the therapist does not withdraw, they accuse him or her of pretending to care. Individuals with BPD are highly vigilant of the most subtle interpersonal cues, minor misrememberings of their history, and contradictory statements, all the result of having been lied to, manipulated, and used by family members whom they trusted and loved.

As a result, the therapist will have to engage in gap work from early on, and in fact most of the treatment's early stages will be in the gap. Essential to the gap work, as described in Chapter 9 ("The Gap: When the Trauma Schema Emerges in the Therapeutic Relationship"), is having enough knowledge about the trauma story to be able to effectively make the link between the current issue and the client's trauma schema. The therapist should communicate to the client that the focus in therapy will be on the impact of the client's traumas rather than the management of the current, provocative crisis.

While the therapist is following the gap procedure, the client may often reject any attempt at sympathy or apology, will be annoyed at the incomplete understanding of his or her trauma history but refuse to fill the therapist in, and will scoff at the therapist's pitiful wish to have been there to help the client. The therapist must proceed in any case in a calm and firm manner.

CONCRETIZING THE CONDITION OF BORDERLINE PERSONALITY DISORDER

It is helpful for a therapist to discuss in the first session the client's diagnosis of BPD and to provide information about the condition and its causes, effects, and challenges (although most clients already have this information and have read profusely about BPD). The therapist needs to discuss that BPD is a long-lasting condition but that it usually dissipates over time, often by one's 30s or 40s. The goal is to objectify BPD and to separate it from the client. Thus, when the client declares that the trauma treatment is harming him or her and is not working, the therapist can attribute that feeling to the client's BPD rather than the client's personal misery. A statement such as this one may be given:

> Borderline personality disorder is an illness that forms during one's teenage years and is either caused by or worsened by childhood sexual, physical, or emotional abuse and neglect. It usually lasts a long time, affecting how the people who have the disorder feel about themselves and their ability to sustain intimate interpersonal relationships. The good news is that even without treatment, it becomes less strong over time, and with treatment, it improves more quickly, so that by one's late 20s or into one's 30s, things are a lot better.
>
> You were betrayed by people who claimed they loved you. In fact, they may actually have loved you, but then they used you, or sexually abused you, or promised to care for you and then changed their minds and abandoned, rejected, humiliated, or ignored you. This led to your having very strong urges to find people to love you and, at the same time, becoming very sensitive to any sign that they will betray you or leave you. This makes you feel at times very angry at them, and at times very angry at yourself, and you may try to hurt yourself or hurt them. You often feel desperate and in need of

help, and you call out for help, and if that doesn't come, you become enraged. That leads people to say that you are simply pretending to be desperate as a manipulation, which makes you even more upset, and knowing how wrong they are, you become willing to go even further, even to kill yourself, or nearly kill yourself.

Having BPD will mean that you will feel all these feelings toward me. You might want to call me in the evening or the middle of the night. You might feel that I don't care or that I am meeting with you only for the money. Then, at different times, you might feel that you can't live without me and that you want me to be your parent.

I know all of this and will not blame you for this. You were mistreated by someone you loved, and that has caused your understanding of love to be mixed up. The key thing for us is that we don't want these problems caused by BPD to interfere too much with our trying to find out and discuss what happened to you, and how you were abused and mistreated, because if we can do that, your BPD will improve, and you will feel a lot better. Any questions?

DISCLOSING THE PERPETRATOR

Even more than in the usual trauma-centered treatment, disclosing and mentioning the perpetrator helps the client with BPD differentiate between past and present and, more importantly, between perpetrator and therapist. The client will resist and become annoyed with the therapist's mentioning the client's perpetrator, in each session, multiple times, but the therapist should gently persist. Therapists of clients with BPD should be able to remain calm and be undisturbed when placed in the perpetrator role. When the client is experiencing the therapist in this role, the therapist should not act on his or her own feelings of anger at this undeserved attribution, and instead should demonstrate deep compassion toward the client. In many cases, the perpetrator is alive and is living with or in close contact with the client. Bringing up the past abuse seems to be pouring salt in the wound and causes distress because the client is still working on establishing a caring relationship with the perpetrator, often his or her parent, who often is not cooperating. Many clients with BPD continue to have conflictual relationships with the people who were responsible for their condition but whom they will not give up, because on a deep level they still love them. In fact, this is the kind of relationship they will establish with the therapist: a conflictual and distressing relationship that they will not give up. It is important to note that unlike victims of other traumas in which the perpetrator has been rejected, the client with BPD holds some love toward the perpetrator and resents attacks on him or her from others, including from the therapist. Therefore, it is helpful to develop the *reparative dream*.

REPARATIVE DREAM

Because of the continued attachment of the client to his or her perpetrator, most clients with BPD understand that their perpetrator's abuse of them was due to their perpetrator's own distress or illness or past traumas. The clients then develop a wish to help the perpetrator or to repair this damage by some action in their own lives, as if to undo or make up for the earlier injury. Although the means by which a client enacts this compensatory wish are often self-defeating, it can be useful to identify it and acknowledge it as a sign of a laudable character trait that, if redirected in a rational manner, could become a basis for a future career or more successful relationships. Many of these reparative dreams involve acts of charity, becoming a good mother, or developing a health-related career. Supporting the reparative dream provides the client hope, reframes his or her suffering as a basis for a future career or contribution, and also distances the therapeutic process from the immediate crisis.

> Sheila is a 27-year-old white woman who is the mother of three children, two of whom have been removed from her by her state's department of children and families. Sheila was raised by her mother in a chaotic, neglectful, and conflictual environment, in which she was sexually abused by two loosely related family members and left alone for long periods of time. The family moved frequently. By age 9 she was unable to behave properly in school, and from ages 10 to 17 she was placed in a variety of group and foster homes, hospitalized often for suicidality, and placed in residential facilities, where she was sexually abused. From ages 17 to 21, she was hospitalized more than 20 times, raped on numerous occasions, and arrested frequently for disturbances of the peace. She was often homeless but maintained a relationship with her mother, grandmother, great aunt and uncle, and other family members, always with great conflict. At age 21, she had her first child, who was removed immediately; at age 22, she had a second child whom she kept for 1 month prior to the child's removal; and at age 23, she had a third child whom she is currently caring for, although she is being monitored by the state's department of children and families.

> CLIENT: Good morning, Doctor.
> THERAPIST: Good morning, Sheila.
> CLIENT: I've got a lot to talk about....
> THERAPIST: I'm looking forward to talking more about your mother.
> CLIENT: Mother...I don't call her "mother." Don't you remember that?
> THERAPIST: I thought you didn't want me to call her your "mom."
> CLIENT: I don't want to talk about her.
> THERAPIST: Your mother is key.

CLIENT: Why is your desk always so messy? No wonder you can't keep any of my information straight. Maybe I should straighten it up before we continue?

THERAPIST: Every time I act in a way that indicates I am not fully attending to you, it reminds you of all the false promises your mother and uncle made to you, so I can understand why it is upsetting.

CLIENT: Don't get off on that trauma stuff again. You're making excuses like usual.

THERAPIST: This is your trauma treatment, so that's what I'm thinking about.

CLIENT: You should think about something else.

THERAPIST: Whenever I make excuses for myself, it's like how your mother responds every time you confront her with what happened as a child.

CLIENT: Excuses, excuses. I'm tired of it.

THERAPIST: There probably was a whopper of an excuse.

CLIENT: Yes, there was. This morning, I was on the phone with her and she was telling me that I was going to lose Samantha [her current child] like I lost the others.

THERAPIST: Tell me more.

CLIENT: So I told her to go to hell, that I'd make it this time, no thanks to her, and she said I always blamed her, and so I asked her if she remembered the time she left me at some strange man's apartment for 3 days, and that after a day he left me alone, and there was barely anything in the refrigerator and I was really scared, and when she came back finally I was crying and she said she forgot.

THERAPIST: She said she forgot you?

CLIENT: And I asked her why she forgot, and she said things had gotten really messed up at her job.

THERAPIST: Messed up at her job?

CLIENT: Yeah, and so this morning she got quiet cuz I think she remembered this, so I told her—actually I yelled at her on the phone—that that was the biggest f—king excuse I had ever heard, and that I would never ever do that with Samantha, as long as I live!

THERAPIST: That was inexcusable.

CLIENT: I was so mad.

THERAPIST: Did you call back?

CLIENT: I did because I was coming here and I needed her to baby-sit Samantha.

THERAPIST: Do you know why you brought up the state of my desk?

CLIENT: It was messy, and you don't care for me.

THERAPIST: It is messy, but I think it reminded you of this memory when your mother used the fact that her job was messed up as an excuse for neglecting you, and you worry that I will neglect you also.

CLIENT: You are a smart ass.

THERAPIST: And this is one way your childhood traumas live on in the present, because you loved your mother so much, and you knew she was in trouble and couldn't handle things, and as a result you were left alone, vulnerable to the guys she depended on and one of whom molested you. You are so vulnerable that you can't trust anyone who offers to care for you, as I do, because you worry they won't sustain the relationship and you'll be left alone to your own devices, and anything that comes close to reminding you of this is a trigger for the memory, only instead of just remembering, you demand that the other person not act that way—that's the BPD part. And once you get a handle on this process, you are going to do a lot better.

CLIENT: That's a nice story, but you left out a lot of details.

THERAPIST: I know, and it's those details you have to tell me about.

CLIENT: I've told you a lot already, and you have forgotten half of them.

THERAPIST: I rely on you to correct me each time I do. But the thing I hear again today, which I hear over and over from you…

CLIENT: You're bored with me.

THERAPIST: …is that down deep you forgive your mother because you know she couldn't have done any better, and you have decided in your heart that you are not going to let anything stop you from being a good—no, a great—mother to your kid and that you would never do anything to your kids like your mother did to you.

CLIENT: It's hard when they take away my kids for mental health issues.

THERAPIST: You did nothing to harm your kids, and if—God forbid—they take away Samantha, you will want to get pregnant again in order to repair this mother-daughter relationship that has gone on in your family for at least three generations.

CLIENT: I think I'm pregnant already.

THERAPIST: Have you abandoned any of your children?

CLIENT: No. They took them away from me, but I see them every week.

THERAPIST: Your mother was impaired.

CLIENT: It's hard for me to talk about this.

THERAPIST: Every time you think about it, your heart gets sick and you ask yourself, "There's nothing I can do about it, so why think about it?"

CLIENT: Yes, why do I have to think about it?

THERAPIST: Because your mother caused you a lot of pain that contributed to your BPD, which is making your life difficult.

CLIENT: (*Smiles.*) You're a know-it-all.

THERAPIST: I don't know it all yet, because you have more to tell me about it—like, I'm interested in your uncle; didn't you say he molested your mother?

CLIENT: No, my cousin.
THERAPIST: Cousin? You mean his own child?
CLIENT: Yes, Martha.

In this session fragment, the client's avoidant strategies include provocative and intrusive comments about the therapist, and attempts to shift the subject away from the trauma material. The therapist remains steadfast in discussing the traumatic material and eliciting more details, referring to the client's story and noting BPD as a thing, and reinforcing the trauma-centered frame several times. He mentioned the client's perpetrator numerous times. He was able to make the link between his messy desk and her mother's excuse of her job being messed up, which the client accepted but, as is typical, was unable to explore further. The goal is not to aim for a stable working relationship with the client, but to continue to gather information about the events and point out how these events and the schemas they produced are interfering with the client's life today.

CONCLUSION

Working with clients with BPD is a challenge for most therapists, but in many instances it is possible to conduct a trauma inquiry and proceed with trauma-centered psychotherapy. Although the condition is generally pernicious and chronic, the client will show improvement in sensitivity to interpersonal slights and better regulation of emotional states over time. As in any trauma-centered treatment, successfully revealing and differentiating the past from the present will significantly decrease the client's inner distress and outer reactivity.

STUDY QUESTIONS

13.1 Is it necessary to believe that borderline personality disorder is caused by trauma in order to do trauma-centered psychotherapy with these clients? Why or why not?

13.2 What are the major challenges to trauma-centered psychotherapy with clients who have borderline personality disorder?

13.3 T/F It is important to establish the trauma-centered frame and collect an initial detailed trauma history as quickly as possible with clients who have borderline personality disorder.

13.4 T/F It is fair to say that the therapist will experience being in the gap with the client who has borderline personality disorder often during the treatment.

13.5 T/F The client with borderline personality disorder is most likely to cast the therapist in the role of victim in the trauma schema.

13.6 T/F The therapist should explain the relationship between borderline personality disorder and trauma often during the treatment in order to concretize and externalize the client's condition, as a way of building an alliance with the client to engage in the trauma-centered work.

13.7 What is the role of the reparative dream in working with clients who have borderline personality disorder?

CHAPTER 14

Trauma-Centered Group Psychotherapy

In this chapter, we apply the axioms, principles, and techniques of trauma-centered psychotherapy to group therapy. We do not presume the use of any particular theoretical orientation or approach to group therapy, but rather provide guidance to group therapists of any kind in integrating a trauma-centered frame into their work. A number of excellent group therapy models are described by other authors (Harris 1998; Klein and Schermer 2000; Lubin and Johnson 2008; Mendelsohn et al. 2011; Ready et al. 2008; Resick and Schnicke 1993).

Group therapy poses particular challenges and offers specific benefits because of having more people in the room. The amount of time allowed for each person to talk is greatly reduced, but this is compensated by the additional time required to listen. Because of various absences, late arrivals, and newcomers, the group environment is much more variable and unpredictable than individual therapy. The avenues for avoidance are exponentially increased in group, and the potential interpersonal triggers of trauma schemas are increased. Hearing the details of others' stories can potentially create a cascade of memories among all group members. The possibility of arguments, emotional displays, and even physical action among members of a group creates a background concern. For clients whose traumatic experiences occurred in group settings (e.g., school, bullying, family, combat, party), the group atmosphere in itself may be a trigger.

Interestingly, the history of posttraumatic stress disorder (PTSD) was propelled by groups such as veteran rap groups and women's consciousness raising groups, in which mutual comfort and solidarity were fostered among fellow victims. However, in the development of treatment for PTSD, group therapy has had a difficult time. In addition to the lack of adequate time for each client's story and the mutual triggering among group members, unique group dynamics emerge that challenge group therapists. These group dynamics are driven by the relatively rigid interpersonal boundaries of trauma victims, leading to atmospheres either of merging and ignoring differences (e.g., we are brothers; only we know what rape is) or of breaking apart as an expression of complete separateness. Both states reflect an inability among trauma victims to tolerate differentiation, or the balancing of similarity and difference. These challenges have been responded to through many different forms of structuring by group therapists (Klein and Schermer 2000).

A common form of structuring is through the *time-limited group*, which usually meets for 12–20 sessions. The presence of a beginning and a pre-established end helps to maintain a focus on the work and minimizes ambiguity. These groups may be organized with *preestablished content*, in which each week a specific topic is introduced and discussed, often with accompanying manuals or written homework. Some group formats minimize open group discussion and consist of a series of *individual interviews* conducted in the group, as an attempt to minimize uncontrolled group interaction. In contrast, *open-ended groups* meet continuously, with members leaving and new members being admitted periodically. The following discussion is designed to be more or less applicable to any of these types of group.

ESTABLISHING THE TRAUMA-CENTERED FRAME

As in individual therapy, establishing the trauma-centered frame is the most important component of conducting a successful group therapy. Either a group is set up explicitly as a trauma group or the focus of an ongoing group is altered. In the latter case, the group leader should inform each group member of the new aims and methods that will be used. Through advertisement, referral information, and the group's title, members should be well aware of the group's content. An individual screening meeting is recommended prior to a client's entrance into either a new group or an ongoing group.

Referral to trauma-centered group psychotherapy is usually recommended after the initial stages of individual trauma treatment have been completed and the client is able to discuss his or her traumatic events in some detail. The main purpose of group therapy is for the client to work on the interpersonal aspects of the trauma schemas in the presence of other clients with both similar and different experiences. Effective group therapy will balance the support provided by other group members with the increased opportunities for differentiation created by the diversity of the group environment (Lubin and Johnson 2008). Clients can transition from individual to group treatment or continue in both, since the goals of each remain distinct.

INITIAL SCREENING MEETING

The purpose of the screening meeting with a client is to ascertain the appropriateness of the referral, based on the standard criteria one is using for the group. Then, the therapist should conduct a trauma history in enough detail to obtain a sense of the client's major trauma schemas. If the client is unable to do the trauma inquiry, then the client is not yet a good candidate for trauma group therapy. The person may either begin or continue in individual therapy to explore and become more comfortable with his or her own trauma material. History of treatment, especially other group treatments, and information about a client's capacity to socialize are also important factors. In contrast to other models, trauma-centered group therapy is not contraindicated when the client is also attending individual therapy, especially if that too is trauma centered. The client who is accepted should be told that he or she will have to discuss his or her traumatic events in the first meeting of the group.

FIRST GROUP SESSION

In keeping with the principle of immediacy, a new member to a group with rolling admission is introduced and asked to talk in some detail about his or her traumatic events at the beginning of his or her first session. Major avoidances are addressed by the therapist, who inquires about details left out by the client. The aim is to provide the other group members with a relatively detailed overview of the client's traumatic events, as well as to establish the norm for direct trauma talk in the group. Immediately following this presentation, the group therapist asks all other group members to summarize their traumatic events and basic personal information. Thus, a new client's first session is completely taken up by a review of traumatic experience by the entire group. Again, avoidances and shortcuts by older members are noted and corrected by the therapist (and occasionally by other group members themselves). In groups in which members are beginning together, the first session (or two) consists of every group member speaking about his or her own traumatic experiences.

The therapist in group sessions, as in individual therapy, will continuously demonstrate personal engagement with the traumatic material and be tolerant of the expression of strong emotion. In the group environment, there is more leeway for therapists to accomplish this without undermining their professional role. Because members are required to speak to the group, discussion calls for an element of a presentational style, which allows for more spontaneous, active, and dynamic interactions among group members. Although the therapist will not condone any physical acting out or violence among group members, displays of emotion are not uncommon, and occasionally someone may have to leave the room for a time. The therapist should not demonstrate fear of these emotional expressions and whenever possible should even positively frame them as being in the service of the work or as serving to gain relief from the years of suppression.

The *structured group format* may follow any number of models existent in the literature. A common structure is a 5- to 10-minute mini-lecture on a preestablished or spontaneous topic related to trauma (often chosen based on the content of the previous session), followed by general discussion among group members, and then a 5-minute wrap-up by the therapist, who summarizes the session and points out links between members' experiences and the concepts presented. A marker board is often used to provide a context of impersonal distance and can be referred to when needed to diminish the intensity of the interpersonal interaction among members (Lubin and Johnson 2008).

The *unstructured group format* may begin spontaneously, or group members may decide to ask someone in the group to fill them in on what has been happening in his or her life, or a volunteer can be recruited to be on the hot seat to answer questions from the therapist and group members for all or part of a session.

The principle of immediacy is extremely important. New group members begin by talking about their trauma, and casual conversation at the beginning of the group session should be curtailed. All members should know that their work is to relate their own experience to what they are hearing from the member who is speaking. Important trauma-related topics should not be put off to the latter part of the group session.

FOLLOWING THROUGH WITH THE TECHNIQUES

In both time-limited and long-term groups, the therapist should continuously apply the trauma-centered techniques of getting the details, decoding current behavior, introducing discrepancy, and disclosing the perpetrator.

Getting the Details

Whenever a group member is discussing his or her trauma, the therapist should inquire about further details when the speaker uses stops, jumps, bumps, labels, or bridges. The therapist should do this each time the member mentions his or her trauma, even though the other members of the group already have heard these details. Repetition of the details provides ongoing exposure to group members. The therapist should be aware of any attempt by group members to establish a norm that "we have already heard that, so we can skip over it." New members can be a useful means of reinforcing the therapeutic norm because they have not heard the details, so members are asked to repeat them "for the new member's benefit." The therapist can also periodically ask the group as a whole whether they remember the details of a member's story. If anyone says that they do not remember (or there is a hesitation), this becomes a reason for the member to repeat them.

Over time, as the details of their traumatic experiences are repeated and become well known, the group members can be helped to identify the trauma schemas of other members, which are then made explicit by the therapist. Knowing these schemas will be helpful if group members are to assist the therapist in decoding other members' current behaviors. In this way, group members should become full participants in the trauma-centered tasks of the treatment. Once a core group of members have learned how to do this, the group will become a powerful therapeutic influence on each incoming client.

Decoding Current Behaviors

The major work of the group is in hearing other members discuss their daily lives and the issues that beset them in the present. A certain amount of advice giving and commonsense problem solving may occur during these discussions, as is typical in many forms of group therapy. However, when the therapist or group members sense the presence of a trauma schema that is influencing a member's behavior, then this should be identified and discussed. Group members should know that this is what they are supposed to do, largely by modeling themselves after the therapists' comments, as well as by direct instruction by the therapist. Decoding proceeds in the same manner as in individual therapy, only with multiple inputs from different people.

Introducing Discrepancy

Once the client is confronted with possible links between the current situation and his or her trauma, the therapist and/or group members can help the person separate the two situations. If the therapist is running a cognitive-behavioral group, specific formats and content may be used to accomplish this task (i.e., identifying faulty cognitions) (Resick and Schnicke 1993). The therapist can ask the group if anyone thinks that the member in question understands the difference between the past and the present. Often, someone will say no, and then that member can be instructed by the therapist to point it out to the member, thereby also stimulating member-member interaction. One technique available in group therapy is called *going around*. When an individual therapist points out the discrepancy between past and present to the client, the client may not believe him or her. In a group, however, having members one at a time point this out to the client becomes far more persuasive.

> CLIENT 1 (*after speaking some time about a situation in his work setting*): So I really don't know if I am in danger of being fired.
> THERAPIST: Given the humiliation you received at school when you were young, I can see why you are concerned about how your boss spoke to you.
> CLIENT 1: Right. You should have seen his eyes! What, you don't think I'm gonna get fired?
> THERAPIST: Not really. Your boss has always supported you. I think you are misreading him. Can I check this out with the group?
> CLIENT 2: I agree. You're nervous because of what happened at school.
> CLIENT 3: Remember, you even told us about how the main bully—uh, Bob?
> CLIENT 1: Robert.
> CLIENT 3: Robert looked at you. You said, "I remember his eyes."
> CLIENT 4: I think you can ask to talk to him. You have in the past.
> CLIENT 5: I don't hear any threat to your job.
> CLIENT 1: Yeah. I don't know. Thanks.

Going around is even more powerful when a trauma schema has been played out among group members.

> CLIENT 1 (*crying*): I feel so worthless. And I always do this, taking up space in the group. It cuts out time from everyone else.
> THERAPIST: Are you sure about that?
> CLIENT 1: Yes. I know people are just tolerating me here....They probably talk to each other between sessions about how selfish I am.
> THERAPIST: Let's go around the group and find out. I want you to ask each group member whether they feel you are selfish or are just tolerating you.
> CLIENT 1: I don't want to bother them.
> THERAPIST: Go ahead, ask.
> CLIENT 1: So don't you think I'm selfish?

CLIENT 2: No. I think you were really harmed by your mother, who said all these things to you even when you were what, 10?

CLIENT 1: Six.

CLIENT 2: Six. Terrible.

THERAPIST: Are you just tolerating her?

CLIENT 2: Not at all. I value your contributions to the group.

CLIENT 3: You offer so many insights. I really rely on you for help all the time.

THERAPIST: Ask again.

CLIENT 1: Am I a burden?

CLIENT 4: I really feel for you. You remind me of me last year....I felt so bad. I think of you as a gentle, good person.

Commentary such as this presents a strong challenge to the distorted ideas trauma victims have and, when combined with the authority of the therapist, helps to alter these schemas.

Disclosing the Perpetrator

Openly discussing the perpetrator is a component of trauma-centered group therapy, as it is of individual therapy. Ensuring that references to their traumatic events do not avoid mentioning the perpetrator—that is, maintaining the relational nature of the trauma schema—will be very helpful when members are triggered by each other and may project onto each other aspects of their perpetrators. Many interpersonal tensions in the group will be caused by displaced perpetrator dynamics. As a general rule, the therapist should try to have the perpetrator of each group member mentioned at least once in every group. This can be accomplished by a technique called the *roll* (Lubin and Johnson 2008). The therapist, while making a point concerning one group member, then goes on a *roll* through the rest of the group, pointing out similarities or differences and mentioning each member's perpetrator(s). The following is an example:

> So Paul, it is interesting—as you pointed out—how the memory of your father beating you was triggered by the police officer you yelled at, just like Susan's memory of her mother is evoked by her daughter, or Sam's uncle keeps coming up in his dreams, or Sharon's rapist seems always around the corner, or Vick's memory of Father Bernard keeps him from going to church.

Frequent and ample consideration of the members' various perpetrators not only will provide opportunities for continued processing of the memories and desensitization to triggers that remind them of their perpetrators, but also will help prevent unnecessary interpersonal tension and conflict.

THE GAP IN GROUP THERAPY

As the group members get to know one another and intimacy increases, group members will themselves be triggering each other. Incredible moments of group confrontation will arise, driven almost exclusively by the intersecting trauma schemas of group members. Given the potential volatility of these schemas, they may lead within a few seconds to harsh words being said, misunderstandings and accusations made, and a spoiling of the supportive group atmosphere. Members who appear to be friendly with each other may rapidly descend into threats or say critical or negative statements. These traumatic reenactments produce the conditions of the gap, in which the participants cannot differentiate between their traumatic pasts and the current group situation.

Attempting to manage these moments simply by asking people to calm down and perhaps apologize will usually fail, and at least be an abandonment of the trauma-centered effort. It is important to remember that these moments are inevitable if the group therapy is being effective in evoking and working through the trauma schemas. They become opportunities for additional healing and growth, all the more so because they are occurring not between the clients' past and life outside the group but between their past and what is happening in a real social grouping. This provides an important opportunity to address the distortions immediately with all parties involved. This is when the work can most effectively be done.

The therapist in such a situation should follow the same five steps detailed in Chapter 9, "The Gap: When the Trauma Schema Emerges in the Therapeutic Relationship": 1) restatement of the problem, 2) linking to the trauma, 3) acknowledgment of harm, 4) pointing out the discrepancy, and 5) recognizing the failure to prevent the traumatic event. The therapist should usually employ the going around technique to enhance the sense of discrepancy.

In the moment that the gap arises within one member, that person will be applying his or her trauma schema not only to self and perhaps to the member who triggered him or her (who becomes the perpetrator) but also to the entire group. Members who support the other person will be viewed as collaborators; the therapist or silent members who stay above the fray will become bystanders. The member in the gap becomes the victim: misunderstood, hurt, and fearful, and therefore justified in striking out. The member who has triggered the member in the gap will also feel victimized, which may lead him or her into the gap and to quickly view the first member as the perpetrator and other group members as collaborators or bystanders.

GERALD: Last week we were discussing whether we could move the group to Monday (*enraged*), and he (*pointing at Larry*) shot me down.

LARRY: What?

GERALD: Shut up. He (*looking at Larry*) treated me like I am nothing, and it makes me so angry because it's just like what my mother did to me my whole childhood, as if I was weak, nothing, shit.

THERAPIST: What comment are you referring to, Gerald?

GERALD: He said, "People like you can meet anytime because you have nothing better to do."

LARRY: I was joking. My God, are you sensitive or what?

GERALD: You see, you do think I'm a ninny.

LARRY: I didn't say "ninny." Where did that come from?

GERALD: Stop shouting at me!

LARRY: I'm not shouting. I just talk loud.

GERALD (*to therapist*): I feel like punching him out.

THERAPIST: So you thought that Larry was putting you down, as having nothing better to do, discounting you?

GERALD: Totally!

LARRY: But…

THERAPIST: One minute, Larry. (*To Gerald.*) I can understand how much that must have upset you, because it is like what your mother did so brutally your whole childhood—calling you weak, nothing, ignoring you—and it caused you so much pain, so much hurt.

GERALD: It did.

THERAPIST: But in this case, I believe you misunderstood Larry, because he said it in a humorous way, and he included himself as someone who is also retired, and not as a way of putting you down, unlike your mother.

GERALD: Really, I didn't hear him include himself. I was so mad.

LARRY: Yes I did. We are both retired, not like these other fellows.

THERAPIST: Are you sure of what I am saying, Gerald?

GERALD: Not so sure.

THERAPIST: So let's go around the group and find out. Ask each member how he took Larry's comment. (*Each confirms having understood Larry's comment as a playful and harmless one.*)

GERALD: Thanks. I really took it another way. Like I'm irrelevant.

THERAPIST: You may have felt irrelevant to your mother, but I don't think you are irrelevant to the group. Why don't you ask them, the group? Yes, ask somebody whether you are irrelevant to the group.

GERALD (*to a member*): So what do you think, do I contribute much here?

ROBERT: Absolutely. You are very active. You're smart.

CARLOS: I listen to your opinions. You are not irrelevant at all. (*Others say similar things.*)

THERAPIST: How your mother treated you was horrible and very damaging to you. I only wish I could have been there to shut her up, but I wasn't. (*Gerald looks over at the therapist.*) I'll bet you wondered why I didn't tell Larry to shut up last week.

GERALD: Yes, I did!

THERAPIST: I guess I was like your father, who just stood by and let your mother put you down.

GERALD: I hadn't figured that out, but now that you point it out, yeah! I wondered if you felt the same thing.

THERAPIST: I don't, but the question is: what did your father think?

GERALD: Well…(*He begins telling the group more about his father, and the group continues.*)

This example illustrates the combined effort of a therapist and group members to help an upset member become aware of an important trauma schema. The same protocol as that used in individual therapy is applied, only with the added benefit of input from a variety of other people, which simultaneously takes the single focus off the therapist and strengthens the impact on the client. Members' diverse feedback disrupts the all-or-nothing schema of the member in the gap, thereby encouraging a more differentiated understanding of what occurred.

DISSOCIATIVE REACTIONS IN THE GROUP SESSION

Another challenging situation is when group members dissociate during the course of a group session. Rather than applying their trauma schema onto the group, these members, when triggered, protect themselves by dissociating, examples of which include appearing to fall asleep, curling up in their chair, staring unresponsively into space, moaning or singing, appearing to faint onto the floor, having a pseudoseizure, or revealing an alternate personality.

These behaviors are disturbing enough in individual therapy, where even experienced therapists have difficulty maintaining a calm, focused response. In a group setting, these reactions—especially when they occur with inadequate warning—will be very upsetting to other group members and may evoke strong efforts to do something such as hold or talk to the dissociating group member. Common feelings among group members are fear over the lack of safety in the group therapy and distress over the inability of the therapist to bring the client back to reality. Therapists can likewise derail the group and demonstrate their own inadequacy by interrupting the flow of the group (thereby abandoning the current speaker) and attempting to bring the client back by various techniques, or worse, calling 911 and stopping the group entirely.

The therapist should inform the group members at the outset (either in their screening session or collectively when the group begins) that these traumatic reenactments and dissociative reactions may occur, and reassure members that these are defensive maneuvers of the client to feel less distressed.

The therapist should tell members that the dissociative state will be temporary and that the group will continue unless the behavior is loud or disruptive.

Once the dissociative reaction has begun, the therapist may choose to speak to the client, attempting to decode the behavior in terms of what is known about his or her trauma. Sometimes, this will help the client return, but even when it does not, it demonstrates to group members that the therapist understands what is going on and has remained in control. This is usually reassuring to group members. Witnessing another member dissociate becomes an opportunity to educate members about trauma and can significantly deepen their commitment to the group work.

In a women's trauma group, after an intense exchange between two members over their relationship, another member, Helen, became pale, closed her eyes, and began to rock in her chair, mumbling to herself. The other group members immediately noticed.

> CLIENT 1: Helen, what's wrong? (*Helen rocks harder.*)
>
> THERAPIST: Helen is having a dissociative reaction now. She is protecting herself. Something probably triggered her memories of her own abuse.
>
> CLIENT 2: (*One of the previous speakers.*) I feel bad. I think my arguing with Pam must have set her off.
>
> CLIENT 3: Yeah. We shouldn't have been arguing like that.
>
> THERAPIST: No, I disagree. The purpose of this group is for all of you to be able to work things out, no matter how distressing. It is just that sometimes this will trigger other members' memories. (*Helen quiets down a bit.*) Did you notice that when I said that just now, Helen quieted down? (*Members nod.*) If you remember, Helen's main trauma was the domestic violence between her father and mother. I wonder if your arguing may have reminded her of her parents' fighting, and she remembered when that led to violence in the home and against her. (*Helen stops rocking.*)
>
> CLIENT 1: Yeah. Helen has told us many times how scared she was. She was young, even 2 or 3 when it began.
>
> CLIENT 2: So what do we do now?
>
> THERAPIST: Helen is protecting herself. She will stop dissociating at some point and return to us, and we can talk to her then about what triggered her and how your argument is different from that of her parents. Why don't we get back into the issue between you two, because I think there is more we can do to understand what is going on. Okay? (*Members agree.*) To start with, did you feel badly that your argument with Pam might have set Helen off?
>
> CLIENT 2: Yeah.

THERAPIST: Does that connect with anything you felt when you were being physically abused by your mother?

CLIENT 2: Well, yes, I really feel bad that my younger sister sometimes got hit after I got into it with my mom…

EXAMPLE OF TRAUMA-CENTERED GROUP PROCESS

The group in the following case example has been meeting continuously for several years. It consists of a core group of four women who have been in the group for over 2 years and three women who have joined in the past 2 years. They range in age from 29 to 52, and all have been traumatized, by childhood maltreatment, sexual assault as teenagers and adults, domestic violence, loss of an infant child, or work-related accident.

THERAPIST: Good afternoon. (*Goes to board and writes, "What is love?" Silence, followed by moans and giggles from group.*) [introducing mini-lecture]

KENDRA: Good question.

FRAN: You expect us to answer that?

JOSIE: I think she does.

THERAPIST: Let's put down some possibilities here.

PAULA: Friendship.

FRAN: Sex.

JOSIE: Understanding each other.

DEBBIE: Caring about the other person.

KENDRA: Willing to sacrifice yourself for another.

BETH: Being one with each other.

PAULA: Warmth in the heart.

THERAPIST: Gia?

GIA: A lie. A trick in order to get something.

THERAPIST: Alright. Who has told you, "I love you"? [highlighting the relational]

PAULA: My mother.

BETH: I can't remember anyone.

KENDRA: My husband, after he beat me.

GIA: Right.

DEBBIE: My father, before he abused me.

THERAPIST: This is not going in the right direction! Surely "love is all you need!" (*Silence.*) Complicated, isn't this?

GIA: I don't know what love is, or if it is ever possible, because my family used it as a way of controlling me, and I have always associated love with being hurt.

THERAPIST: Say more.

GIA: (*Tells group more details about her controlling father, domestic violence in the home.*)

DEBBIE: That must have been confusing.

GIA: I'll say. Whenever I get a warm feeling inside, I become anxious, worried that something bad will happen.

THERAPIST: Something bad did happen. Does that mean it will happen again? [identifying a trauma schema]

GIA: I don't know.

THERAPIST: Is there anyone in this group you feel close to, have had warm feelings toward?

GIA: Yes, most everyone. Beth.

THERAPIST: Ask her how she feels about you. [going around]

GIA: Beth, what kind of feelings do you have about me?

BETH: I have loving feelings for you. I feel so sad that you had to go through what you did. I can see how love and fear got mixed up, and how that has to get in the way of becoming intimate with anyone now.

KENDRA: Yeah, like me, Gia has never married or hooked up with anyone for long.

BETH: But I really like you, Gia. I think you are an awesome person.

THERAPIST: (*To Beth.*) Beth, do you see the look on Gia's face?

BETH: Yes.

THERAPIST: What do you think she feels, listening to what you said?

BETH: I don't know. How did you take what I said, Gia?

GIA: The words sound good, but I suddenly feel nauseous. I don't mean to offend you.

BETH: No, no, I know.

THERAPIST: Let's assume the nausea is a real feeling. And let's assume it's not about Beth. What does the nausea remind you of, Gia? [identifying a bump]

GIA: We were having dinner, and my father demanded that my mother pass him the butter, and she hesitated too long, so he took his fork and stabbed it into her hand. She went running upstairs to her bedroom, there was blood all over, and I ran to the bathroom and threw up.

PAULA: Where was the love?

GIA: I had just said grace, and thanked God for loving us.

JOSIE: That's sad. Gia, you did not deserve that. (*Gia cries.*)

FRAN: I agree.

THERAPIST: When abuse or violence occurs within a family, it's common for feelings of intimacy to become mixed in with fear, anger, and betrayal. Beyond the physical effects of sexual abuse or violence, this is one of the major injuries that occurs, and it can impact a person's life for a lifetime if unaddressed. Thinking about it, almost all of you have had similar experiences where someone who said they loved you, or who did love you, harmed you terribly. I am thinking of your mother, Debbie; or your husband, Josie; or your father, Fran. [roll]

FRAN: My father…

THERAPIST: Remind us of his name? [mentioning the perpetrator]

FRAN: Frank. I was named after him…promised me the world, bought things for me, and then, you recall, when I became a teenager, he'd get sloshed and take me out driving in the car and unload all his miseries and complaints about my mother.

BETH: Wasn't there one time he fell asleep on you in the car?

FRAN: Yeah, good memory. For the new members, you probably don't know, but one time he parked the car in a Home Depot parking lot, maybe 11 P.M., and we sat there for an hour as he moaned about his pitiful life.

PAULA: How old were you?

FRAN: Only 14, so I couldn't drive the car or anything. I couldn't wake him up either, so we sat there until 1:00 A.M., when he finally woke up.

JOSIE: Where was your mom?

FRAN: At home, watching TV.

KENDRA: Watching TV? What did she think you and your dad were doing?

FRAN: I don't really know. Later she told me that she was glad he spent time with me because then he got off her case.

PAULA: That's like sacrificing your kid. Did he ever touch you?

FRAN: No…He groped me a few times. Mostly he was drunk and just said I was his beautiful daughter, the light of his life, his love.

KENDRA: Sick. (*Fran looks upset.*)

THERAPIST: Kendra, did you see what came over Fran's face? [noticing a bump]

KENDRA: No, uh, yes. What? Are you upset, Fran? Did I insult you, your father?

FRAN: It's just that he's the only one who ever said those things to me. I guess part of me wanted to hear them, liked what he said, even if he was drunk and with me instead of my mother.

THERAPIST: So that was Frank, your father. What he did was not appropriate. How has Frank shown up in your more recent relationships? [decoding]

FRAN: Oh, boy. All of them, really. Last one was this man—I think I told you guys about it a couple of weeks ago—real nice at first, met him at AA, sober a couple of years. We began dating, and I really liked him until he started coming on to me, and I sort of told him to back off, and he took offense and switched on me, becoming very critical, like my dad was of my mother. The whole thing made me sick, and I switched AA groups to get away from him.

JOSIE: What about that other guy you met at Thanksgiving?

FRAN: He was too nice. (*Others laugh.*) Yeah, if they are too nice, I have this thought that they don't really care about me.

BETH: I know what you mean: someone who might really treat me well is obviously just pretending.

THERAPIST: What do you mean, Beth?

BETH: When I have a really normal, nice conversation with someone, it doesn't seem real.

JOSIE: Do you think that's because down deep some of us don't think we deserve to be treated well?

BETH: Maybe. I know I don't.

THERAPIST: What's it mean to be treated well? Anyone.

PAULA: Like we do in here. We listen. Everyone gets to talk about what's on her mind. We get a lot of support here.

THERAPIST: Then why don't you or any of you feel that it's fake or unreal? (*Pause.*)

DEBBIE: Because it's not about the surface stuff. We talk straight, the hard parts, we argue, it's a mess in here (*others laugh*), not all prettied up and nice, that's what feels unreal.

THERAPIST: I hear what you are saying. But Debbie, you know what a mess is!

DEBBIE: (*Pause.*) Yes, I do.

FRAN: What do you mean? I'm sorry, but I don't remember if you've talked about that since I came to the group.

DEBBIE: My mom...

THERAPIST: Remind us of her name. [mentioning perpetrator]

DEBBIE: Eleanor, such an elegant name, was a heroin addict, and I grew up with her going from one tenement to another, or friends' or junkies' homes, while she tried to get her next fix. Most of the time I was left behind in a filthy, messy apartment, with almost nothing to eat.

KENDRA: Did she say she loved you, too?

DEBBIE: No, actually, she told me I was trash, worthless, and that I was only a burden to her....She abandoned me when I was 8, and that's when the state took me.

JOSIE: No confusion there, right?

DEBBIE: Guess not, though she sends me letters for Christmas each year and writes "I love you" on the card, which I find really odd and I suppose confusing.

BETH: What do you tell yourself?

DEBBIE: I say that it was because she was an addict and that covered up her real feelings for me.

PAULA: But...

DEBBIE: But I don't remember any expression of love or kindness from her for the 8 years I lived with her, so, got me!

THERAPIST: Eleanor. [mentioning perpetrator]

DEBBIE: Eleanor. (*Begins to cry.*)

PAULA: (*Reaches for some tissues and stands up to give one to Debbie.*)

THERAPIST: Paula, in addition to a tissue, perhaps Debbie might benefit from being asked why she is crying. [supporting emotionality]

PAULA: Oh, is that okay? (*Members nod.*) Debbie, what's on your mind?

DEBBIE: Eleanor, or Ellie, was the name of my daughter who died last year of cancer. (*Silence. Two other women begin to cry.*)

PAULA: Oh my God. You named her after your mother?

DEBBIE: (*Nods.*)

(*Silence.*)

THERAPIST: Debbie, did you love your daughter? [emotionality]

DEBBIE: Yes, yes! (*Crying very hard.*)

THERAPIST: Then you know what love is, real love?

DEBBIE: Yes, I do.

THERAPIST: How about other members of the group: have you discovered what real love is in your current life, despite what happened in your pasts? In fact, let's go around on this one. How about you, Josie? [going around, introducing discrepancy]

JOSIE: I love my son. He's 2 now. I feel our relationship is pure, separates me from my father.

BETH: I have my cats; that's real love for me.

KENDRA: I think I have found it with my mother now. It's weird, since we were not close when I was growing up, given everything that was going on, but she has really been there for me this year during my divorce, and we go out for coffee and have a good time. She looks at me lovingly; it's good.

FRAN: I don't have anyone, but I feel loved in here, from each of you. I have never had that feeling. That's why the group has been good for me. I hope it will give me strength to find someone in my outside life to love.

PAULA: My husband. He loves me.

GIA: I don't have anyone who I feel really loves me. I know I have high standards. I just don't feel comfortable yet letting anyone in, anyone close.

THERAPIST: Thank you. (*Stands and goes to the board.*) So what is love? The answer is that it's complicated. Intimacy brings with it conflict, and many traumatic events occur with intimates, which lead to confusion. And they were the ones who said they loved you then. But we also got into the question, maybe the more important question, of who loves you now. And finding a way, the courage, to open yourselves up to another person, knowing that it involves a risk, so you can create a loving relationship now, despite what happened to you, is the path toward healing. And I think each of you did a great job today providing more details about what happened, and about the people who caused you harm, and how you are thinking about them. See you next week.

In this group session, the therapist began with a short exercise that led quickly into a general discussion and then individual contributions from several group members. Using techniques such as the roll and going around, the therapist entered the discussion when necessary to encourage further revealing of details, decoding of behaviors, pointing out of discrepancies between the present and past relationships, and naming of perpetrators. The group members worked collaboratively to identify similarities and differences in their thoughts and experiences. This group has incorporated the therapeutic norms of a trauma-centered group process. Groups such as this one can be very effective agents of change, healing, and ongoing support for traumatized clients.

STUDY QUESTIONS

14.1 When should the client be referred to trauma-centered group therapy?

14.2 T/F The group setting itself might trigger clients who were traumatized in group environments.

14.3 T/F Clients are not likely to be triggered by the stories of other group members.

14.4 T/F It is possible to conduct trauma-centered therapy in structured or unstructured groups, and in time-limited and open-ended groups.

14.5 T/F Each group member should describe his or her major traumatic events in their first group meeting.

14.6 T/F Groups provide greater opportunities for introducing discrepancy, because each group member can share his or her own unique experience that will vary from the client's.

14.7 T/F It is not necessary to inform the group members in the beginning about possible dissociative reactions and how they will be dealt with.

CHAPTER 15

Trauma-Centered Couples and Family Psychotherapy

The application of trauma-centered psychotherapy in couples and family therapy can be a very powerful intervention in the lives of trauma victims. Because trauma schemas are relational (axiom 4), the effects of prior trauma permeate the victim's social relationships, especially with intimates such as spouse and family. Because of the frequency of contact among members of a family, habitual patterns of behavior become established and reinforced, and thus trauma schemas in one individual can alter the communication patterns of an entire family, without any recognition of their source.

In this chapter, we describe how trauma-centered psychotherapy can be applied in couples and family contexts. The challenge we face in this discussion is the degree of variation among important factors in these contexts: which person or persons have been traumatized, the family constellation, and the method of family therapy being employed. The trauma-centered approach can be used in any of these contexts. The reader is referred to a number of excellent sources for specific models of family and couples trauma treatment (Figley 1989; Johnson 2002; Johnson et al. 1995; Monson and Fredman 2012).

Trauma-centered family psychotherapy should be conducted by a clinician who is well trained and experienced in couples and/or family therapy. A clinician may employ any of a variety of useful methods of family therapy, such as transgenerational, structural, strategic, systemic, and narrative approaches, among others (Goldenberg and Goldenberg 2000). Trauma-centered psychotherapy can be used with any of these methods, either as part of the family therapy from the beginning or for a temporary period of time within an ongoing family therapy. Most families have problems that extend well beyond the trauma of its individuals. In some settings (usually institutional settings), more than one therapist can be present, which allows for more opportunities to work with the family and its subparts. However, this chapter is written with the assumption that one clinician is conducting the family therapy.

VARIATIONS IN TRAUMATIC EXPERIENCE WITHIN FAMILIES

Perhaps the most common arrangement seen in family therapy is when one family member has been traumatized, either recently (e.g., a teenage daughter having been raped in school) or in the past (e.g., a mother who was severely maltreated as a child, a father who served in Vietnam). This arrangement is common in foster or adoptive families, where a child was abused in his or her biological home. A second common arrangement is when the entire family was traumatized by the same event (e.g., the sudden death of another family member, a motor vehicle accident that they all experienced, a house fire). A third arrangement is when multiple family members have been traumatized but by entirely different traumas.

An important question is whether these traumas have been revealed or not. In some cases, one version of the traumatic event, but not the entire story, has been revealed or is known by other family members. In other cases, the parents and the traumatized child may know, but the siblings have been kept in the dark. In some families, these secrets may be due to avoidance, whereas in other families, the secrets are maintained by forceful strictures against telling, based on either religious, moral, or personal grounds. In most of these cases, the complete story has probably not been revealed (axiom 3).

VARIATIONS IN THE FAMILY CONSTELLATION

Significant variations exist in the family constellation that may present to the family therapist. All relevant family members may be adults (e.g., elderly parents with adult children), or any combination of adults and children can be present. The ages of the children are relevant for inclusion: Children younger than 6 years generally are not appropriate for trauma-based family therapy unless a child that young is the victim. Latency-age children (ages

6–12) may be appropriate for inclusion in family therapy sessions, depending on each child's personality and behavior (e.g., some children this age will not be able to concentrate on the discussion). Generally, teenagers (ages 13 and older) will be expected to participate. Every family is different, of course, and aunts, uncles, grandparents, boyfriends and girlfriends may all be appropriate participants.

Attendees at family therapy sessions should generally include everyone 1) who is willing, 2) who may be affected by the trauma, 3) who has been involved in the family conflict, and 4) who can behave appropriately in the meeting. Obviously, the clinician will have to decide on attendees based on many unique factors in each case. There is often quite a bit of change in who attends sessions on any given day or over time, because various family members may have schedule conflicts or the therapy needs might change. For example, what begins as couples therapy may soon transform to family therapy, with either children or parents brought in, or family therapy may devolve into couples therapy.

RECURSIVE NATURE OF POWER DYNAMICS IN FAMILIES

Many common denominators in group dynamics exist in families despite the broad range of variations. Families, even healthy families, are an intense tangle of intimate and conflicting power dynamics (Goldenberg and Goldenberg 2000). Because so much is at stake and because the family members spend so much time together and know one another's behavioral patterns so well, communication among them occurs on multiple levels simultaneously. Each member is deeply aware of the strengths and weaknesses of the other members. *Familiarity breeds contempt* because being in close proximity allows each person to see how everyone else is behaving based on his or her own self-interest. It should come as no surprise that human beings act in their own self-interest. Much of the time, cooperative and altruistic behaviors coincide with the self-interest of the individual. However, in most families, traumatized or not, members can recognize the difference between the overt behavior and the underlying motivations of the others, based on previous experiences: when a child happily does his chores, the others suspect he is planning to ask for something; when a husband brings a big bouquet of roses to his wife, she believes he is trying to make up for his many business trips; when a child cries, other family members view it as "crocodile tears" and assume that the child is manipulating to get something. Because of the recursive nature of family interactions, each person's behavior is understood by its perceived motivation, and the responses of the others in the family to this behavior are also known and interpreted, and the responses to this interpretation by the others are also well known. This cascade of interpretations descends to a version of the core question "Do you love me?" Unfortunately, for many, the answer to that question is "Not quite enough." Most of the time, the family members conduct their interactions on the surface of this onionlike structure. The rules governing these interactions are maintained by the power dynamics of the family system and those authorized with power. In general, those in power want the family to operate smoothly and therefore will attempt to compartmentalize problematic areas. Secrets will be maintained. Differences will be minimized. Sadly, these family secrets are usually known by everyone; the meaning of being labeled a secret is most often that one is not supposed to talk about it.

In family therapy, however, family members will have the time and the purpose to revisit the underlayers of their interactions. This is why family therapy in general can be experienced as a threat to the established authority structure of the family, and well-trained family therapists know how important it is to identify those family members who hold the power and to negotiate with them as the family therapy proceeds. Otherwise, these gatekeepers will prevent the family from returning to future sessions.

THE SITUATION IN TRAUMATIZED FAMILIES

With the presence of trauma among one or more family members, the family dynamics often become fraught with even more tension. The fear or shame (axiom 1) contained within the traumatized member will be sensed by all members. The need for avoidance (axiom 2) of this fear or shame is likely to permeate family interactions. Even when the traumatic event is public and known, over time the family will discuss it less and less, yet the effects of the family's avoidance will continue and subtly shape aspects of the interaction of family members, as they circumvent the shadow of the trauma in the room. Strong forces toward compartmentalizing the traumatic experience may be brought to bear. Minimization of its impact may be repeatedly applied. The result is that many aspects of the trauma may remain incompletely known (axiom 3), even though family members think that they know about it.

Over time, the trauma schema held by each traumatized member will enter the recursive communication structure of the family, as repeatedly the member responds to others' behaviors according to his or her schemas (axiom 4). The others in turn will respond to the member's behavior, shaping their responses unintentionally along the lines of the member's perpetrator.

This interaction may occur on the surface or farther down in the underlayers. Wherever it lies, when the family members interact from that place, the presence of the trauma schema will be reenacted within the family. Other family members will be treated as if they were the member's perpetrator, bystander, or collaborator. These family members, in their outrage at being misunderstood, will act in ways that indeed mirror the roles of perpetrator, bystander, or collaborator. All of this will take place without any awareness of the original traumatic event. Because this process is one of mutual invalidation (e.g., "You are helping me only because you plan to ask me for something later," "You are crying only to get sympathy from me") based on the awareness of the others' self-interest, the victim member will feel that his or her traumatic experience is being ignored or belittled. Later, in family therapy, when the victim does disclose more details of his or her trauma, some family members may actually invalidate these disclosures as manipulation. Figure 15–1 illustrates the situation in traumatized families before treatment.

For the effects of a family member's trauma to be disclosed and effectively processed, the family members in power will need to loosen their grip on the compartmentalization within the family. This is likely to open up other areas of conflict within the family not directly related to the one member's trauma, such as marital conflict. Because the trauma schemas have become integrated into the larger family dynamic, the therapist may be confronted with a mixture of current and past issues that may overwhelm the family. The family therapist needs to be aware of this challenge in order to help those in power tolerate but also contain the problems that will emerge.

Because a family's communication patterns have adapted so deeply to the trauma schemas of its members, changing them will be extremely difficult. In group therapy, the members' trauma schemas are also projected or displaced into the group interaction, but because group members are relative strangers to one another, they are less entangled with one another and are more likely to be able to provide discrepant information to the member. In family or couples therapy, the members will have a more difficult time differentiating the traumatic root of the behaviors from their perceptions of the member's personality. Likewise, it will be difficult for the traumatized member to believe that the other family members have acted against him or her as an unintended replay of the trauma rather than acting as who they really are. After all, they were not even traumatized. Through the displacements of the trauma schema into the family interactions, great harm has been done to the entire family: the arguments, misunderstandings, yelling, and slamming of doors have actually occurred, often many years after the neglect, abuse, rape, or combat originally altered the individual. After so much has taken place, how is the therapist to persuade the family that they

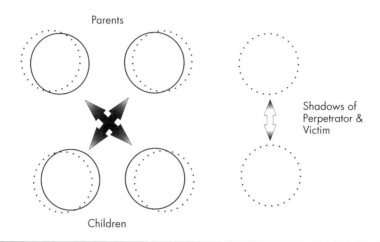

FIGURE 15–1. The situation of the family before treatment.

Family conflicts are infiltrated by the trauma schemas.

are not to blame for all of these bad behaviors and that only the original perpetrator is responsible? To this daunting task, we now turn.

SETTING UP THE TRAUMA-CENTERED FRAME

As in individual and group therapy, establishing the trauma-centered frame
is the first step in family or couples therapy. If the family or couple states at
the beginning of treatment that they are there because of a trauma that one
of them has experienced, then establishing this frame is more straightforward. Often, however, this is not the case. The therapist can choose to conduct a brief trauma inquiry on each participant as part of the first meeting,
which is recommended as standard practice, and if trauma has occurred, the
therapist can then proceed to set the frame. Otherwise, if a traumatic experience of a member is revealed in the course of couples or family therapy, then
the therapist can decide whether or not to proceed with a trauma-centered
approach.

Establishing the frame with the family requires that the therapist tell the
members 1) that for the next period of time, the family therapy will focus on
the impact of the trauma on the family's or couple's current problems; 2) that
they will be discussing the details of the trauma; and 3) that this will be uncomfortable and that at times members may think that the trauma is not relevant or that other problems have come up that need to be discussed first, but
that it will be important to continue to focus on the trauma until a full un-

derstanding of how it plays itself out in the family interaction is obtained. These points should be said explicitly, and agreement from all parties should be obtained. The therapist will be reminding the family members of this discussion whenever they balk at further exploration of the trauma.

GOALS OF TRAUMA-CENTERED COUPLES AND FAMILY PSYCHOTHERAPY

In this section, we discuss the four goals of trauma-centered couples and family psychotherapy. The goals are briefly described in Table 15–1. Regardless of what method of family therapy the clinician is employing, these four goals can serve as the foundation for the trauma-centered couples or family psychotherapy.

Identify and Share the Specific Traumas

For trauma-centered family therapy to proceed, everyone should know which traumatic events have occurred. There are many ways this information may be gathered. One or more of the family members may be in individual therapy, with either the therapist or another clinician. This therapy may or may not be trauma centered. Some family members may not have been told about the trauma. Once trauma-centered family therapy has been initiated, the relevant traumatic events should be shared with the entire family or couple during the first session (principle of immediacy). It is usually a good idea for the therapist to conduct a trauma inquiry of each person in the family, either by asking the family if there are any other traumatic events that anyone thinks could be impacting the family or, more comprehensively, by meeting alone with each member of the family and asking him or her. These meetings can be brief enough to get the basic information and to decide whether these traumatic events should be subjects of the treatment. What is important is to have all of the relevant traumas revealed to all members of the family in treatment, at the beginning of treatment.

Share the Details of Each Trauma With the Family

The family or couple should be told that the goal of the treatment is for them to share the details of their traumatic events with the other parties. There are several challenges to this goal. First, the other family members are likely to think that they already know the details of the trauma, but more likely they do not, because rarely has the victim member gone into the minute but important details. Second, if there are children in the family ses-

---

TABLE 15–1.   Goals of trauma-centered couples and family
                psychotherapy

Identify and share the specific traumas

It is important that each person's traumas are openly shared among family members. The family therapist addresses the intricate means by which avoidance of this task has been maintained in the family.

Share the details of each trauma with the family

The therapist aims to have some of the most upsetting details of the traumatic events shared among family members so they can be reminded of how deeply the person was affected.

Learn how the trauma schemas are affecting current behaviors

The therapist points out the similarities between problematic behaviors in the present and aspects of the family member's traumatic experience, highlighting the impact of trauma schemas on current family interactions.

Collectivize family members' relationship with the trauma

The therapist aims to transform the family from blaming each other for their current problems toward viewing themselves as a group that has been harmed by their members' traumatic experiences, requiring a collective commitment to working with one another against the trauma's pernicious influence.

---

sions, the parents may have a strong wish to euphemize, minimize, or shape the information. Unfortunately, successful trauma-centered family therapy is not built out of euphemisms. The clinician will have to decide (with the parents) whether the children can hear the details. If not, then they should be excluded from the treatment sessions. Third, family members, including the victim member, will challenge the need to go into the details. The therapist will need to explain the rationale for this goal. One way of doing this is to explain that 1) an injury to one member of the family or couple is an injury to the whole; 2) the injury has affected everyone; 3) as a result, the perpetrator has become a member of the family; and 4) knowing the details of what the perpetrator has done will help the family, as a whole, fight back.

Learn How the Trauma Schemas Are Affecting Current Behaviors

A large part of the therapy will consist of decoding current behaviors in the family as reenactments of the trauma schemas. This process is significantly easier when the traumatic events are recent rather than remote, because then family members are more likely to appreciate the impact of the trauma. The clinician is faced with the challenge of convincing the family members that what they have viewed as bad habits of one another are in fact driven, at least in part, by trauma schemas built out of events long ago. The challenge for the therapist will be to help them perceive these behaviors differently, through the process of introducing discrepancy between past and present. The deep and multilayered adaptations of the family members over years will make establishing this sense of discrepancy difficult. However, persistent and detailed decoding can surprise the family and ultimately open the members to the possibility that the trauma is currently active.

Collectivize Family Members' Relationship With the Trauma

In the beginning of treatment, family members often view themselves as the caring supporters of the victim member, within whom lies the memory of the regrettable trauma. Generally, everyone views the trauma as being within the victim and therefore possessed by the victim. The goal of trauma-centered treatment is to shift this perception, so that the victim is viewed as being a member of the family, in which all members have been injured by the perpetrator, who is located outside the family. To accomplish this task, 1) the victim has to share the details of the trauma so that everyone has intimate knowledge of the event; 2) the family needs to realize that everyone in the family has been injured by the event, which requires that the perpetrator be brought into the family interaction so that the traumatic event is shared among the family; and 3) collectively the family needs to expel the perpetrator. Figure 15–2 illustrates the goal of family treatment: to extract the perpetrator-victim schema from the family interactions.

SPECIFIC TECHNIQUES OF TRAUMA-CENTERED COUPLES AND FAMILY PSYCHOTHERAPY

In this section we present four techniques used in trauma-centered couples and family psychotherapy. These techniques are briefly summarized in Table 15–2.

Being Active and Maintaining Control

Although the principle of being active and maintaining control is well supported by most schools of family therapy, it is especially true for trauma-centered family therapy (Goldenberg and Goldenberg 2000). The family or couples therapist should not ease back and allow the family to interact on their own, for within minutes they will descend into their familiar habitual pattern of interaction. They then will feel that the therapist is too

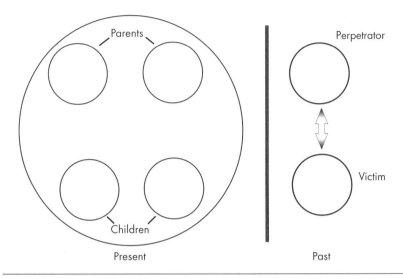

FIGURE 15–2. The situation of the family after treatment.

Trauma schemas have been extracted from the family interactions.

weak to impact the family (i.e., the other members of the family that each member wants changed), and they will become hopeless. They then will blame the therapist for this hopelessness. In the traumatized family, the therapist will quickly be viewed as a disinterested bystander who will be of no help to them. The principle of engagement requires that the family therapist be active, strong, and engaged in the discussion. It is also important for the family therapist to stay in control of the discussion. Family members will interrupt one another as a means of controlling or shutting down or managing the level of stress in the meeting. As one member begins his or her oft-repeated point, the others may be quick to point out his or her real motivation or contrary facts in order to invalidate what is said. The family therapist should not let that happen, and therefore needs to indicate from the beginning that he or she will allow each person to have his or her turn and to speak without being interrupted. The therapist will often have to tell other group members, "One moment—you will have your turn" or even just put out a hand to indicate that they are not to speak yet.

Meeting With Individuals

In family therapy, the clinician generally does not want to meet separately with individual members, because they tend to share details and then try to

---

TABLE 15–2.   Specific techniques of trauma-centered couples and
family psychotherapy

Being active and maintaining control

The therapist needs to direct the sessions and remain in control of the
interactions to prevent the couple or family from descending into well-worn
patterns of conflict.

Meeting with individuals

Unlike in typical family therapy, the therapist at times may need to meet alone
with one or two family members, especially when it is important to hear specific
details about traumatic events that the family members have yet to agree to
reveal. When the family reconvenes, the therapist places gentle pressure on the
individual to share with the whole family what he or she talked about privately.

Using circular questioning

The therapist asks family members questions that they do not have the authority
to answer, in order to dislodge well-established patterns of communication and
control in the family, and to unearth family dynamics more efficiently.

Using third-party questioning

In this variant of circular questioning, the therapist conducts a conversation
about a family member, in his or her presence, with another family member.
The purpose is to help family members tolerate the feelings and perspectives of
one another without interfering or suppressing them, and to elicit corrective
information from the traumatized family member when the conversation
inaccurately characterizes the traumatic event.

---

swear the therapist to secrecy. The other members then develop concerns
that the therapist is in collaboration with someone else, and soon the therapist's neutrality is severely compromised. There are times in trauma-
centered psychotherapy, however, when this good advice can be abrogated
because of the more important need for the details of the trauma to be
known. Thus, when the clinician senses that individual members do have
information about their traumas that they are reluctant to share, spending
some individual time with them during the family session (i.e., having the
family wait in the waiting room or another room while the clinician meets
with the individual for 10–20 minutes) may be indicated. After the clinician
and individual have talked, the family returns and the family session proceeds. In this case, prior to the individual meeting, the clinician makes it
clear that whatever the individual shares about his or her trauma should be
shared with the whole family. In the individual meeting, the clinician sets
an expectation that what is discussed will be shared, and then in the family
meeting, the clinician asks the individual to share that information. The clinician does not out the information himself or herself. Sometimes, partic-

ularly with children, the individual might ask the clinician to tell the rest of the family what he or she had said, and in most cases this is fine. The goal is to get the information out to the whole family and to support a new norm of openness within the family. If the individual declines to share the information, then the clinician will engage the other family members in wondering why the individual does not want to share it. This scenario occurs when the victim member is so frightened of telling the details to the family that he or she needs the engagement of the therapist to facilitate the process (principle of engagement).

Using Circular Questioning

Although circular questioning was developed in strategic and systemic family therapy (Selvini Palazzoli et al. 1978), its application in trauma-centered psychotherapy is extremely helpful. There are a variety of definitions of circular questioning, but it is best understood in comparison to direct questioning. In *direct questioning*, the therapist asks a person about a topic that the person has the authority to answer (e.g., "What is your favorite color?" "Do you love your wife?" "How do you feel about what your son just said?" "Were you sexually abused by your uncle?"). The problem with direct questioning in family therapy is that people often respond according to what is in their best interests, which may not be either completely truthful or may be in anticipation of the response from another family member. For instance, when a husband is asked, "Do you love your wife?" and he replies, "Oh yes, of course!" while his body retracts and he turns his eyes away from her, neither his wife nor the therapist may completely believe him. However, he has the authority to answer that question, so if the therapist were to explore this matter further, he or she might appear to be questioning the husband's authority. Most therapists will hesitate to do this, and therefore the discussion hits a dead end. This often occurs when the therapist asks a young child about his or her trauma, "Do you remember being hit by your dad?" and the child responds, "No," when everyone knows he does remember. Checkmate. It is somewhat impolite to counter this with the child and say, "Oh yes, you do remember."

Circular questioning, in contrast, involves asking someone a question about a topic that he or she does *not* have authority to answer (e.g., "What is your mother's favorite color?" "Does your wife love you?" "How does your son feel about what you just said?" "Does your son remember being hit by his father?"). Family members often know the real (or better) answer to these questions because of their intimate contact with the other member; however, they are less likely to give the expected or appropriate answer, and are more likely to reveal a more truthful view that reflects the underlayers of the family's relationships. The therapist then follows up this question by asking the other member a similar circular question (not a direct question such as, "So do you love your husband?").

> THERAPIST: Does your wife love you?
> HUSBAND: Well, hard to tell sometimes, one day yes, the next no.
> THERAPIST (*to wife*): What does your husband mean by that answer? What is he trying to say?
> WIFE: He thinks I am having an affair.

By continuously asking each family member about the inner workings of the others' feelings and thoughts, the clinician can much more effectively avoid dead ends and the appearance of challenging members' authority.

In response to a circular question, a family member will often answer, "I don't know," either out of reluctance to speculate or embarrass the other member or because he or she truly does not know. In this case, the clinician responds by asking that person to ask the other the same question (which will be in direct form).

> THERAPIST: Does your wife love you?
> HUSBAND: I don't know.
> THERAPIST: Ask her.
> HUSBAND (*to wife*): Do you love me?
> WIFE: Of course I do, dear.

Then the clinician follows up with the first person by asking a circular question.

> THERAPIST: So, what do you think, does she love you?
> HUSBAND: I…guess so.
> THERAPIST (*to wife*): Why does your husband only "guess so" when you said you do love him?

Circular questioning avoids dead stops and allows the clinician to keep the conversation going, which is useful in the trauma-centered approach, where attempts to stop the conversation are frequent. Circular questioning also helps to maintain the neutrality of the therapist, because he or she is working through the family members and never (or rarely) stating his or her own opinion or asking direct questions.

Using Third-Party Questioning

Third-party questioning, a technique related to circular questioning, is a discussion between two people about another, in the presence of the other. In normal social etiquette, this is improper behavior. People are not supposed to talk about another person in their presence, although it is common to do so behind the person's back. Nevertheless, people are usually curious about what other people say about them behind their backs. Third-party questioning in the family therapy context is tolerated because of this curiosity.

The major use for third-party questioning is when a family member is intent on stopping the discussion either by not cooperating or by denying obvious truths. This is common among traumatized children younger than 12. Once the person has indicated that he or she will not cooperate with the exploration of the trauma or other aspects of the therapy session, the clinician can turn to another family member or spouse and carry on a conversation about the other person but remain ready to reengage the person when he or she wants to reenter the conversation. The person usually speaks up when he or she feels that what is being said is wrong. Traumatized people do not tolerate error well, and if they hear others speaking about the trauma incorrectly, it is almost impossible for them to stay silent. In this way, many recalcitrant children are brought back into the conversation.

> THERAPIST: Chris, can I ask you about your memories of being hit by your biological father?
> CHRIS: No.
> THERAPIST (*to foster parent*): Chris does not want to talk about being hit by his biological father.
> PARENT: I can see that.
> THERAPIST: Why do you think that is?
> PARENT: I think it makes him sad, you know. It wasn't good.
> THERAPIST: I understand it went on for a long time. Do you know how long?
> PARENT: I think the social worker said 3 years.
> CHRIS (*interjecting*): Four.
> THERAPIST: Oh, 4 years. Not good. (*Still to parent.*) Do we know if Chris was ever bruised badly enough that he had to go to the hospital?
> PARENT: I'm not sure. He doesn't like hospitals, though.
> THERAPIST: How do you know?
> PARENT: Every time we go by St. Francis Hospital, he gets upset.
> THERAPIST: Perhaps he was remembering a bad time in the hospital.
> CHRIS: My dad said he was going to leave me there.
> THERAPIST (*to Chris*): You mean as a threat?
> CHRIS: Yeah. If I got him angry again.
> THERAPIST: Bad.
> CHRIS: Yup. Bad.

The following is another example of third-party questioning from a couples therapy session.

THERAPIST (*to husband*): Now, if you don't mind, I'd like to ask your wife some questions, and I'd like you just to listen for a while. Is that okay?

HUSBAND: Sure.

THERAPIST: So, Martha, it seems your husband is really reluctant to share with you all the details of his experience in Vietnam.

WIFE: Yes, appears so. I just know a little bit.

THERAPIST: I think we know that what he went through there is affecting your relationship now.

WIFE: Big time. For sure. He even says it.

THERAPIST: What's his reluctance?

WIFE: Maybe it's too gruesome.

THERAPIST: Let's work on this. He told you about the time he and his squad entered this village, and a lot of villagers were killed.

WIFE: Yes, these things happen. He said he felt guilty about it.

THERAPIST: Okay. What did he do that might have made him feel guilty?

WIFE: Kill women and children? (*Husband begins to look extremely uncomfortable.*)

THERAPIST: Yes. Did you notice the reaction of your husband just now?

WIFE: Yes.

THERAPIST: What was that?

WIFE: He seems upset, wide-eyed.

THERAPIST: Seems we are in the territory. You understand that it is okay for him to get upset about these memories. They could hardly be pleasant.

WIFE: I understand.

THERAPIST: He is not going to be hurt by becoming upset about them.

WIFE: Okay.

THERAPIST: You came into couples therapy after he left you for a month and then told you he was thinking of leaving you, despite the fact that the two of you have had such a good relationship.

WIFE: Yes, it was so upsetting because I was pregnant with our first child.

THERAPIST: When did he leave?

WIFE: The month?

THERAPIST: In terms of the pregnancy?

WIFE: When I started to show.

THERAPIST: If that was a trigger for him, if that triggered a memory from Vietnam that freaked him out, and if that memory was from his time at the village, any ideas what that might mean happened there? (*Husband is now looking away and tearing up.*)

WIFE: Oh, could he have killed a pregnant woman? (*Husband erupts in tears, shaking.*)

(*Therapist indicates to wife to go over to comfort him, which she does. They are in a close embrace, although husband seems to be holding back just a bit.*)

HUSBAND: Yes, I killed her....I didn't know at first. We just shot up the hut. (*Crying.*)

WIFE: I'm so sorry, honey. I love you. You were doing your duty. You didn't mean to hurt her.

HUSBAND: It was stupid...horrible... (*He stops crying and looks panicked.*)

THERAPIST (*to wife*): Do you see this?
WIFE: Yes.
THERAPIST: Ask him what he is remembering.
WIFE: Honey, what are you remembering?
HUSBAND: I can't tell you.
THERAPIST: Tell him it is okay for him to tell you, that you will not be hurt.
WIFE: Please tell me, sweetheart.
HUSBAND: (*Erupts again in tears.*) When I...went into the hut...she had been hit in the abdomen....I saw...the fetus. (*Cries and holds onto his wife now with a full embrace.*)
(*Pause.*)
THERAPIST (*to husband*): So when your wife started to show, all you could think about was this woman and her baby, and how you killed them?
HUSBAND: Yes...yes...yes.
WIFE: That was then, honey. I know you would never hurt me. I love you.
HUSBAND: I love you, so much. How could I have done that?
THERAPIST: You were a soldier.
WIFE: You were a soldier.
THERAPIST (*to husband*): Looking at your wife, do you believe her that she loves you and trusts you?
HUSBAND: (*Looks at her.*) Yes.
THERAPIST: How is she doing with this information?
HUSBAND: She seems okay.
THERAPIST: I think so, too. (*To wife.*) It seems you have an answer to the question why your husband left you when he did.
WIFE: Yes I do. And I want him. (*They stay in a close embrace.*)

In this session fragment, the use of the third-party conversation allowed a productive decoding of a traumatic memory, circumventing the hesitation of the husband. Notably, the therapist followed the principle of incompleteness and was alert to hear more from the husband even after being told he had killed a pregnant woman. The truly horrific memory was yet to come: seeing the fetus out of its mother's belly.

METHOD OF TRAUMA-CENTERED COUPLES AND FAMILY PSYCHOTHERAPY

We recommend four steps in trauma-centered couples and family psychotherapy:

1. Identify and name the traumatic experiences within the couple or family.
2. Reveal and explore the details of these traumatic experiences and have them shared among all family members.
3. Examine current conflicts among family members from the lens of these

traumatic experiences and schemas, and decode the links between the past and the present. Significantly, both the behaviors of the victim member and the responses of the other members to those behaviors will be decoded in terms of the trauma schemas, so that family members can see that their own behaviors have been influenced covertly by the traumatic event.

4. Make palpable the ongoing influence (i.e., presence) of the perpetrator to family members, to help them reorganize their relationship against him or her as a collective.

These steps occur in an overlapping manner, as details of the traumas emerge over time, and decoding and discussing the perpetrator can begin early on. The goal of convincing the family members of the impact of the trauma is the most central aim of this work. Once they have been convinced, they will be more able to bond with the victim member in a collective stance against the trauma and perpetrator and collectively mourn the losses that occurred.

Case Example 1

This family consists of a 14-year-old girl (Teresa), her biological father (Mike), her stepmother (Maria), and a 7-year-old half-sister. Teresa was abused during visits with her biological mother from ages 4 to 9, after her parents divorced. The father, who knew she was being neglected but not abused, had attempted to stop the visits but was unsuccessful in court. Five years ago, the mother finally left the state, and Teresa had no more visits with her. A hearing for termination of parental rights, with the intent of the stepmother's adopting her, was in process. Teresa had been verbally and physically aggressive at home, oppositional, and binge eating. Her father had locked up the refrigerator and the kitchen cabinets. Teresa hoarded food in her room, which was a complete mess, with food and clothing strewn everywhere. Her behavior in school was fine, however, and she was doing well academically. Several previous therapists had implied that the parents were doing something wrong for her to be upset only in their home, which distressed them greatly. She was referred to the therapist after a brief hospitalization for suicidality. A decision was made not to include the sister in the family meetings due to the graphic details likely to be disclosed. The first two sessions were focused on hearing the details of what happened with the biological mother from the father's point of view and then Teresa's. In the second session Teresa declined to provide any more details.

> THERAPIST: Let me summarize what we know so far: Teresa visited with her mother almost every week for 3 years. During that time, she spent a lot of time waiting at her mother's job while

her mother worked, and where she was not fed for long periods of time. We think that she was physically punished on several occasions because she came back into your home with bruises and once with a broken arm. Your attempts, Mike, to stop the visits failed. Teresa has indicated there is more to the story, but she isn't yet comfortable enough to talk about it. To remind you all, it is important that as many of the details as possible are shared, because whatever happened to Teresa is influencing the whole family today.

MARIA (*to Teresa*): I hope you will be able to share more of the story.

MIKE: I hope so, too, although I don't think her behavior is all about her mother—after all, it was 5 years ago. (*Teresa fidgets.*)

MARIA (*to therapist*): She is a teenager after all.

THERAPIST: The only way to know is to find out about the details. (*To Teresa.*) Teresa, I know you are hesitant to share details about what your mother did, but I have a question: I assume all that time you were at your mother's house, you were hoping that your dad would come to take you home? Is that right?

TERESA: Yeah, he never came.

MIKE: I always came!

TERESA: When you were supposed to.

THERAPIST: You mean at the end of the visit.

MIKE: Oh, I see, yeah. I wasn't allowed to pick her up early.

THERAPIST: Teresa, you have heard from your dad that he feels that he did everything in his power to stop the visits. Do you believe him?

TERESA: No.

THERAPIST: Why not?

TERESA: He doesn't care, really.

MIKE: That's not true.

THERAPIST: He doesn't care. Are you angry about that?

TERESA: Yes (*in a little girl's voice*).

THERAPIST: He should have come to get you?

TERESA: He should have come.

THERAPIST (*to parents*): How many times has Teresa run away?

MARIA: Four times this year.

THERAPIST: Any pattern to them?

MARIA: Yeah, she runs away usually when there is a family activity. We scramble all over, it disrupts what we have to do, and then a couple hours later she calls us and tells us to pick her up.

MIKE: The last time, after we got the call, she was at a pharmacy, I think. I drove right there, was there within 15 minutes, and she was gone. Couple hours later we get another call from a library, and I was mad, because she was making our lives miserable on purpose, so I said she'll have to wait a little longer. She started screaming, "I hate you" on the phone, and I couldn't get her to calm down.

TERESA: You told me I was selfish.

MIKE: You were being selfish. Anyway, I got in the car and picked her up, and she wouldn't talk to me the entire night, and frankly that didn't matter to me.

THERAPIST: So, do you see any connections between this behavior and her experience with her mother?

MIKE: Not really, other than the fact that she was abused by her mother so she is taking it out on me.

THERAPIST: Well, let's put ourselves in Teresa's situation: she is being neglected or worse by her mother on these visits, and she hopes that you will come early to pick her up and get her out of there, and you don't, so she feels angry at you and wonders if you care enough for her.

MIKE: All right.

THERAPIST (*to Teresa*): So far so good?

TERESA: Yes.

THERAPIST: Years later, these memories are reactivated for some reason, so Teresa behaves in a manner that is affected by her traumatic events.

MARIA: How is that?

THERAPIST: She runs away. What does that force you to do?

MIKE: Pick her up.

THERAPIST: Pick her up, which is what she had wanted you to do when she was at her mother's. If you don't pick her up, then it proves to her that you don't care. If you do pick her up, then…

MIKE: I did pick her up, but then she made it worse by playing this cat and mouse game!

THERAPIST: Apparently another way of testing how much you care. This time you waivered, which may be why she started screaming at you on the phone.

MIKE: I see. But you think this is all about that?

THERAPIST: We are exploring. I have another question. (*To Teresa.*) Any connection between a pharmacy and your mother's visits?

MIKE: She worked in a pharmacy.

THERAPIST: So Teresa asked you to pick her up from a pharmacy. How about a library?

MIKE: We usually made the transfer at a local library.

THERAPIST: Interesting coincidence wouldn't you say?

MARIA: That's weird. Did you do that on purpose, Teresa?

TERESA: (*Shrugs shoulders.*)

THERAPIST: So whether she was aware of this or not, her recent running away was a kind of replay of her experience years ago with you and her mother. If that is true, that is how trauma creeps into the present.

MIKE: (*Stares at therapist.*)

THERAPIST: I want to meet alone with Teresa for a few minutes, if you don't mind waiting.

MIKE: Sure.

The therapist talked alone with Teresa, who with some initial reluctance revealed that her mother locked her in a work closet at the pharmacy for hours. The closet was a mess. She was not given any food or water. She was also put in her mother's car on the weekends when the mother was having sex with a boyfriend in the house, even during the winter. She was often hit and yelled at also. Mike and Maria were invited back to continue the family session.

THERAPIST: Teresa was able to give me some more details about her mother's abuse. Would you like to share some of them with your parents?

MIKE: Not really.

THERAPIST: I think they need to know these things.

TERESA: (*Shrugs shoulders.*) You do it.

THERAPIST: You are willing to have me share it with them?

TERESA: Yes.

THERAPIST: Teresa told me that her mother locked her in a closet at the pharmacy when she was working, often without food or water, for hours.

MIKE (*in genuine distress*): That's terrible! (*Face becomes red.*)

MARIA: That's horrible. (*To Mike.*) What's wrong, honey?

MIKE: It makes me so mad. I knew bad stuff was going on, but I couldn't do anything about it.

MARIA (*to Teresa*): There was no food there?

TERESA: No.

MARIA: Where did your mother keep her lunch?

TERESA: In the refrigerator.

MARIA: What refrigerator—the pharmacy's?

TERESA: (*Nods.*) But it was locked.

MIKE: I could kill her.

THERAPIST: That is not the only thing that happened to her.

TERESA: She kept me in her car when men came over to the house.

THERAPIST: For a long time also?

TERESA: A couple of times overnight. It was cold.

THERAPIST: What were you feeling?

TERESA: I wanted my dad to come and get me. I thought I was going to die.

MIKE: What were men doing at the house?

Teresa: (*Shrugs shoulders.*)

THERAPIST: Tell them what you said to me, Teresa.

TERESA: Having sex.

MARIA: How did you know that if you were in the car?

TERESA: (*Becomes very red, upset, kicks her feet, puts her hand on her head, says nothing.*)

THERAPIST (*to Mike*): Do you see her reaction?

MIKE: I do.

THERAPIST: She seems to know her mother was having sex with men. I think she said men, right?

MARIA: Right.

THERAPIST: How would she know about the sex? Any ideas?

MIKE: God forbid. (*Becomes tearful, tense.*)

THERAPIST (*to Teresa*): Teresa, is that because at other times you saw your mother having sex?

TERESA: (*Nods. Shakes feet up and down and open and shut.*)

THERAPIST: Is there more? (*Teresa ignores this.*) I think there is more.

TERESA: They had sex with me. (*Bursts into tears. Mike bursts into tears and shouts "No!" Teresa runs over and jumps into Maria's lap, who comforts her. Mike comes over and hugs both of them. They all weep for several minutes.*)

THERAPIST: I am very glad that you were able to get that out, Teresa. (*Everyone sits back in their places.*) So we have a lot of information here. Each of Teresa's memories is linked to one of her disruptive behaviors now. She runs away so you can come and pick her up. She raids the refrigerator so you will put a lock on it like her mother did. She hoards food in her room, which is a big mess like the closet at her mother's workplace. There must be a connection also to being locked in the car, but we don't know what that is yet.

MARIA: She will not stay in the car if Mike leaves to buy something at a store. She panics.

THERAPIST: There we are. Being left alone in a car without Mike reminds her of the time she was left alone in her mother's car.

MIKE: I can't believe all this.

MARIA: It's amazing. I had no idea.

THERAPIST: Being sexually molested by her mother's male friends?

TERESA: Not friends.

THERAPIST: More on that later; "not friends" is also going to be connected. We have time to look at all this. Instead of fighting with each other, you can join together to deal with these terrible memories. It will take time, but you did a fine job today. Thank you, Teresa, for letting us know some of what happened to you.

MARIA: Some?

THERAPIST: There's more, isn't there, Teresa?

TERESA: Oh, yes.

THERAPIST: So I will see you next week.

In this session, the use of individual meetings, circular questioning, and third-party questioning was helpful in eliciting the trauma-related information. The therapist was persistently attending to the parents' uncertainty about the impact of the trauma. As more and more details were decoded and linked to specific aspects of the traumatic events, the parents became more convinced and open emotionally to their daughter's pain.

Case Example 2

Sandy, a 10-year-old girl, is the first child of a 26-year-old single mother who has borderline personality disorder and who has had significant difficulties raising her child. The child has spent much of her time being cared for by her grandmother. Sandy shows periodic aggressive and disorganized behaviors at home and school, and at times demonstrates sexualized attitudes, oppositional behaviors, and periodic depressive episodes when she feels that she is not worth much and feels that her mother does not love her. These behaviors became much worse after Sandy disclosed to her grandmother that she had been sexually molested (involving vaginal stimulation but not intercourse) by a cousin once in his home. She had been referred to the therapist based on this trauma. Sandy currently lives with her mother and half-brother but stays often with her grandmother when the conflict with her mother becomes too heated.

In the first few meetings with Sandy and her mother, it became clear that the grandmother was an essential part of this family system, so she was invited to join. The mother, in a separate meeting with the therapist, confided that Sandy had been the product of a rape and that from her birth, Sandy has reminded her mother of her perpetrator. The rape derailed her performance at school, causing her to drop out and leading to other difficulties in life. The mother said it tears her apart when Sandy says she does not feel that her mother loves her, "because I'm not sure I do. Her presence brings me back to the rape....I just freeze when I'm around her." She had not told Sandy this secret for fear of harming her further. This dynamic was made more intense when the mother and a boyfriend had a baby boy, on whom the mother showered warmth and love, proving to Sandy that her mother was not a cold person in general, but cold only to her.

> THERAPIST (*to grandmother*): I am glad that you could come.
> GRANDMOTHER: You're welcome.
> THERAPIST: Last week we were talking about the impact of the molestation by Sandy's cousin.
> GRANDMOTHER: That was terrible.
> THERAPIST: Have you talked to Sandy about how she felt about it?
> GRANDMOTHER: Yes, of course,…a little.
> THERAPIST: How does Sandy feel about it?
> GRANDMOTHER: Well, terrible, I guess. (*Looks over at Sandy.*)
> THERAPIST: You aren't sure?
> GRANDMOTHER: Not really.
> THERAPIST: Ask Sandy.
> GRANDMOTHER: Sandy, how do you feel now about what happened to you last winter?
> SANDY: Not much.
> THERAPIST: What is Sandy trying to say?
> GRANDMOTHER: I don't know.… She doesn't want to talk about it now.
> THERAPIST: She was at her cousin's house?

GRANDMOTHER: Yeah, I had a meeting, and so I usually bring her over to my sister's house.

THERAPIST: Where was Sandy's mom? (*Sandy fidgets and turns away.*)

GRANDMOTHER: Out and about.

THERAPIST: Did you see what Sandy just did?

GRANDMOTHER: Yes. I think she's sensitive about the fact that her mother isn't always around.

SANDY: She's never around.

MOTHER: You know I'm around when I can be (*sharply*). I keep my eye on you, check in with Nana every day.

SANDY: (*Yells.*) You're never around. You hate me!

MOTHER: (*Yells.*) Do *not* talk like that to me, young lady!

GRANDMOTHER: Calm down, calm down!

THERAPIST: Sandy, are you upset that your mother was not around that day when you were molested?

SANDY: Yes.

THERAPIST (*to mother*): It seems Sandy is upset about that day in particular. Perhaps she has an idea that if you had been with her, she would not have been harmed. (*Sandy nods.*) And that you have not been with her for a long time…

SANDY: My whole life.

THERAPIST (*to grandmother*): Does Sandy think that her mother is not around because she doesn't care for her? (*Sandy nods.*)

GRANDMOTHER: I believe so. She says it all the time.

THERAPIST: And is there a reason that her mom has kept her distance all these years from Sandy?

GRANDMOTHER (*tearing up*): Yes. (*Sandy gets quiet.*)

THERAPIST: A good reason?

GRANDMOTHER: A good reason.

THERAPIST: Why has she not told Sandy the reason?

GRANDMOTHER: Because she loves her and doesn't want to upset her. (*Mother begins to tear up.*)

THERAPIST: Let's check this out. Could you ask your daughter why she hasn't told Sandy yet?

GRANDMOTHER: Honey, why haven't you told Sandy?

MOTHER: I don't want to hurt her any more than I already have.

SANDY (*in a little girl's voice*): What happened, Mommy?

MOTHER: (*Looks with anxiety at therapist.*) What should I do?

THERAPIST: Your daughter believes that you have stayed away from her because you do not care for her, and that is not correct, and that thought is causing her to be upset and act out in school and your home. This is where we face our traumas, together, everyone in this room.

SANDY: What happened, Mommy?

MOTHER: So you remember I told you that your father was my boyfriend and that he decided that he couldn't help out and so we…

THERAPIST: Sandy, would you like to hold your mother's hand?

SANDY: (*Moves instantly to hold her mother's hand, and the mother begins to cry as she speaks.*)

MOTHER: So he never was in your life and because I was so young when I had you, I had to give you to Nana to help out so I could try to finish school, even though I didn't.

SANDY: (*Nods.*)

THERAPIST: (*To grandmother.*) How is she doing?

GRANDMOTHER: I think she's doing fine.

THERAPIST: Should she keep going?

GRANDMOTHER: She should keep going. Keep going, sweetheart.

MOTHER: Anyway, that wasn't true. (*Becoming more upset.*) Your father was someone I barely knew and he...he...raped me, beat me up (*Sandy starts crying*), and he got arrested and put in jail for it, but all these years I guess you remind me of that—of my rape—and I guess I just close up around you, and we fight instead.

SANDY: (*Crying, goes to sit on her mother's lap and hugs her tightly. Grandmother holds out her hand to comfort her daughter. They maintain this for several minutes.*) I'm so sorry, Mommy.

MOTHER: No, Sandy, I'm sorry. It's not your fault. You were a beautiful baby and are a beautiful girl now too. It's me. It's all my fault.

THERAPIST (*to mother*): Why do you think it's your fault?

MOTHER: Because I did things just to spite my mother. I was just not a great kid, wanted to do things my way. (*Cries again.*) I'm sorry, Mom, I should have listened to you.

GRANDMOTHER: Yes, you should have, but you were not to blame for being raped.

THERAPIST: That is right. What was his name?

MOTHER: Richard.

THERAPIST: Full name.

MOTHER: Richard Salem.

THERAPIST: Richard Salem is to blame. He raped your mother, and that is why she thinks of him sometimes when she is with you; this is why she gets tense and you haven't known why, up until now. This is why she seems nicer to your half-brother, because he doesn't remind her of the rape.

SANDY: I see.

THERAPIST: Richard Salem has harmed this whole family. All of you.

SANDY: (*Hugs mother tighter.*) He hurt my mommy.

THERAPIST (*to Sandy*): Now I have a question. Why did your mother give birth to you anyway?

SANDY: I don't know.

THERAPIST: Ask her.

SANDY: Mommy, why did you have me anyway?

MOTHER: Because I love you, you were my baby.

THERAPIST: Could you say that again?

MOTHER: Because I love you, you were my baby.

THERAPIST (*to Sandy*): What do you think? Does she mean what she is saying?

SANDY: Yes!

THERAPIST: Ask your grandmother why your mother had you anyway.

SANDY: Nana, why?

GRANDMOTHER: Because she felt that she had been hurt by Richard, but you were the good thing that came out of it. . . . You were hers, and she loves you. (*She cries, and Sandy goes to her to console her.*)

SANDY: I love you, Nana. (*Quiet.*)

THERAPIST: So let's review all this. Sandy, your mother was raped by a man named Richard Salem who was arrested and jailed for the crime, but your mother decided to have you because you were her baby and she loved you. However, she was only 16 and not very mature, so she couldn't really raise you well, and so she gave you to your grandmother to help, but then they got into arguments over you.

SANDY: Which they still do!

THERAPIST: Which they still do. Your mother was traumatized by the rape and feels that it ruined her life, so you have always been a reminder of that, even though it's not you but Richard Salem who is to blame. This is why she tenses up and sometimes doesn't show a lot of warmth to you, which you, not knowing the truth, have assumed means that she does not love you.

SANDY: Which is not true.

THERAPIST: Which is not true. Right, Mom?

MOTHER: It is definitely not true.

THERAPIST: Any questions?

SANDY (*to mother*): Can we go to McDonald's?

MOTHER: You know that— (*catches herself*). You manipulative little pumpkin!

SANDY (*to the therapist*): That's a yes!

In this session fragment, the therapist's use of circular and third-party questioning, reassuring the family that it is better to reveal the truth, and naming of the perpetrator were helpful in exposing how their current interactions were tangled up with history. A burning secret was opened up for discussion, and the mother and grandmother were shown that Sandy was capable of listening and benefiting from hearing it. Pointing out the rewards of open communication is key in helping families reorient themselves in more productive patterns.

Case Example 3

The importance of mentioning the perpetrator by name cannot be overestimated. Without being reminded about the original cause of suffering for members in the family, the family soon reengages in the same recriminations and accusations that have characterized their conflicts for months or years, casting each other in the role of perpetrator. Because of the rapid pace of family or couple interactions and the intensity of their relationships, concretizing the presence of the perpetrator may be helpful. This is accomplished by telling the family that the perpetrator has insinuated himself or herself into the family so intimately that it is just like he or she is now a member, so it is only fair that the person be given a seat. An extra seat is pulled into the circle of chairs in the session. Sometimes, it is useful to have one of the members, especially a child, write the perpetrator's name or draw a picture of him or her on a sheet of paper and pin it to the back of the chair.

> Amy and Brian are a couple in their 30s who have come to treatment because of the deterioration in their relationship. She feels that he is either distant and uninterested, or needy and bothersome. He feels that she is a hypochondriac, with too many anxieties about her body and health. One of their common arguments occurs when they are planning to go out to dinner: they decide to go out for a romantic dinner but cannot agree on a restaurant because she is "picky about the food" and he "doesn't like to drive far." They end up yelling at each other, and she retreats to the bathroom. He becomes impatient and yells at her to get out and then insults her about her hypochondriasis. They end the evening with one of them saying, "Okay, go by yourself!" or "Okay, go with someone else!" The following transcript picks up about 15 minutes into the first session.

>> THERAPIST: This argument you have about dinner seems to be indicative of the problems you have been having in the relationship? (*Both nod.*) Okay, if you don't mind my asking, has either of you had any traumatic or frightening or especially bad experiences in your life?
>> BRIAN: Not really. Got into a few fights in high school. Teased in middle school a couple of times.
>> THERAPIST: Any sexual abuse or being inappropriately touched?
>> BRIAN: No.
>> THERAPIST: Any sudden deaths or losses?
>> BRIAN: No. My grandmother died last year but after a 3-year decline.
>> THERAPIST: Any other event?
>> BRIAN: Nope.
>> THERAPIST: How about you, Amy?
>> AMY: Not really.
>> THERAPIST: Any neglect or physical abuse, severe punishment?
>> AMY: No.…There was one incident.

THERAPIST: Tell me about it.

AMY: I was in college, and a boy I was dating got rough and he sort of forced himself on me.

THERAPIST: Does Brian know about this?

BRIAN: Yeah, she told me. Real jerk.

THERAPIST: Can you tell me some of the details about it?

AMY: I guess. Is this really important?

THERAPIST: I think it can be. These events have a way of influencing us.

AMY: Well, we had been dating a few times, and he seemed nice enough.

THERAPIST: His name?

AMY: George. Anyway, we were having dinner at this restaurant— I can't remember the event, but he had wanted to go out to a good restaurant and buy dinner for me, and I said sure. Anyway, we drank quite a bit of wine and I said I had to go to the bathroom and so I did.

BRIAN: You didn't tell me this part.

THERAPIST: Continue, Amy.

AMY (*showing discomfort*): Anyway, I was in there a little too long or something and when I opened the bathroom door, there George was.

THERAPIST: What was the bathroom like?

AMY: It was very small, only one stall, you had to lock the outside door. Anyway, George was right there, and he wasn't smiling and…pushed me back into the bathroom.

THERAPIST: You opened the door and there he was, not smiling. Then what happened before he pushed you back into the bathroom?

AMY: (*Upset.*)

BRIAN: Honey, what happened?

THERAPIST: Brian, do you see that Amy is getting upset?

BRIAN: I do.

THERAPIST: Have you heard the details of this experience before?

BRIAN: I thought I had, but maybe not.

THERAPIST: Perhaps you might hold your wife's hand. (*He does.*) Go on, Amy.

AMY: He grabbed my breast and squeezed it and then pushed me back into the room.

THERAPIST: Go on.

AMY: He was very rough and pushed me against the wall and I tripped and fell down on the toilet seat. He had this weird look on his face and he said, he said, "You barely ate your dinner, you selfish bitch. Now you are going to make up for that." And he took out his…

THERAPIST: Penis?

AMY: Penis, and pulled off my clothes and had sex with me.

BRIAN: Shit.

THERAPIST: That is terrible, Amy. George pulled off your clothes, and then what happened?

AMY (*becoming upset*): He pulled off my panties and put them into my mouth, I guess so I wouldn't scream.

THERAPIST: Then what happened?

AMY: He pulled me up over the toilet seat and entered me from behind.

THERAPIST: Anally or vaginally?

AMY: Vaginally.

THERAPIST: Did George have to hold you?

AMY: Yes, and he kept hitting me in the back with his fist.

THERAPIST: Was he saying anything to you?

AMY: Yeah, "you piece of ass," "I'm going to leave you here, and I don't ever want to see you again."

THERAPIST: What else did he do?

AMY: (*Again, upset.*) Not much.

THERAPIST: (*Silently looks at her.*) Not much?

AMY: (*Bursts into tears.*) He grabbed the back of my head and rammed my head against the toilet. I almost blacked out, then he pulled me back and opened the toilet seat and pushed my head into the bowl (*cries*).

BRIAN: Oh my god!

AMY: I thought I was going to drown or die. He then let go, kicked me, and told me to wait in the bathroom for 10 minutes before coming out. I washed myself up and tried to look okay— I think my forehead was bleeding—and then I went home to my apartment and stayed inside for 3 days.

BRIAN (*overwhelmed*): Sweetheart, I had no idea! Oh my God! (*Gives her a long hug.*) I want to murder that bastard. I will!

THERAPIST (*to Amy*): I really appreciate your telling us about this experience. It was quite a horrific one. Can I have you check in with Brian to see if he is okay?

AMY: Are you okay? Do you think I am a monster?

BRIAN: Yes, no, I am enraged that someone could do that to you! And he is the monster.

AMY: I love you.

BRIAN: I love you. (*They embrace again.*)

THERAPIST: So let me review what we have done here. Amy revealed that George brutally raped her on a date in college. She minimized how frightening and violent it was to you, Brian, so you have had no idea how much it has influenced her. But it has influenced her, and next week let's try to examine the specific ways that that experience is alive now in your relationship and may be causing some of the problems you have mentioned. How does that sound?

BRIAN/AMY: Fine.

The next session they arrived in an upbeat mood. They said that they had had a great week with no arguments and had felt very intimate with each other. The therapist noted this and pointed out how George had insinuated himself into their lives, only Brian had not known about it. To help illustrate this, the therapist said that with their permission he would like to set a chair for George in the session. They laughed and said, "Sure." The therapist moved a chair next to Amy.

> BRIAN: That makes me mad.
>
> THERAPIST: That there is an empty chair for George next to your wife or that George raped her years ago?
>
> BRIAN: Both. I could kill him!
>
> THERAPIST (*to Amy*): Looking at him now, what do you think your husband is feeling.
>
> AMY: Helpless, he wasn't there and couldn't have been there.
>
> BRIAN: Helpless. Exactly. I think you are going to have to get rid of this chair. I can't take my eyes off of it.
>
> THERAPIST: Have there been times you feel helpless around Amy recently?
>
> BRIAN: Yes, all the time; she has so many anxieties and things, and I've tried to help her out, but nothing works!
>
> THERAPIST: So there are some obvious links between what happened to Amy and your arguments at home. They often occur around going to a restaurant. You accuse her of being a picky eater, like George did. She goes into the bathroom and doesn't come out, even though you yell at her, but she doesn't want to come out because that's when George attacked her.
>
> BRIAN: Yes. I have even said to her, "What's wrong with you? You got your ass stuck in the toilet?"
>
> THERAPIST: So the traumatic event from 15 years ago is being reenacted between the two of you, without your knowing it.
>
> BRIAN: I am so sorry.
>
> AMY: I didn't know this either, but it is so clear. I'm still so afraid of him. (*Unconsciously puts her hand out to rest it on the chair.*)
>
> THERAPIST: George [naming the perpetrator]. (*To Brian.*) What's going on with Amy now?
>
> BRIAN: I don't know.
>
> AMY: What do you mean?
>
> BRIAN: You just put your hand on George's chair.
>
> THERAPIST: Did you hear her say that she was still frightened of George?
>
> BRIAN: So why did she reach out to touch him? You should reach out and touch me, honey!
>
> AMY: I don't know.
>
> THERAPIST: People will do anything for people they are terrified of. Do you remember reaching out for George during the rape?
>
> AMY (*thinking*): Yes, I think I reached back with my hand to stroke his thigh because I thought that might make him less angry with me.
>
> BRIAN: That's enough. (*Gets up and moves the chair out of Amy's reach, into a corner of the room.*) It's like he's kidnapped my girl.

AMY: (*Giggles.*) You haven't called me that in years!

BRIAN: I didn't know I was competing for you with someone else.

AMY: I didn't either. But now that I know, I want you to win.

BRIAN: Damn right.

THERAPIST: George is a shadow. We have to pull him out into the light, so he has less power.

BRIAN: I will have to keep my eye on him.

THERAPIST: Sounds like a plan. Now let us go over again what happened to Amy. Could you hold her hands again, Brian?

BRIAN: (*His hands are trembling.*) Yes, damn it, I hate that thing! (*Referring to the chair.*)

THERAPIST: Amy, what's going on with Brian?

AMY: I don't know. I really feel your presence. You are really here. I feel protected.

THERAPIST: How does that feel?

AMY: Good. I must still feel unprotected. Over the past 6 months, with Brian becoming more angry and distant, I think I have felt even more vulnerable.

BRIAN: You are right, and I haven't particularly felt like protecting you because I had no idea there was something or someone who was threatening you. But now I know! (*He stands up, and they embrace.*)

The rest of this session was spent reviewing again the details of Amy's trauma and decoding a number of specific links between it and the couple's current interactions.

THERAPIST: So, I think you see how this works. I encourage you to periodically talk about George's assault on Amy, to remind yourselves of who the real problem is. Paradoxically, the more that you allow George to remain a presence in your lives, the more passionate you will remain with each other, because this will give Brian a reason to want to protect you, Amy, and for Amy to be more available to you, Brian. Call me if you want to schedule any further sessions.

The couple did not require any further sessions, and a year later the therapist received a card thanking him and saying that all was well.

CONCLUSION

Couples and family therapy can be a very powerful means of affecting not only the traumatized individual but also people in his or her immediate social system, who have been drawn into patterns of communication shaped by the person's trauma schemas, thereby sustaining those schemas. Although many clients expect or request individual therapy, the clinician should keep open the possibility of couples or family therapy, which can be an extremely effective means of intervening in trauma-related disorders.

The basic goal is to open up the family communication to include details of each member's traumatic experiences and to make others aware of how influential these experiences continue to be within the family. Through the use of specific techniques, in particular circular questioning and third-party questioning, the process of revealing the impact of the trauma schemas on the family can be hastened. At heart, the method intends to expose and desensitize the family to discussions about the traumatic events, taking the pressure off the traumatized individual and disseminating the stress throughout the entire family. Although the traumatic events remain a burden, as a shared one the load on each person will become more manageable.

STUDY QUESTIONS

15.1 Why is it likely that trauma-centered therapy with the client's partner or family will be helpful?

15.2 T/F Quite often, family members think that they know about the trauma, when in fact they have not been told most of the details.

15.3 T/F Quite often, the roles of the trauma schema (victim, perpetrator, bystander, collaborator) are being played out among family members without their awareness.

15.4 What are the main goals of trauma-centered family treatment?

15.5 T/F It is not necessary for the therapist to be active and maintain control of the family/couples sessions.

15.6 T/F The therapist should never meet individually with any family member, because that would make other family members feel the therapist was aligning with another member.

15.7 T/F Circular questioning is asking a question to a family member that he or she has the authority to answer.

15.8 T/F In third-party questioning, the therapist discusses the behavior of a family member with another member, while the first person is present.

15.9 Why is it so important to externalize the perpetrator in trauma-centered family therapy?

CHAPTER 16

Adjunctive Methods

A number of adjunctive methods can aid the trauma-centered psychotherapist in getting details, revealing trauma schemas, decoding behavior, providing discrepancy, and disclosing the perpetrator. These aids concretize in physical form the process of exploring the effects of trauma and therefore may be recommended in specific situations and with specific clients. These methods include narrative, pictorial, ceremonial, and role-play methods (Table 16–1).

The methods described in this chapter are appropriate for any clinician and do not require specific training in art, drama, or narrative therapy. However, for readers interested in reading more about arts therapies in the treatment of trauma, many books are available (Adams 1997; Cohen et al. 1995; Johnson et al. 2009; Malchiodi and Perry 2014; Sajnani and Johnson 2014; Schauer et al. 2011; Sloan et al. 2012).

Generally, one should consider using the methods described in this chapter with 1) clients who request such methods, 2) children who do not use words well, and 3) anyone who will benefit from the concretization of their thoughts and feelings. Even though these methods can be used with anyone, they are unlikely to offer any particular additional advantage for clients who can effectively process their feelings verbally. This comment should not be construed as discouraging clinicians from receiving or enjoying or processing the artistic creations of their clients, be they poetry, visual art, music, songs, or crafts. Our focus in this chapter is on methods that specifically further the goals of trauma-centered psychotherapy.

TABLE 16–1.   Adjunctive methods used in trauma-centered
               psychotherapy

Narrative approaches

Editing the text—The therapist engages in a trauma inquiry through editing of
the client's written narrative.

Two-story method—The client is helped to develop two contrasting explanations
of his or her traumatic experience or illness when the client has uncertainty over
what might have really happened.

Mailbox—The client writes letters to perpetrators, lost loved ones, or himself or
herself at an earlier age; places them in a mailbox in the office; and then reads
the responses written by the therapist.

Artwork techniques

Two-dimensional grid—The client draws a series of pictures about his or her
traumatic event, varying along a timeline (one dimension) and close or far
perspective (second dimension).

Conversational art—The therapist and client pass one sheet of paper back and
forth, creating one drawing of the traumatic event, through which the therapist
attempts to help the client bring forth additional details, and accompanying
feelings, about the event.

Self-portrait—The client draws a series of self-portraits from different
perspectives related to his or her complex set of feelings about the traumatic
experience and his or her perceptions of how others reacted to them.

Perpetrator portraits—The client draws a series of portraits of the perpetrator
from different perspectives in order to elucidate the client's traumatic
experiences and to aid in the desensitization to reminders of his or her
perpetrator.

Photographs and videotaping—The client takes photos of relevant scenes related
to his or her trauma, videotapes his or her testimony, or prepares a film as a
means of concretizing his or her traumatic experience and communicating it to
others.

Therapeutic ceremonies

The therapist helps the client develop a ceremony to let go of real or symbolic
reminders of his or her trauma and to mark the transformation of his or her
suffering into new, productive activities and relationships.

Role-playing techniques

Telephone—The therapist utilizes an (unconnected) telephone to organize
simple role-plays between the client and significant people in his or her life,
especially those linked to the traumatic event, such as the perpetrator and the
client's family members.

Memory box—The client places a written description of a memory he or she does
not want to share with the therapist in a lockbox in the therapist's office.

These adjunctive methods are helpful in the same way that standard verbal techniques are helpful: they provide opportunities for exposure to the traumatic memories, which furthers desensitization. Producing physical objects or artifacts allows clients to remain exposed to their memories, because verbal processes can seem to evaporate shortly after a session ends. Also, these methods, by using concrete objects, support the establishment of discrepancy between past and present; for example, a picture of the trauma drawn by the client is not the same as the trauma. One's mental image of the trauma is more easily confused with the traumatic event.

Many of these approaches may be familiar to the reader in their pure form: as activities engaged in by the client as the therapist watches from the side. However, because trauma schemas are relational, a relational use of these methods, which facilitates a conversation between the client and the therapist, may be a preferred approach.

NARRATIVE APPROACHES

The basic instruction for a narrative approach is for the client to write his or her trauma narrative on paper or computer. Speaking and writing are different activities. Writing allows for editing and more careful review; it seems more final, more solid than speech. Many trauma clients write in their diaries without suggestion by the therapist. This may be because writing is a form of testimony, and the desire to let the world know of the truth—to be able to tell the untold story and to "break the silence"—is strong. Thus, encouraging the client to write out what happened can in itself be helpful. However, in a trauma-centered psychotherapy context, this is usually insufficient (Schauer et al. 2011). The aim is to address the inevitable avoidance and to get as many details as possible.

Another narrative approach is for the client to audiotape or videotape his or her trauma narrative. The advantage with this format is that wider opportunities exist for the client to share the product with other people and for the client to participate in the presentation of the material. Many clients have used these media in advocacy and performance venues as part of their recovery process. Audiotaping is also used in primary exposure treatments such as prolonged exposure (Foa and Rothbaum 1998), but not specifically for presentation to other audiences.

Editing the Text

One narrative technique that can be a useful adjunct to the trauma inquiry for certain clients involves editing the text. The client writes out (on paper, e-mail, or flash drive) a narrative of his or her traumatic memory. The clinician then inserts commentary into the narrative at the same points he or she might if the client were speaking: at the bumps, jumps, stops, bridges, and labels within the text. The text, slowly expanding, goes back and forth between them, as the narrative becomes more and more detailed. In the following example, the client's original text is in regular type, the therapist's inquiries are in parentheses, and the client's additional responses are in italics.

We were walking out of Walmart. It was a beautiful sunny day, and I couldn't remember where I parked my car, so Jennifer and I wandered from row to row. (Did you have groceries, a cart?) *I had a shopping cart, and Jennifer had a bag.* Suddenly, I heard the screech of a car braking several rows away from me (What did the screech sound like?) *It was just a short, high-pitched squeak,* and at first I didn't think much about it. (What were you looking at then?) It came from behind me, *and I was looking at a red convertible and thinking how nice it would be to have one of those.* Then I realized that Jennifer wasn't with me. (What did you do with your packages?) *I left the cart in the middle of the row and turned around.* People were running toward the accident. (The accident?) *It was weird. I didn't know what had happened, but my body just seemed to move.* I felt dizzy. It couldn't be. (What were you thinking?) *The thought came to me that Jennifer had been hit by the car and I remembered when she was 6 and she ran out into the street and was nearly hit by a car and how I told myself then that I would never let her be in danger again.* I ran too and hit the side of a car and fell. (Fell on what? Did you hurt yourself?) *I scraped my knees really badly; in fact, there was blood but I felt nothing.* I heard screams. (Screams?) *Yes, I don't really know. Maybe loud talking. Actually no, I was screaming.* When I got there, Jennifer was lying on the ground with a lot of people hovering over her. (What did she look like?) *She was lying on her back in a funny position, like a rag doll, flat on the ground, and her face was bruised and she was bleeding profusely from her forehead. Her eyes were closed.* She was unconscious. (What do you mean?) *A man was trying to wake her up by slapping her on her face, and I remember I got very mad at that.* I don't remember what happened next. (What did you do when you saw Jennifer lying on the ground?) *I think I kicked the man, and then someone restrained me.* Vague memories of the ambulance. (Say more.) *I see the inside of the van and the emergency medical workers attending to Jennifer. Someone was holding me down. They gave me a shot. I must have been hysterical. I could see Jennifer's head, which they had bandaged up, and it was bloody....* It's all my fault.

A variant on this editing technique brings in the presence of the perpetrator. The clinician states that he or she will be responding in the role of the collaborator to the client's story. In this approach, the therapist's "edits and queries" will be challenging or negating ones, as if from the perpetrator's point of view. This activation of the perpetrator will mimic the actual situation inside the client's head, as he or she has hesitated to speak about what happened, as if at the behest of the perpetrator. This activity will externalize this confrontation with the negating influence of the perpetrator and allow more processing to occur. The therapist generally should write from the perspective of the collaborator, who is on the side of the perpetrator, and not directly in the perpetrator's voice. This type of intervention usually brings forward very strong emotions from the client, which are contained by the written word and delay between responses, but which nevertheless may break out into a rageful response when it seems that the perpetrator's perspective has gained any momentum.

> He took me over to the corner of the room. (Why were you there in the first place, if not to have sex?) *We were dating. I had no interest in being raped.* He pushed me down on the floor, rammed his finger into my rectum, and grabbed me very hard around the neck, and I thought he might be cutting off my circulation, and then pulled off my panties and tried to enter my vagina with his penis, which was not erect enough at first, so he yelled at me, grabbed me harder on the neck, and fingered my anus for several minutes. (Isn't this just a bit more rough sex than usual?) *I wasn't turned on, I was resisting him. He was hurting me.* Finally, he hit me in the small of my back and I cried out, which seemed to turn him on enough to be able to enter me. As he thrust himself into me, every once in a while he hit me again, hard, on the back, and then on the head. I cried, and then he laughed. (You never said "Stop" or "You are hurting me"?) *He was entirely self-absorbed and not with me at all. He didn't even care when I threw up.* I got sick to my stomach and threw up, but he kept pounding away. It was horrible. I felt like a slab of meat. (You were no slab of meat to him. He probably loves you!) *That's disgusting....He has no idea what love is.* I kept thinking what he was going to do to me after he finished. How long would I be dead before anyone would find me. (You are being dramatic.) *He was out of control. Crazy. That's what I was thinking.* Anyway, after about 15 minutes, he finally stopped. He put his clothes back on, spit on me, and left the apartment. (He was angry at you.) *Yes he was. And he raped me.*

This collaborator approach, although provocative, can greatly enhance the processing of traumatic memories by some clients, who are called to bring forth ideas and details in their own defense.

Two-Story Method

The two-story narrative technique can be useful when the client is unsure whether his or her memories are correct and when other people have questioned the veracity of those memories. If the therapist also has some doubt about the client's memories, the situation is particularly challenging (see Chapter 17, "Strains on the Therapist"). In the two-story method, the client is asked to write his or her story from two perspectives: 1) as if the story were absolutely true and 2) as if there were another explanation, such as mental illness. As in the legal system, which provides an arena for both sides of an issue to be presented in the best possible light, the client is asked to make every effort to be convincing in both texts. The clinician acts as the client's coach in helping to build a case for each view. In the end, the client and clinician jointly assess the credibility of the two descriptions. The following are examples from one client.

Version 1

> When I was about 3 years old, I remember being taken by my father to his shop at the lumber yard. I sat in the main office sometimes and sometimes in the back office. On several occasions, after the yard closed and everyone else had gone, I witnessed my father cutting up a dead body into pieces and putting them into a bag. He then put the bag in the trunk of our car, and he would drive me home and drop me off with my mother. He drove away for an hour or so and then came back and we had dinner. Looking back on this, I now know he was working with the Mafia, and his job was to dispose of some of the bodies. That was his job. His buddies often came over to the house and drank and laughed all night, or he would receive strange phone calls and then have to leave the house suddenly. I was really scared of him, and especially so because he hit me all the time and told me not to talk so much. He told me that I needed to be quiet. Now my parents deny all of this and have had me hospitalized whenever I start talking about it, saying I have bipolar disorder or psychosis. But I don't. I remember these things. They happened. Even if no one believes me.

Version 2

> When I was 16, I developed bipolar disorder and was hospitalized several times. I was apparently psychotic, and once took off all my clothes and walked down the street where I lived, knocking on neighbor's doors and shouting that my father was killing people. In my first hospitalization, I woke up one morning remembering that I had witnessed my father cutting up dead bodies in his lumber yard when I was very young, age 3 or 4. This was a symptom of my bipolar disorder. I also remembered many incidents of my father being drunk and hitting me and my mother, but both of them have said that it didn't happen. My dad has not had a drink in a long time, and both of them seem like normal, happy people now. I'm sure he was no angel when he was younger, but my memories are probably not true. I have a mental illness.

Following the preparation of the two reports, the client is asked to read them aloud and then to discuss his or her feelings about them. Then the therapist asks to read the two reports aloud to the client. Hearing the therapist read the two versions often helps the client to gain confidence in his or her own story as well as to acknowledge that a degree of uncertainty remains in his or her memories. Coming to an understanding that there are multiple perspectives on his or her traumatic experiences, despite the fact that a true event occurred, is a significant accomplishment for the trauma client and usually is associated with the attainment of a much greater level of equanimity.

Mailbox

The therapist prepares a mailbox out of a shoebox by cutting a slit in the top and printing "mailbox" in big letters on the side. The mailbox is kept on the therapist's desk or bookcase. When an issue arises during therapy in which the client expresses a desire to speak to, write to, or ask a question of a relevant person (e.g., perpetrator, family member, absent or dead person), the therapist asks the client whether he or she would like to write a letter to the person and send it through this special mailbox. The client may look at the cardboard box with a questioning look, and the therapist can then say, "Who knows? You might get a response!" The client writes his or her letter to the person, whether dead or alive and whether in or out of the client's life, making a statement or asking a question. The therapist then provides a real envelope, and the client addresses it and puts it into the mailbox. The therapist can inquire about how the client felt about writing the letter.

During the week between sessions, the therapist writes a response to the letter, acting in the role of the particular person, and puts it in an envelope addressed to the client and then into the box. When the client arrives for the next session, the therapist says, "I think you've got mail!" The client opens the mailbox and reads the letter. After discussing the letter, the client may want to carry on the correspondence. Throughout, the therapist playfully denies having anything to do with the letter and acts as if he or she is hearing the contents for the first time. This is underscored for the client when the client opens and reads the letter and the therapist says, "What did he (she) say?" or asks to read the letter.

This playful separation of the therapist and the other person allows the client to open up some of his or her feelings about that person. Most clients will show a certain amount of excitement that naturally comes from receiving and opening a letter to them. The therapist can choose to respond to his or her letters in a neutral way, not taking any particular stance, or can choose to stretch the client by presenting strong responses from the "person" (e.g., more rejecting, asking for forgiveness, avoiding or taking responsibility, attacking the client), based on what might enhance the therapeutic process.

FIRST WEEK

CLIENT: I hope he rots in hell.

THERAPIST: If you could, would you want to write him a letter where he is, in hell?

CLIENT: That would be sweet.

THERAPIST: Look, I have a special mailbox that sends letters anywhere you want.

CLIENT: Right.

THERAPIST: Here, write him a letter and we will send it, and maybe next week when you come, he will have written back!

CLIENT: Okay. (*Writes letter.*)

THERAPIST: Do you want to read it to me?

CLIENT: Sure. "I hope you…"

THERAPIST: Start it with, "Dear Robert," like a real letter.

CLIENT: "Dear Robert, I hope this letter finds you suffering in hell. Dying of cancer was a really great way to get sympathy and distract people from what you did to me and sis. I can't believe you got away with everything….I remember, though, everything you did to me. Every minute of your touching me and drinking and stupidity. I'm writing I guess because I'd like to know if you're sorry. If you cared at all. Sincerely, your niece, Sarah." That's stupid, he doesn't care. Why do I want him to feel sorry?

THERAPIST: Good question. At one time you looked up to him, even loved him, and then he betrayed that trust and harmed you and the relationship. Do you think he'll write back?

CLIENT: Yeah, he will. Some bullshit though.

THERAPIST: Let's see! (*Client places letter in envelope and into the box.*)

SECOND WEEK

THERAPIST: Hi. So I think you've got mail.

CLIENT: No kidding (*smiles*).

THERAPIST: Smiling because you got a letter? (*Offers her the box.*)

CLIENT: (*Takes the letter out and reads it.*)

THERAPIST: What did he say?

CLIENT: You know, you wrote it!

THERAPIST: I did not (*smiles*). That would be mail tampering. Read it to me.

CLIENT: "Dear Sarah, thank you for your letter. I can't believe your letter made it down here. Yup, I'm in hell and it's bad, not like you'd think, but bad. Can't tell the days from the nights. Thanks for your thoughts about my cancer. I suffered so much. Glad to have all the family support—yours too! In terms of feeling sorry, I can't say I know what you mean. Did you think I did something to you? Touching you or drinking? Freckles, I don't think that happened. Maybe you imagined something? Maybe someone else? Anyway, have to go now. Write again if you want! Love and hugs, Uncle Robert."

THERAPIST: That was something. (*Silence.*)
CLIENT: I guess I should have expected that. (*Tears up.*)
THERAPIST: Is it okay for you to have wanted him to say he's sorry?
CLIENT: I don't know…Yes.
THERAPIST: You think so because you are a caring, healthy person. He was not.
CLIENT: I feel so bad to have opened myself up to him and have him reject me, again.
THERAPIST: Why don't you write him back and tell him, straight out.
CLIENT: Okay. (*Writes letter and puts it into the box without showing it to the therapist.*)

"Dear Robert, Your denial that you did anything to me hurt me a lot. I opened myself up to you because somewhere inside me I loved you, and I can't get over the fact that you did not care for me, that you abused me and sis, and that you hid behind your cancer as a way of avoiding me. But I do not hate you anymore. I am sad for you. You lost me and yourself and God. And I lost you. But I am doing well, and life is good for me now. Goodbye. Do not write me back. S."

THIRD WEEK

THERAPIST: Hi. How are you doing?
CLIENT: Good. I really felt good last week writing that letter.
THERAPIST: What did you say to him?
CLIENT: I said that I wasn't angry at him anymore. That I felt sad for him, and I said goodbye to him and not to write me back.
THERAPIST: Oh. I hate to say this, but you got a letter.
CLIENT (*a little annoyed*): I told him not to write back!
THERAPIST: Since when has he listened to you?
CLIENT: (*Thinking.*)
THERAPIST: What would you like to do?
CLIENT: I'm not opening that letter from him. I'm done.
THERAPIST: You could write, "Return to sender" on it and send it back?
CLIENT: Great idea! (*Takes letter out of box, writes "Return to sender" on it, and puts it back in the box. Sighs.*) That's that.
THERAPIST: Yup! (*Smiles, pauses, and continues the session.*)

For this client, the mailbox provides a distanced way of dialoguing with her perpetrator, allowing her to reveal her underlying care for her uncle, and dealing with the fact that she will never receive an apology from him. Paradoxically, the mailbox creates a sense of immediacy and encounter that would not have the same sense of surprise if it had been discussed or even role-played with the therapist. The focus remains on the client's relationship with her uncle and not on what the therapist might think.

This technique can be used with a client of any age, depending on whether the therapist believes that the specific client will enjoy it. Some teenagers are very interested in writing letters, and even young children understand the concept of writing a letter and often get excited about the idea of receiving personal mail. The therapist needs to be comfortable with taking the time to respond in writing to the client.

ARTWORK TECHNIQUES

Two-Dimensional Grid

In the first phase of the two-dimensional grid technique, the therapist begins by asking the client to draw a picture (using pencils, crayons, markers, pastels, or watercolors) of his or her traumatic event. This request may occur when during the trauma inquiry a particularly powerful scene is described that might lend itself to visual rendering. After discussing the picture, the clinician asks the client to draw another picture of the trauma, either a few moments before or a few moments after the initial picture, to provide a sequenced rendition of the event. This is repeated in both directions until a series of pictures extends from before the beginning of the traumatic event through to the end of the event. If the clinician notes a jump between two pictures, he or she may ask the client to draw the moment in between, in order to capture the avoided experience. The collection of pictures can be laid out on the floor like a cartoon or triptych, or they can be stapled together in order from front to back. This chronology then provides the backbone for the next phase.

Choosing a picture from the middle near the climax of the event, the clinician either points out or lightly circles with a pencil a smaller area of the picture and asks the client to "zoom in" and draw another picture of just that piece, now greatly expanded. This is the visual equivalent to the verbal technique of getting more details. The same process can be repeated with the new drawing, so that the pictures zoom in to smaller and smaller areas of the event, perhaps to the face of the perpetrator or another visual detail that the client fixated on. These detail pictures are then placed vertically below the initial sequence of pictures. Likewise, the clinician can ask the client to zoom out from the original picture and view the trauma scene from further away. These pictures are placed above the initial sequence. This process can be repeated for any or all of the pictures along the entire chronological continuum, resulting in a two-dimensional array of pictures of varying detail, from beginning to end. The result of such a project can be quite stunning. The purpose is to locate the most intense moments (in time) and sights (in space) of the traumatic event.

Figure 16–1 is an example of a two-dimensional grid. The first picture drawn by the client is the picture in the middle (labeled 2), depicting his father coming into the room to beat him when he was a teenager. The client then drew the picture labeled 1, which was of a few moments before, as the father was driving into the driveway with his car, signaling the client that he might be beaten. The picture (labeled 3) was then drawn, depicting the client lying on the floor after he had been beaten. The therapist then drew a small circle around the father's hand in picture 2 and asked the client to zoom in on it; the client then drew the fourth picture (labeled 4), showing his father's fist. The client reported that it was this image that showed up most often in his dreams and nightmares.

Conversational Art

In the conversational art technique, the clinician begins by asking the client to draw a picture of anything he or she likes, perhaps a squiggle or an abstract form. The client is told ahead of time that the exercise will involve the client and clinician working together on the same sheet of paper. The client then hands the clinician the paper, and the clinician draws on it in a way that is consistent with, is supportive of, and mirrors what the client has drawn. For example, if the client draws a flower, the therapist draws a similar flower or a garden bed around the flower. Then the clinician gives the picture back to the client, who draws more as he or she wishes. The next time the clinician has the picture, he or she draws lines, colors, or shapes that offer some challenge—are at some tension with—what the client has drawn. For example, in a drawing where mostly pastel colors are drawn, the clinician might use a dark brown or black marker to draw a shadowy figure in the corner or another shape pushing up against a particularly pretty part of the picture. The aim is to represent a slight challenge to what the client is drawing, without spoiling or ruining the picture. How the client responds in his or her next turn at drawing will indicate the client's basic attitudes toward threat: to wall off, try to erase, ignore, or lose interest are all possible protective responses. The client may also respond in more adaptive or creative ways, integrating the discrepant images into a coherent whole. Throughout this process, the clinician and client carry on a conversation about what is happening in the picture, as well as how the client's drawn responses are linked to current behaviors in the client's life.

Unlike methods of art making where the therapist observes the client drawing and inquires about the client's thought process, conversational art allows the therapist to join the conversation in a manner that can influence and challenge the client. The therapist can identify and challenge the cli-

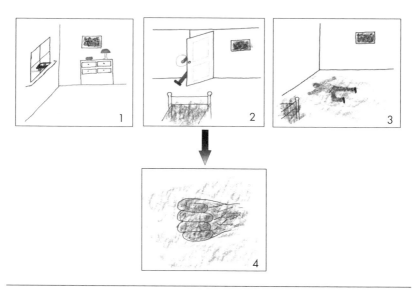

FIGURE 16–1.   Example of a two-dimensional grid.

ent's avoidant behaviors and can then introduce graduated levels of imaginal exposure to images related to the traumatic events. The developing picture on the paper becomes a concrete representation of the shared relationship between client and therapist, which many clients appreciate.

A particularly powerful extension of this technique that the clinician might use is called *harming the picture*. In this exercise, the clinician asks the client to draw a picture of a positive memory or a scene that is peaceful for him or her. The clinician initially contributes to the picture by adding details that fit in with the feeling of the picture or enhance the peaceful feeling. When it appears that the client has begun to invest in this picture, the clinician then explains that the next part of the exercise will involve his or her adding something to the picture that will significantly interfere with or mess up the picture, serving as a metaphor for what the traumatic event did to the client's life. Then the clinician, in his or her next turn, does something to the picture that ruins it, such as by drawing a large black spot, drawing a big X over an image, covering something over, or smudging an image with a finger. Even worse things can be done: ripping part of the picture, crumpling it up to wrinkle it, or cutting a hole in the middle. Even though these actions may evoke a playful wringing of hands, how the client reacts when he or she gets back the ruined and spoiled picture will be important. How he or she handles this moment will reveal many of the client's trauma schemas, adaptive strategies, and resiliency. The client may adapt by making the X or black spot into something that fits in with the original drawing; may wall it off with pretty colors; may fold the paper into an origami object or airplane; or may refuse to work on it anymore, throw it away, rip it up even more, or declare that he or she did not like the picture to begin with. These attitudes can easily be linked to feelings of resiliency, defensiveness, hopelessness, or wanting to give up on their lives after the trauma.

Figure 16–2 illustrates a drawing by a 35-year-old female client, whose trauma was witnessing her brother being shot and killed several years before. She initially drew a bucolic scene with hill, tree, and two children holding balloons. The therapist added a sun. Then the client put in a house and two children on a teeter-totter. The therapist added smoke from the chimney. Then the therapist gave the client instructions for the harming-the-picture technique and blackened over the boy with the balloon. The client handled the intrusion by enclosing the clinician's black spot within a pretty pink fence. In their discussion, this was easily linked to her adaptive strategy of appearing happy to her husband despite having many anxiety symptoms. The therapist then used the zoom technique, asking the client to draw the black area from close up. The result, shown in Figure 16–3, is an image of her brother's face just before he was shot. The client was then able to describe in much more detail and with deeper emotion the moments that led up to that horrific event. Later, she showed her husband both drawings, which led to his greater understanding about what his wife had been dealing with.

Self-Portrait

In the self-portrait exercise, the client is asked to draw a self-portrait of himself or herself in the present. Then the client is asked to draw a self-portrait at the time of the trauma (during the worst moment). If the client has other important traumatic events, he or she is asked to draw a portrait for each event. The portraits from the past are then placed in a pile, with the earliest portrait on top. The current portrait is placed on the bottom facing the other direction, so that when the client holds up the stack, with all the past portraits facing him or her, the current self-portrait will be facing the therapist. The therapist then explains that the client is showing his or her present face to the therapist while simultaneously being aware of all the past faces from his or her traumas. The therapist can ask, "Whom will you let me speak to?" and the client, if he or she wishes, can place a portrait on the table and carry on a conversation with the therapist about what, for example, the child experienced, and so on with the others. The client often holds one portrait to the last and is reluctant to share it. The irony is that by having drawn it concretely in front of the therapist, the client knows that

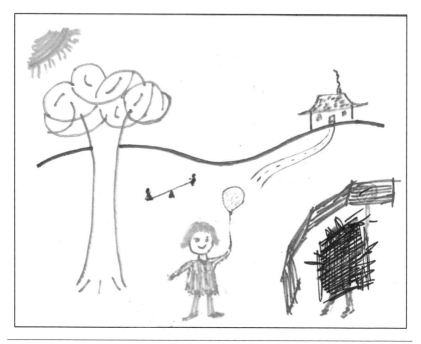

FIGURE 16–2.   Example of conversational art utilizing the technique of harming the picture.

the therapist knows that it is there—this is precisely the situation that is desired in trauma-centered psychotherapy. Some clients may want to use these portraits from time to time to aid them in talking about their various traumatic memories.

Perpetrator Portraits

In trauma work, the tendency is for most attention to be placed on the victim. The result is that the perpetrator is often overlooked, and this is a mistake. Having the client draw a portrait of the perpetrator is a powerful, challenging activity that can significantly aid in facing the cause of the client's suffering. The initial attitude is often that by drawing or thinking or speaking about the perpetrator, one gives attention to, pays homage to, and therefore maintains the power of the perpetrator. Actually, however, by keeping the perpetrator unchallenged in the shadows, his or her power remains. The client should be asked first to draw the perpetrator as the client remembers him or her during the traumatic event. Other portraits of the perpetrator at other times, perhaps when he or she was not abusive, can

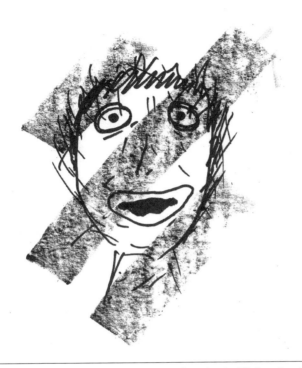

FIGURE 16–3. Example of conversational art utilizing the technique of zooming in on the blacked-out figure depicted in Figure 16–2.

then be requested. As noted in Chapter 15, "Trauma-Centered Couples and Family Psychotherapy," a portrait of the perpetrator can be displayed in each therapy session (individual or family) as a reminder of his or her presence. The basic question that such a portrait raises is this: What is there to do about him or her? The person may be dead, or jailed, or living with the client. An effective exercise is for the clinician to place a blank sheet of white paper on the table next to the perpetrator's portrait, along with a few paper clips, some tape, scissors, and markers. The therapist then says to the client, "Using these materials, do something that makes sense to you about this portrait." Whatever the client chooses to do or attempt to do will enhance the discussion about his or her recovery.

Photographs and Videotaping

Some clients may be interested in bringing in photographs of themselves, their families, or their surroundings from the time of their traumatic events.

Others may want to go out and take photos of the places where the events took place. All of these can aid recall and ground the discussion in concrete stimuli. In one remarkable case, a client videotaped an actual interview with her father, from whom she had been alienated nearly her entire life, on the circumstances of her early life with him, including asking him on tape if he had sexually abused her. All of these methods stimulate clients to move into productive and creative action regarding their trauma stories, and thus tend to engender feelings of empowerment in addition to the desensitization.

THERAPEUTIC CEREMONIES

When concrete objects have been produced, whether they are written texts, artwork, or photos, the issue of disposal arises. Many clients will want to keep and preserve their representations of themselves and their traumatic events. However, others have a desire to destroy these items. It may be useful to organize this process within a ceremonial frame. The typically chosen disposal techniques involve 1) burying, 2) burning, or 3) shredding. The clinician can offer help in structuring a brief ceremony in which the client prepares a statement explaining why he or she is disposing of these memories (usually referencing moving on, progressing, or leaving them behind). The client then decides whether to invite anyone in his or her social network to join in the ceremony. Other people may wish to speak as well. From a trauma-centered perspective, these ceremonies have more therapeutic value if 1) they include some of the details of the trauma, 2) the perpetrator is specifically mentioned or represented, and 3) the remains are not completely destroyed but are transformed into something of value.

In one possible type of disposal ceremony, the therapist and client gather outside with close family members (e.g., spouse, child, parents) during the client's normal session time. The client brings a sampling of objects (e.g., diaries, drawings, poems) to destroy. A script similar to the following, which involves burning of materials, can be used.

> THERAPIST: We are here to honor the progress toward recovery of (name), who has experienced the traumatic event of [named] when she was (mention age) years old. She was harmed by [name the perpetrator], who changed her life forever. (*Turns to client.*) You have worked very hard to confront and process these memories; to transform your relationship to the perpetrator of your trauma [name perpetrator again]; and to find new people, activities, and interests in the world that are meaningful to you. Please tell us of your journey.
> CLIENT: (*Says what she wishes.*)
> THERAPIST: You now wish to transform your diaries of your suffering, to allow them to pass on in new ways into the world.

CLIENT: Yes, I do. (*All watch as material is burned.*)

THERAPIST: Nothing will eliminate the memories of the traumatic event you experienced; however, your experience can inform you and help you in your future work, as these ashes will feed the ground in which they are placed. What is your hope?

CLIENT: (*Says what she wants about how the ashes will help something else grow. Clients often know where they want the ashes to go: under a newly planted tree, in their backyard at home, etc. A client, perhaps with the help of family and therapist, digs the hole, places the ashes in it, and covers them with the ground.*)

THERAPIST: May the remnants of your [name the trauma: e.g., sexual assault, loss of your child] be forever changed—no longer repeating themselves over and over again, but feeding new growth, just as these ashes of your former diaries will feed the growth of [name the place or tree].

In some situations, such as when therapists are not comfortable or are unable to go outside, the client can be asked to burn the material himself or herself and to bring the ashes to the office in a jar or canister. Some clients use the pieces of their diaries or drawings to make a new artwork, such as a collage that shows something more hopeful about their future. One client took pieces of her clothing and fashioned a quilt that she gave to a homeless shelter. It is often useful to allow brief comments by the other people who attend the ceremony, as a way of celebrating the client's success.

Johnson (2012) and Lubin and Johnson (2003) have written more extensively about healing and therapeutic ceremonies for traumatized people.

ROLE-PLAYING TECHNIQUES

Telephone

Many clinicians are not comfortable role-playing with their clients. However, the use of a telephone or cell phone is an excellent adjunctive technique for clients who prefer a more concrete form of processing and one that many therapists find palatable. Talking on the phone is such a normal function in society today that for most people, talking on a pretend phone will feel somewhat comfortable. One of the major advantages of the use of the telephone in individual therapy is that it introduces a third person with whom the clinician can carry on a conversation when the client comes to a halt. When the individual therapy process is decentered, impasses can sometimes be avoided.

Another advantage of using the phone is that the therapist does not need to role-play other characters; the therapist continues as himself or herself and stays true to what he or she is thinking about the client. The questions asked of a pretend person on the other end of the phone are the same ones that would be asked of the actual person. The telephone helps to concretize the speculation of the client and therapist about the traumatic events and the other important people involved.

For role-playing with the telephone, the clinician needs to have available a telephone or cell phone that does not actually work (e.g., a cell phone not turned on, a telephone that is not connected). We describe several exercises involving use of the telephone.

THERAPIST CALLS SOMEONE

When the client is talking about someone else relevant to his or her traumatic experience (e.g., family member, witness, perpetrator) and the client refers to some ambiguity about what that person thinks or feels, the therapist says, "Well, let's find out. I'm going to pretend to call him now. Do you know the number? (Clients rarely do.) That's okay, I can look it up." The therapist then pretends to dial a number and talk to the person (who might actually be in jail, dead, living with the client, or in an unknown location). The therapist asks that person several questions about how he or she experienced the event and then responds as if the person answered. Occasionally, the therapist can respond as if the person is asking a question and then turn to the client and say, "He wants to know how you are doing?" or "She thinks that what you said is incorrect." Sometimes, a lively discussion occurs, supported by the element of humor in this situation. The trauma victim, however, is usually so engaged in processing memories that he or she brings to this activity a great deal of authentic feeling.

Quite often, when the therapist is acting as the conduit between the (pretend) person on the phone and the client, the conversation will heat up to the point that the therapist can say, "I can't answer that; why don't you talk to him?" and hand the phone to the client.

This technique is helpful in carrying on a third-party conversation when there is no third party. When the client gets stuck or is reluctant to continue a trauma inquiry, the therapist can pretend to call another person who was present at the traumatic event or perhaps another therapist or police officer who might have information.

In the following case example, the client is an 8-year-old girl who was abused by a neighbor who was babysitting.

> THERAPIST: So the babysitter took off your clothes and her own clothes?
> CLIENT: (*Nods.*) Yes.

THERAPIST: Were you scared?

CLIENT: No, she said it was a game.

THERAPIST: I see. Then what happened?

CLIENT: (*Hesitates.*) She hurt me.

THERAPIST: How did she hurt you?

CLIENT: (*Shakes head.*)

THERAPIST: It's hard to talk about this. It must have been pretty bad.

CLIENT: (*Nods.*)

THERAPIST: Does your babysitter know what she did to you?

CLIENT: (*Nods.*)

THERAPIST: If it's okay with you, I'm going to make a pretend call to her on this pretend phone! See, it doesn't work for real, but I am going to call her up anyway and ask her, okay? (*She nods and smiles.*)

THERAPIST: (*Dials.*) What's her first name?

CLIENT: Rachel.

THERAPIST: Hello? Rachel? Hi, this is Dr. Jones and I am here with Angelina. Yeah, and we are talking about what you did to her when you were babysitting her. Yeah. Can I ask a few questions? Great, because this isn't a real phone call, you can tell me the truth! All right, so Angelina was saying that you introduced her to a game where she and you took off your clothes, and then you hurt her, but Angelina is having a hard time talking about it. Yeah. So how did you hurt Angelina? Oh…That's terrible. Did you slap her? (*Angelina shakes her head.*) Did you pinch her? (*Angelina nods.*) How many times? Two times?

CLIENT: Five times.

THERAPIST: And did you pinch her in her private parts? Yes? (*Angelina looks down.*) And did you put your finger in her private parts? No?

CLIENT: Yes she did!

THERAPIST: Wait a minute, Angelina said you did. Are you lying to me, Rachel? (*Angelina nods.*) Please don't do that. And did you ask Angelina to touch your private parts? Yes? (*Angelina looks down.*) With her fingers? (*Angelina looks upset.*) Uh-huh, and anything else? (*Angelina starts fidgeting.*) Rachel, did you ask Angelina to touch your private parts with her mouth? (*Angelina starts to cry.*) That was very bad, Rachel. Did you have to hold her head down? No?

CLIENT: Yes you did!

THERAPIST (*to Angelina*): She's lying to me; I think you will have to tell her yourself. (*Hands the phone to Angelina.*)

CLIENT: You pushed me down and held my head and told me to lick you like it was cherry pie! You liar! (*Hangs up the phone.*)

THERAPIST: She lied to me.

CLIENT: What a liar.

THERAPIST: I'm so sorry that happened. And I'm glad that you helped me get the truth out from her. Thank you. I assume that's not all that she did… (*Angelina then proceeds to talk more about the event.*)

In this example, the client's anxiety about continuing to talk about the traumatic event is circumvented by the presentation of the perpetrator as a third person in the interaction. The fact that this was a completely imagined conversation was not an obstacle to the client, whose interest in getting the facts right overrode the artifice of the role-play. The concrete nature of the telephone provided enough sense of reality to engage the client effectively. The therapist did not act as a drama therapist with special theatrical skills, but instead spoke naturally as if the perpetrator was present, using the questions appropriate to the standard trauma inquiry.

Making a pretend telephone call to a third party is also useful when the client wants to know what the therapist thinks that person's views are, even though the therapist may never have met him or her. The therapist really has no basis to guess but often does. Using the dramatic frame of the telephone often provides the therapist with more flexibility to explore the possibilities.

CLIENT: Do you think my mother believes my story?
THERAPIST: I don't know. Let me call her. (*Dials the phone.*) Hello, Ms. Smith. This is Dr. Davis, and I am here with your daughter in a therapy session, and she was wondering whether you believe her story about being sexually molested by your nephew.…Uh-huh…Really?…Why do you think that?…But she has a lot of details…I know…Of course it would be upsetting.….All right, I appreciate your talking to me.… You're welcome, anytime. Bye. (*The therapist then turns to the client.*) Well, she seems to have a lot of doubt about it. It is her nephew, you know.…
CLIENT: But I'm her daughter!
THERAPIST: Absolutely, and she said that, so actually I am of the mind that she does believe you but cannot bring herself to acknowledge it because it would mean she would have to change her behavior around the rest of her family.

In this session fragment, the therapist is able to communicate two sides of an issue with a diminished focus on whether these views are the therapist's personal views. The dramatic frame creates a useful distance that maintains a focus on what the mother might feel, as opposed to what the therapist thinks.

INCOMING PHONE CALL

The incoming phone call variation is best used once the phone has been used several times and the novelty has worn off. When the client is talking, the therapist suddenly makes a "ring, ring" sound and looks over at the phone and then turns to the client and asks, "Do you want me to answer this?" or "Is she calling us back?" If the client says no, the therapist moves on and then a few moments later says "ring, ring" again. Human beings have a number of irresistible urges, one of which is to answer a ringing phone, even if it is pretend, so it is likely that the client will want the therapist to pick up the phone or even do so himself or herself. The therapy is enhanced either if the client wants to answer the phone and an ensuing discussion takes place with the third party or if the therapist and client mutually agree to ignore the call and let it ring, representing the client's feelings about making contact with that third party. When the therapist represents the phone call as coming in from the other person, the independence and freedom of the perpetrator, so feared by the client, can be strongly evoked and then dealt with in the session.

CLIENT MAKES A CALL

Eventually, the client will know that making a (pretend) call is an option in therapy and may ask to call someone he or she is talking about. These moments are very interesting, because the client will speak, and the therapist will not be privy to what the other person is saying. Once the phone call is completed, the therapist should ask, "So, what did he (she) say?"

The following is an expanded example of the telephone technique with a 10-year-old boy who had experienced severe physical abuse by his biological father from age 4 to 8, prior to the boy's removal from the family home. He has been in a reasonably caring foster home for 2 years and has demonstrated occasional aggression and provocative behaviors at school.

> THERAPIST: So let's spend some time talking about what your father did to you.
> CLIENT: I've talked about this a lot before. He hit me.
> THERAPIST: I understand that it began when you were about 4?
> CLIENT: (*Sullen.*) Yeah, about then.
> THERAPIST: What was your first memory of being hit.
> CLIENT: He was drunk and yelling at my mom, and I started crying and he came over and hit me on the face.
> THERAPIST: What did you do then?
> CLIENT: I don't remember.
> THERAPIST: Over the years, how often was he violent with you?
> CLIENT: He hit my mom every day.
> THERAPIST: How often did he hit you?
> CLIENT: (*Hesitates.*) A lot.
> THERAPIST: Do you remember the worst time?
> CLIENT: I don't want to talk about it.

THERAPIST: I understand, it's got to be upsetting, but that is what we are here to do. I'm sorry this happened to you.

CLIENT: They were having a fight in the living room and he hit my mom hard, and she screamed. She ran up the stairs to her bedroom. I came out of my bedroom to see what was happening and to stop my dad from coming up the stairs to hurt her again. He came up anyway and slugged me hard in the chest, and then he pushed me down the stairs to get by me.

THERAPIST: That's terrible.

CLIENT: I broke my shoulder. That's what made the state remove us.

THERAPIST: Were you frightened?

CLIENT: (*Nods. Looks sad.*)

THERAPIST: You have had time to think about this. Why was your dad this way?

CLIENT: Drank too much, I don't know. He did it when he didn't drink too. I don't really know.

THERAPIST: Did you ever ask him?

CLIENT: No, I stayed away from him.

THERAPIST: You see this phone here? It's not real, but sometimes I use it to call up people. Mind if I call him up now and ask him?

CLIENT: Whatever, okay.

THERAPIST: Where is he?

CLIENT: West Haven.

THERAPIST: Know his number

CLIENT: Yeah. 203-555-9387.

THERAPIST: (*Dials it.*) Hello, this is Dr. Jones from the Health Center. I'm here with your son, and I asked him why you hit him and his mother, and he wasn't sure. Do you mind if I ask you directly?… Great…Anger problems…From childhood?…I see…Better now… Anger management classes are good, yes.… Oh, that's nice.…Well, thank you, I may need to call you again, if that's all right?…Okay, bye.

CLIENT: What did he say? He took anger management classes and he's okay?

THERAPIST: Exactly. Said he had anger problems from his childhood but that he has worked on it, and he is better.

CLIENT: I don't believe it.

THERAPIST: Is he a smooth talker?

CLIENT: Yes. He wants to visit me, and that's what he says, that he is all better. But I don't want to see him.

THERAPIST: He caused a lot of damage to the family.

CLIENT: Yeah.

THERAPIST: Have you told him that you don't want to visit him?

CLIENT: No.

THERAPIST: (*Picks up phone.*) Why don't you tell him now and get it over with? I'll make the call.

CLIENT: No, I don't think so.

THERAPIST: Great thing about this is that he's not really on the other side of the phone. (*Client smiles.*) Let me talk to him first. (*Dials.*) Hello,

Mr. Smith. This is Dr. Jones again, yeah. I have your son here, and he'd like to say something to you…Yeah, that's right…Frankly, neither he nor I think you have fully realized the damage you did to your family…No, a couple of anger management classes just doesn't do it…That's right…So, if you don't mind, let me put your son on, and I'd like you not to interrupt him, okay? (*Hands phone to client.*) Here.

CLIENT: Hi, Dad…I wanted to tell you that I don't want you to visit me… I'm not ready, I guess…I know you love me (*rolls eyes at therapist*), but I don't want you to visit now, okay?…I got to go now, Dad…Bye.

THERAPIST: (*Looks at client.*) So, what did he say?

CLIENT: The same old thing…He's sorry and wants to visit.

THERAPIST: How did he take what you said?

CLIENT: I don't think he listens to me.

THERAPIST: Was his tone respectful?

CLIENT: He didn't argue with me.

THERAPIST: That's good.

Memory Box

The memory box is a small wooden or metal box that has a lock or combination lock on it. Written on it in large letters is the phrase "DO NOT OPEN!" Inside, the therapist will initially have put some small objects or paper, enough so that if the box is picked up, the client will hear something rattling around inside. When the client comes to a memory that he or she is having a hard time discussing or if the client says, "I don't want to talk about that" or "I never want to tell anyone else about that," the therapist will offer the client the opportunity to write the memory on a piece of paper and place it into the memory box, and then lock it. The box stays in the therapist's office in view of the client and can be referred to during future sessions, especially in working on the client's ambivalence around disclosure or discussing his or her traumatic memories. The therapist also playfully decides with the client about who shall keep the key to the lock. The client may also bring in small objects that remind him or her of certain memories that he or she wants to put into the box.

CLIENT: I'd rather not talk about that.

THERAPIST: Okay, but the rule around here is that you have to put memories you don't want to talk about into the memory box, see? Over here. It's got a lock and says, "DO NOT OPEN!" Agreed?

CLIENT: Guess so.

THERAPIST: Write down the memory you don't want to talk about on this paper, and we can put it in the box.

CLIENT: (*Starts writing but then stops.*) I have a photo of myself in my wallet. Can I write it on that?

THERAPIST: Certainly. (*Client does.*) Okay, here's the key.

CLIENT: (*Laughs.*) Awesome. (*Picks up the box and hears a rattling sound.*) Heh, what's that?

THERAPIST: Probably some of the other memories you haven't told me about yet.

CLIENT: Really? How'd you know about them?

THERAPIST: Experience.

CLIENT: (*Opens the box, looks in, and places the photograph in the box and closes it.*)

THERAPIST: You are sure you don't want to talk about it now.

CLIENT: Yes, I'm sure.

THERAPIST: Then lock it up.

CLIENT: (*Does so. Holds the key in her hand.*) What now?

THERAPIST: The box stays here, safe and locked. "DO NOT OPEN."

CLIENT: I never told you that it started earlier, when I was age 6.

THERAPIST: I didn't know that, but you are breaking the rules. Can't talk about it if it's in the box.

CLIENT: (*Looks at box warily.*) I'm not going to be able to get it off my mind when I come here, knowing it's in that box.

THERAPIST: Only one way to solve that problem.

CLIENT: Open the box.

THERAPIST: That's right.

CLIENT: Okay, but in my own time. All right? (*Smiles at therapist.*)

In this session fragment, the box serves as a useful device to concretize the client's avoidance, but by becoming a constant reminder of her avoidance, the box undermines it. Avoidance works best if the act of avoidance itself is also covered up. The box represents the therapist's respect for the client's need to avoid, yet at the same time serves as an enticement for her to reveal. The therapist can take a mildly paradoxical stance whenever the client begins to reveal a memory, by hesitating and gesturing toward the box, stimulating the client's urge to speak out.

This technique, like the mailbox technique described earlier in chapter (see section "Narrative Approaches"), can be used with a client of any age, if the need arises and if the therapist thinks the client will enjoy it. The technique is particularly useful for teenagers, who often enjoy being in control and locking the therapist out of their private spaces.

CONCLUSION

The adjunctive methods discussed in this chapter are not necessary in order to conduct trauma-centered psychotherapy. However, with certain clients, these techniques will be helpful in overcoming avoidance and encouraging more detailed remembering. Younger clients often enjoy these techniques, but quite a few adults have surprised us with their enthusiasm as well. The playful, concrete, and distanced elements of these techniques may be effective with certain clients. These techniques can also be helpful to therapists, by engaging them in more playful and active modes of interacting with their clients.

STUDY QUESTIONS

16.1 When might a therapist suggest a written narrative approach to a client?

16.2 T/F In the two-story method, each story should be written to be as credible as possible.

16.3 T/F In the two-story method, the goal is to tolerate the ambiguity of not knowing for certain the truth of the traumatic experience.

16.4 What is the main rationale for using the mailbox method?

16.5 T/F In the two-dimensional grid, the goal is for the client to identify and express the moments of greatest distress in his or her traumatic memories.

16.6 T/F In the two-dimensional grid, the client moves forward or backward in time, and zooms inward or outward in proximity, from the first picture.

16.7 What are the advantages of the therapist participating in the conversational art method?

16.8 T/F The purpose of the technique of harming the picture is to flood the client with emotion.

16.9 T/F The aim of perpetrator portraits supports the goal of disclosing the perpetrator.

16.10 T/F The use of photographs and videotaping often increases the vividness of the client's recall of his or her experiences, and therefore aids in the desensitization process.

16.11 What reasons do clients have to desire to dispose of their autobiographical materials?

16.12 Why is the use of the telephone usually more comfortable for the therapist in role-playing with the client?

16.13 How does use of the memory box address the client's avoidance?

CHAPTER 17

Strains on the Therapist

Every career has its strains, monotonies, and challenges; indeed, many people choose demanding careers for the stimulation and challenge provided over the many years of working life. Trauma-centered psychotherapy is not unique in this regard: it has both deep rewards and perils. These have been well described in a number of excellent texts on trauma work (Dalenberg 2000; Figley 1995; Pearlman and Saakvitne 1995; Wilson and Lindy 1994). In this chapter, we discuss these strains (Table 17–1) not so much in the context of helping the therapist develop self-care strategies, but rather in relation to how they play out in the clinical interaction with clients, consistent with the focus of this book. Part of the job of a trauma-centered therapist is to know how to manage and tolerate these strains. Indeed, there would be deep irony in a trauma therapist's complaints about hearing too much horror, just as there would be in a surgeon's complaints about seeing too much blood. For therapists, managing the stresses of work is best achieved through competence at the tasks they are expected to perform.

NOT UNDERSTANDING THE CLIENT: COMPASSION FATIGUE

A common effect of trauma is that the victim becomes separated from the web of life and relationships. For the victim to feel protected from further invasion or injury, his or her cognitive and interpersonal boundaries become highly demarcated and rigid. The client will often say, "No one can

---

TABLE 17–1.   Strains on the trauma-centered psychotherapist

Not understanding the client: compassion fatigue

Conducting psychotherapy in which an empathic connection between client and therapist is constantly interrupted by trauma schemas can over time cause intense strain and fatigue in the therapist, which must be attended to so that the therapist can continue to provide excellent care.

Not believing the client: false memory and credibility

Extreme or exaggerated descriptions of traumatic events can cause the therapist, who is charged with supporting and believing in the client, to doubt the credibility of the stories. This can lead to intense distress and confusion in the therapist.

Hearing too much: vicarious traumatization

Being exposed to descriptions of intense, horrible events on a frequent basis can cause significant strain in the therapist, which can lead to the development of symptoms of stress such as emotional numbing, reliance on substances, irritability, and sleep disturbance.

Wanting to harm the perpetrator: retaliation and rage

Listening to acts of interpersonal violence while being in a relatively helpless position to do anything about their prevention can cause the therapist to experience intense rage and desire to retaliate, which may interfere with his or her therapeutic tasks.

Wanting to rescue the client: advocacy, charity, and adoption

Experiencing helplessness in relation to the past traumas of clients, therapists may become activated to fulfill their clients' needs in the present, which may interfere with their work as psychotherapists.

Having to be there: emergencies and phone calls

Responding to the many outside-of-session emergencies that some clients experience can cause states of intense distress and then avoidance in therapists. The therapist must have a plan to handle these common demands of trauma treatment.

---

understand what happened to me." Indeed, no one else was present, in that exact location, perceiving the same stimuli, and thinking the same thoughts.

The fundamental basis for the role of the psychotherapist has been an idealized and corrective figure: the good-enough mother, the empathic and genuine listener, the one person who can understand. The attraction of this role is often a reason that people are drawn into the field. A good session is when the client and therapist have reached across the divide, bridged the gap of understanding, and achieved an alliance, a bond, and a working relationship.

However, as the trauma-centered psychotherapist approaches the inner areas in proximity to the client's trauma schemas, the therapist comes to the unfathomable cliff, where he or she will stand and witness the client, again, falling into the chasm, as the therapist stands by helpless to alter the outcome. As discussed in Chapter 9, "The Gap: When the Trauma Schema Emerges in the Therapeutic Relationship," these moments may be a sign that the treatment is progressing, not so much in bridging this gap but rather in recognizing its origins and engaging in the mourning process. Thus, trauma-centered psychotherapy is not based on the establishment of empathy, but rather on engagement with the truth.

For therapists who are unaware of this difference, working with traumatized clients becomes burdensome and distressing. As their attempts to connect with, understand, and help a client initially seem to succeed and then suddenly falter and occasionally fail, therapists can become frustrated or despondent that their every effort has been thwarted by the very person asking, even demanding, their help. This phenomenon in the therapist has been termed *compassion fatigue* (Figley 1995; Pearlman and Saakvitne 1995). Compassion fatigue develops if a therapist is not aware that this strain is an expectable part of the treatment process and that there are methods, such as those described in this chapter, to successfully handle it. Working with traumatized clients does not need to lead to severe compassion fatigue. With proper preparation and an understanding that empathic failure is an expected element of trauma treatment, the therapist can successfully navigate these sometimes troubled waters.

In the following excerpt from a group therapy session, the therapist did not know how to handle the empathic divide.

> A group of veterans on an inpatient unit was gathered by a therapist. The group consisted of all Vietnam-era veterans on the unit who were deemed to need a support group. The first group meeting began with the therapist making a heartfelt statement about the Vietnam War and its terrible effects on the veterans and the nation, and about the inadequate homecoming received by veterans who had risked their lives, and the lack of support from the VA. He said that he was pleased to be in the room with all the era vets, that he assumed they had much to say, that he felt they could benefit from sharing their experiences and feelings with one another, and that it was a privilege for him to listen.
>
> ALAN: Are you a vet?
> THERAPIST: No.
> ALAN: You probably got out of the draft.
> THERAPIST: No, I wasn't called.
> JESSE: You'd probably have gone to Canada anyway, right?
> THERAPIST: I'm here to listen to your experiences. I wasn't there.
> CARL: That's right, you weren't there, so what are you doing here?
>   I think the vets should meet alone.
> THERAPIST: I can understand your feeling that you want to…

CARL: You don't understand shit.

DOUG: Well, I'm an era vet, and I served in the States; though I was put down and shit on for being a vet, I never saw combat, and I just want to say that you combat vets deserve a lot of praise for your courage, even though you got dumped on so bad. (*Silence.*)

THERAPIST: Thank you, Doug. All the veterans who served during that time suffered from what was going on in this country. (*Eyes roll.*)

CARL: Are you comparing holing up in Fort Dix with what we went through?

THERAPIST: No, I…

EVAN: Do you know what it's like to have nightmares about your buddies' heads being blown off in your face? Do you?

THERAPIST: Well, I…

EVAN: No, you don't. (*Silence.*)

THERAPIST: Perhaps you could tell us.

EVAN: I was in a combat engineers unit north of Saigon, and though I wasn't in the bush, we had lots of close calls. You have no idea what it's like when those mortars come down on you (*eyes fill with tears*).

THERAPIST: Do other people know what Evan is talking about?

LEN: No, I don't, cause where I was, I dreamed about being back in the rear where he was; mortars, shit, that's nothing.

EVAN: He's right. I had it easy compared to him.

THERAPIST (*to Len*): You were a soldier in the bush?

LEN: We call it a grunt, yeah; 2 weeks at a time.

THERAPIST: Do you want to tell us about it?

LEN: Are you kidding?

THERAPIST: Why not?

LEN: Don't mean much. Yeah, I saw plenty of bad stuff, plenty more than these candyasses in the rear or in Saigon, or Fort Dix for chrissakes. You just can't understand what it was like. But I just saw the regular stuff, not like Greg (*pointing to a man across the room*). He spent months on long-range patrols. He's the only guy here who has got anything worth saying, to my mind. (*Long silence. All look at Greg.*)

THERAPIST: Greg, could you tell us what it was like? (*Silence.*) On those army patrols?

GREG: Marines.

THERAPIST: Oh, I'm sorry. I assume what Len told us was true—that you saw a lot of violence in the bush. I assume it's a constant burden. Tell us about it.

GREG: (*Eyes fill with tears.*)

THERAPIST: We are here.

GREG: I don't remember much. I don't know. It's all pretty much of a blur.

THERAPIST: I know. It's hard.

GREG: You don't know.
THERAPIST: Tell us!
GREG: (*Just looks out, very upset.*)
JESSE: You're just getting him upset for nothing. This is a waste of time. I am leaving. (*He leaves the room, followed by most of the other veterans.*)

The group, 10 minutes into its 45-minute session, ran into a dead end. Each person in the group, in his turn, was deauthorized and fell silent; each one represented himself as having no basis for his experience; each one deauthorized himself as a credible witness to the others. The only hope was Greg, who as a Marine with intense combat experience could speak to the group about Vietnam. When he deauthorized himself, declaring himself a failed witness to his own experience, as his tear-filled eyes reached out for and simultaneously rejected the therapist, the group disappeared into the gap. The therapist, not knowing what to say, stayed silent.

In this session, the therapist, filled with the romance of the rescue and thinking himself the hero overcoming the culture's attack on these veterans by offering himself as their compassionate witness, became the perpetrator: the self-serving, inadequate, uninformed authority who had sent them over to war, led them incompetently, and stigmatized them when they returned. Importantly, it was not the details of the horrific combat events that distressed the therapist in this example; it was the sense of failure in the therapist's mission to help his clients and their view of him as incompetent, despite his passionate intentions. Although there are plenty of occasions when a client's story may be especially disturbing, the therapist's burnout and fatigue may more often be caused by not being able to handle the gap when it arises with one's clients. Being screamed at, threatened with litigation, demeaned, and rejected by clients for whom one cares deeply and with whom one has worked for a long time strikes the therapist in the heart.

Therapists should not put themselves in this position by attempting to maintain a connection with clients at all costs. Rather, a therapist needs to prepare for those moments when the gap arises and the client glares at the therapist and perceives him or her as another betrayer or perpetrator or incompetent rescuer. According to the principle of incompleteness, the therapist should remain at all times in a state of being partially uninformed. Rather than nodding and saying "yes" or "uh-huh" or worst of all "I understand," the therapist should say something like the following: "I didn't understand exactly what you were saying; tell me more." "You're kidding, how could that be?" "I can't imagine how that felt!" "I'm not getting the full picture; what did you do just before that?" "Really?" Once the gap emerges, the therapist should avoid defending himself or herself, being silent, or apologizing, and proceed immediately with the protocol outlined in Chapter 9 on the gap.

In the following example from an individual therapy session, the client and therapist had been working together for 3 years and the therapist was under the impression that he had done an excellent job and knew the client intimately. They are in the middle of a session.

> CLIENT: Sally and I had lunch in the city, and the restaurant was right next to the tenement that my mother lived in.
>
> THERAPIST: What a coincidence. Did that bring up thoughts about your mom?
>
> CLIENT (*becoming instantly enraged*): She was NOT my MOM! She left me when I was 1. She is my MOTHER. Don't you remember ANYTHING?
>
> THERAPIST (*astonished and upset*): I'm sorry. It was…just…habit. Mother.
>
> CLIENT: Habit, my ass. I don't think you listen to me at all. Don't you remember that I said that I can never refer to that woman as my mom because of what she did? Do you remember?
>
> THERAPIST (*hesitantly*): Yes, but we talked about it over a year ago.
>
> CLIENT (*very angry*): What else have you forgotten about what I told you? Do you remember anything about my mother?
>
> THERAPIST (*feeling very threatened now because he could not remember many details, and he felt that he was about to be quizzed*): I…
>
> CLIENT: What details do you remember? Tell me?
>
> THERAPIST: Well, your mom—
>
> CLIENT: Mother! You did it again! Why are you doing this to me? You are hurting me!
>
> THERAPIST: I am so sorry. Your anger is making me anxious, and I'm used to saying mom, not mother.
>
> CLIENT: I can't stay here.
>
> THERAPIST (*now truly fearful that he will say mom again*): Your mother left you when you were a baby…
>
> CLIENT: No, she disappeared! When I was 1. What happened?
>
> THERAPIST: Your uncle, her brother, came over to the apartment to take you.
>
> CLIENT: NO! That was weeks later. What happened THAT DAY? I TOLD you. Do you take notes? Are you there?
>
> THERAPIST: Peggy, you're right, I can't remember everything we talk about. We have been meeting for 3 years.
>
> CLIENT: What's the point of my talking to you if you don't remember anything? This is stupid…useless.
>
> THERAPIST: Peggy, you are upset. Surely being reminded of your mother at lunch with your friend is part of this.
>
> CLIENT: You are not listening to me. You don't remember anything I've been saying. I am completely alone.
>
> THERAPIST: Are you afraid that I am going to abandon you like your mother did?

CLIENT: Cut out that analytic crap. I can't stand this anymore. I'm leaving!
(*She stands up and rapidly exits, slamming the door.*)
THERAPIST: (*Feels humiliated, frightened, self-critical, angry at the client, concerned that he could not remember the details, and worried about her.*)

Encounters like this one are not uncommon with traumatized clients. The therapist mismanaged the gap because he was thrown into a defensive position and attempted to fix the broken connection with the client, who roundly defeated his efforts. Her deep sense of being abandoned and betrayed needed to be acknowledged and lived through, not repaired, for in that moment, it was irreparable.

NOT BELIEVING THE CLIENT: FALSE MEMORY AND CREDIBILITY

Psychotherapy as a field is based on good will and sincerity, and it maintains the view that people are essentially good. Therefore, when a client comes to a therapist for help and pays money to be heard, the basic assumption is that the person is telling the truth as he or she knows it. Sometimes, the stance of believing the clients is so strong that the therapist comes to believe that the clients are telling the truth, as it is. Because many clients complain that the other people in their lives do not believe them, it is a natural impulse for the therapist to fulfill the role of the person who *does* believe them. The clients then feel supported, and the client-therapist alliance appears to be stronger. The economics of practice also support this tendency to believe, because the effect of telling clients that they are lying, exaggerating, or being self-serving is likely to reduce a therapist's caseload.

Lawyers also are employed to support the client's view of a situation and to advocate for him or her. Unlike psychotherapists, however, lawyers come into contact with those very people who do not support or believe the client. Quite often, the lawyer learns that indeed clients are lying and exaggerating and are basically self-serving. As a result, many lawyers become quite cynical about human beings—a character trait that the public dislikes about lawyers.

Essentially, the basic arrangement in psychotherapy is one in which some collusion occurs between therapist and client to assume that the client is telling the truth. After all, clients normally report stories in which they are in the role of the burdened one, or the victim. It is far less common for clients to report incidents in which they had an ethically questionable role, such as aggressor, betrayer, or perpetrator.

This dynamic is magnified with clients who have been traumatized, or who at least claim to have been traumatized. When a client tells a therapist of some horrendous abuse, the last thing a therapist will say is that he or she does not believe the client or that the client is being histrionic, even when the therapist believes this. Thus, therapists are placed in a situation of lying to the client and of holding that disbelief or doubt inside themselves.

Therapists often have reason to doubt clients' stories. There are clients whose stories are so unbelievable and outrageous that few people would believe them; these include many clients with dissociative disorders or clients reporting cult or satanic ritual abuse. There are clients who report credible acts of abuse but who are so upset and distressed by them that the therapist feels that their sense of injury is entirely out of proportion to the event. Because many times the point of greatest horror in a traumatic event is when the client is *anticipating* the next act of the perpetrator, when that act does not occur, the client's report of abuse or trauma may seem to lack credibility. When clients are children or teenagers, tremendous doubts about their veracity may be raised in the absence of physical evidence. Additionally, when clients are retelling their trauma stories and they near the period in which at the time they were completely overwhelmed with fear, their narratives becomes disrupted, fragmented, and often contradictory, not because they are lying, but because at that time their cognitive capacities to perceive and record events were severely impaired. In fact, if a trauma narrative was instead smooth and integrated, the therapist might question its authenticity or severity. As Tim O'Brien (1990) so elegantly noted, a true trauma story is one that does not sound believable. Indeed, in work with a traumatized client, arriving at a point at which the therapist feels some ambiguity or doubt in the factual truth of the account is to be expected and may be a sign of the true impairment caused by the traumatic event.

In any case, if the therapist maintains a basic assumption that the client will be truthful, then doubt is a sign of a problem. Because it is very hard to express doubt or disbelief within the constraints of a psychotherapeutic relationship, the therapist is forced to hold these doubts inside and then to euphemize or lie to the client. A critical point at which the therapist's lack of support may be revealed is when the client requests a letter to a lawyer, insurance company, or school asking the therapist to support the story. The therapist not infrequently delays or forgets, and then may finally write a general letter that the client feels is inadequate.

Therefore, it is best for the therapist not to hold the basic assumption of client truthfulness and instead to embrace the alternate assumption that doubt, disbelief, and a question of credibility will be an expected, endemic, and continuing aspect of a trauma-centered psychotherapy. The therapist should be prepared and trained to handle this.

For the situation in which the client's story is essentially credible but becomes fragmented as the client approaches the fine details, the therapist understands that this is expected and that as the desensitization process progresses over time, what can become clearer will be.

For situations in which extreme or outrageous incidents are told, the therapist assumes that if these are not true, they are derivatives of other true events, and that by pursuing the trauma-centered inquiry further, eventually the therapist will hear the more credible events. By closely observing the client for symptoms of arousal and distress, the therapist can map out the path to the true story. It is unlikely that made-up or false events can cause actual symptoms, so if symptoms exist, they are likely caused by real events, but perhaps not the events being initially described.

> A 32-year-old single woman entered treatment. She had been diagnosed with bipolar disorder and hospitalized many times for manic episodes, during which she roamed the streets naked and knocked on people's doors to warn them of impending disasters. She claimed to have been horribly abused by her parents, reporting sexual abuse by her father while her mother looked on and being taken as an infant to her father's butcher shop where she witnessed him cutting up and then grinding human bodies as part of his role in a Mafia ring. She reported being younger than 1 year when the latter happened. Her parents viewed these claims as psychotic and as a basis for hospitalizing her, and the admitting doctors concurred. In person, she was earnest and sincere, not particularly angry at her parents, but upset that no one believed her and that her parents had been able to fool everyone around them. The therapist proceeded with the trauma history even though it seemed unlikely that some or all of these events really occurred.
>
> During the course of the trauma inquiry, when she described the scene in the butcher shop, she showed little arousal and little disturbance in her narrative. When she described the sexual abuse by her father, which she believed had occurred when she was 6 or 7, she became much more upset, and her reporting was much more fragmented and confused. Whenever the therapist probed deeper into this story, she often suddenly shifted to the shop scene, suggesting to the therapist that that memory served some protective function, covering a detail in the sexual abuse event. Eventually, she remembered one time that her father was bathing her and rubbing her vaginal area, and her mother came into the bathroom and told him to stop, saying, "Your daughter is not a piece of meat." She remembered thinking at the time of her father and his butcher shop and wondering whether he would chop her up too. Several months later, she told the therapist, "Do you think my memory of watching my dad cut up bodies wasn't exactly real?"

Other examples help to clarify the usefulness of pursuing the trauma-centered inquiry until a more credible story is revealed. The previous example of the 50-year-old businessman who was in a train accident and became flooded with anxiety and posttraumatic stress symptoms, even though he was uninjured, illustrates this point well (see Chapter 2, "Axioms of Trauma-Centered Psychotherapy"). Despite having an initial response of skepticism—wondering how he could be so disabled from such a minor if unfortunate incident—the therapist engaged in the trauma inquiry and discovered that the client had experienced a prior, and much more devastating, traumatic event (a plane crash). Another example of severe symptoms with no discernible stressor is that of a Gulf War veteran who had a panic attack at work on the anniversary of the invasion. He was teased at work and even accused of trying to get out of work, as a result of others' skepticism regarding his illness. Once the therapist uncovered the cause and encouraged the client to explain the situation to his fellow workers and employer, the man received strong support from them.

On occasion, clients do consciously pretend and lie about what happened to them, either out of a need for sympathy or for secondary gain such as in a legal proceeding. In these cases, it is usually correct for the therapist to tell the clients that he or she does not believe them and that therefore there is no basis to conduct psychotherapy with them for that particular purpose. However, treatment may continue for other purposes.

> A 44-year-old woman was arrested for having sex with a 15-year-old boy whom she had groomed as a friend in her role as an administrative assistant at a high school. She had two children of her own. Under the pretext of helping him study, she picked him up after school and drove him to various activities and stopped for food. In the car, they fondled each other and then went back to her house, where they had sexual intercourse on multiple occasions. After she was accused, she referred herself for treatment of posttraumatic stress disorder due to *his* behavior, claiming that he had initiated the sexual contact and had threatened to tell the school officials if she did not comply. After a review of the case and consulting with other authorities, the therapist determined that the client was in fact responsible for the abuse and was denying her own participation to employ the therapist's support in her upcoming court case.

> THERAPIST: I need to inform you that after talking with you about what happened and reviewing the reports from your attorney, I have determined that you were responsible for this situation. You were the adult, and he was a child. I also do not believe that your symptoms of depression or anxiety are due to being traumatized by him, but instead are being caused by your fears over the possible outcome of the upcoming court case against you. I wanted you to know my assessment so that you have the chance to seek out treatment elsewhere if you wish. I recommend that you do not try to defend yourself but admit the responsibility for your actions and accept the consequences. That

would be the right thing to do. You are welcome to stay in treatment here with me, so we can work on what led you to do this and to deal with your fears about being punished. I assume that you did this out of some desire that relates to experiences you had in your own childhood, and if that is the case, then there is work to be done so that you come to a better understanding of what happened here, and to lower the chances that you will repeat this behavior in the future.

The woman accepted these terms and continued in treatment until she was sentenced to a short jail term. She indeed did have an incest history, and her actions with the boy were reenactments of her own previous experiences.

In trauma-centered psychotherapy, the therapist's target is not the traumatic event itself, which cannot be changed, but the trauma schemas that developed as a result of that event. In many cases, the outrageous or unbelievable events reported by the client are best seen as examples of his or her trauma schemas, not the events themselves. Viewed this way, the therapist can develop a better picture of how the client is perceiving the world. These event schemas, then, are derived from other events that actually happened, although the client either has chosen not to report them or does not remember them.

Therefore, in addition to embracing the inability to comprehend the client fully, the trauma-centered psychotherapist needs to embrace doubt. It would be more comfortable if truth could be easily established and the grounds for treatment were solid, but unfortunately this is not the case in trauma work. This issue is discussed in a number of thoughtfully written books, particularly that by Constance Dalenberg (2000). Doubting the client should be characterized not as an impediment to treatment but rather as an opportunity to enhance the clinical work.

HEARING TOO MUCH: VICARIOUS TRAUMATIZATION

Significant attention has been given to *care for the caregiver* and specifically *vicarious traumatization*, which is the sympathetic stress response in the clinician due to listening to horrendous stories of violence, sadism, and cruelty. Saakvitne et al. (2000) provide excellent advice on how trauma therapists can best care for themselves.

The focus of this book, however, is on the skills and competencies required of a trauma-centered psychotherapist, and perhaps the most important of these skills is the ability to listen carefully to these horrific stories and not lose focus on the primary tasks: to get the details, decode the behavior, introduce discrepancy, and disclose the perpetrator. Therefore, any self-care activity that interferes with these tasks is not recommended. Self-care activities that help the therapist relax at home and maintain mental and physical health are excellent. Self-care activities that support any form of avoidance of the material, slowing down of the therapy process, or dampening of the client's emotional expression in order to titrate the therapist's stress, are not recommended, because they interfere with the actual work. Surgeons are also professionals who are subject to intense stresses from their work, and they too require self-care. However, slowing down surgical procedures or not taking as many risks during surgical procedures are not useful for self-care. The purpose of recommended self-care strategies (e.g., rest and relaxation, balancing activities, professional support and supervision, personal therapy) is to maintain the therapist's resilience to do the important work of trauma-centered psychotherapy. Not pursuing upsetting details of the inquiry during sessions and attempts to calm clients before they become emotionally upset, when done to relieve the therapist's own distress, are maneuvers that impair and undermine the effectiveness of the therapy process.

One of the most powerful sources of resilience comes from the respect and even at times awe that therapists develop for clients who have lived through unbelievable misfortunes and, despite difficulties, continue to fight on. This *vicarious resilience*—that is, drawing strength from clients' lives—may be particularly effective in that instead of *compensating* for the stress of work through alternative activities, therapists discover something positive within that stress. Becoming and remaining in touch with one's vicarious resilience brings one closer to the client, who is hopefully attempting to achieve the same goal: to discover something positive within his or her own tragedies. This approach emphasizes the collaborative relationship between therapist and client, who have metaphorically jumped out of the airplane, strapped together. The therapist's challenge is a reflection of the client's. Therefore, whenever possible, finding ways of drawing strength from the work and the client, rather than away from the work and the client, will help the therapist achieve better results and greater capacity to face the traumatic material.

WANTING TO HARM THE PERPETRATOR: RETALIATION AND RAGE

Over time, therapists hear horrendous stories about how people harm other people. Not infrequently, these are relatively well documented and established as true. In too many cases, the perpetrators of these crimes remain at large, living freely and sometimes well. The therapist may experience a version of a client's sense of helplessness in achieving justice, and the anger that such helplessness stimulates can become a desire for retaliation or retribution.

In the vicarious traumatization literature, the effort to suppress these desires over time is viewed as a burden on the therapist (Pearlman and Saakvitne 1995). From a trauma-centered perspective, the therapist has to question not only what he or she does for self-care, but also how his or her reaction plays out within the clinical interaction with the client.

Perhaps the fundamental wish underlying these retaliatory fantasies is the desire to get rid of, or eliminate, the perpetrator. Unfortunately, within the trauma grid, the perpetrator is a permanent member and can never be eliminated from the trauma schema. The reason for this is that the traumatic act is a moment in time at which the perpetrator's and victim's lives, bodies, and minds intersect in a swirl of violence or domination. These moments are of such intimacy that perpetrator and victim can never be separated from each other. Unfortunately, this means that the perpetrator becomes a permanent member of the victim's life and family. In cases of incest, quite often the victim will live many years in contact with or in proximity to the perpetrator. However, even if the perpetrator is dead, in prison, or far away, the client will continue to be haunted by his or her memory of their time together. Without a concrete representation of the perpetrator, the victim remains on alert for his or her reemergence.

Adolf Hitler, for example, will forever be a part of German culture. Although most representations of Hitler have been erased, the German government is constantly on the lookout for the reemergence of neo-Nazi groups. In the Berlin memorial to the Holocaust, there are representations of the dead Jews as unmarked cement coffins in a graveyard. The perpetrator is not to be found. Only the results of the disaster are represented, not the cause.

The intimate possession of the client by the perpetrator, even if long past, is deeply disturbing to all those who now care for the client, including the therapist. Although the client claims that "no one can understand me because nobody else was there," the underlying message is, "except him, because he was there with me." Spouses and family members feel as though their loved one has been stolen, forever.

The therapist's fantasy of wanting to retaliate against the perpetrator is understandable. From the client's point of view, the therapist has arrived at the scene of the crime too late. The damage has already been done. The therapist then feels helpless, and that sense of helplessness can transform into a wish to retaliate. When retaliatory fantasies arise in the therapist, however, it is best to consider the possibility that they are a reflection of an aspect of the traumatic event that has yet to be revealed. If so, that aspect usually involves the perpetrator, whom the fantasies intend to destroy. The sheer power and domination, and sometimes competence, intelligence, and skill, of the perpetrator can be intimidating and daunting. The client's helplessness in the face of this force will be distressing but important to be able to discuss and process.

> A 16-year-old boy began treatment for having been sexually abused by a teacher when the boy was age 10. The male teacher sodomized the boy several times and then rejected him, causing the boy to become symptomatic with anxiety and suicidal ideation and to demonstrate increasing acting-out behavior in school and his foster home (he had been removed from his birth parents for neglect when he was age 7). When the boy was 17, the therapist received a panicked call from the foster mother who said that the boy was suicidal; he had just reported to her that he had visited his former mentor that morning to say good-bye (because the boy was going to leave for college), and the mentor, who was also a priest, had taken him to his house and had sex with him and then told him to keep it a secret. The mother had called the regional bishop of the church and reported the incident, but he brushed her off, saying vaguely that he would look into it. The Department of Children and Families case worker for the boy had just confronted the mentor/priest with the boy's report, and he had completely denied it.
>
> The therapist was very upset by this turn of events. He looked online for information about this priest and discovered that he was a member of a small, independent reformed Catholic church. The priest was in charge of the church's daycare and religious school program, which focused on young boys. The church had just moved to a new address, which happened to be 50 feet from the therapist's clinic. The therapist became enraged and filled with retaliatory thoughts, such as posting a notice on the door of the church that the priest was a pedophile and no one should allow children near him; calling him on the phone and saying, "I know what you have done"; or entering the church at the time of a service and outing the man before his small congregation. The thought that a pedophile had set up his place within a stone's throw of the clinic felt intolerable to the therapist.
>
> Although in some sense the desire for retaliation is understandable, retaliation is not the job of the trauma-centered psychotherapist, and after the incident too much time was taken in therapy sessions with the client jointly being upset and enraged (and therefore helpless) about the priest. When the client then reported he had also had sex with a male prostitute, on purpose, the therapist realized that he was not doing the work of understanding and decoding the client's behavior. Once the therapy was back on track, the key element in the trauma schema turned out to be the "saying good-bye" part, which referenced an act of sexual molestation by the client's own biological father shortly before he was removed from his parents. The client's departure to college had triggered his conflicted feelings about losing his father.

The following example about abuse in the Catholic church had an entirely different outcome.

A 50-year-old lawyer attended the funeral of a colleague at the Catholic church he had attended as a child. During the service, he had a flashback of being sexually abused by a priest when he was 11–12 years old. The abuse included multiple acts of sodomy, masturbation, and frotteurism, which occurred in various locations of the rectory. He could not get these images out of his mind, and he called the church to report his memories. Rather than respond like so many other churches to such a claim, the residing bishop invited the man to come to meet with himself and the church leadership. They listened as the man described his sexual abuse, and then the bishop responded by taking full responsibility for the crime, telling the man that they believed him, saying that acts such as these are crimes and are not part of Catholicism, that the church will pay for any treatment the man required, and that they understood that he may want to sue them for other damages and they would not fight that. The man was referred for therapy, which lasted 1 year. During that time, the therapist requested to accompany the client into the rectory to provide in vivo exposure to the rooms in which he was abused. The church agreed without resistance and cleared the rectory so that the client and the therapist, alone, could wander through the building and sit in the rooms as a means of aiding his remembering and mourning. The client was completely cured. The client did not sue the church despite a clear opportunity to benefit financially. The reason for this is that the church accepted the role of perpetrator and made itself available to the client in that role, which lowered the client's anxiety over the whereabouts of the perpetrator and provided a mechanism for him to mourn, with the church, the events that took place. Neither the client nor the therapist was troubled by retaliatory fantasies against the church.

This latter example highlights the point that a therapist's retaliatory fantasies may mean that not enough time has been spent discussing and disclosing the perpetrator within the trauma-centered psychotherapy, which has allowed the displacement of feelings onto other people in the client's (or therapist's) world. Therefore, retaliatory fantasies in the therapist might be better handled by renewed attention in the therapy sessions to as yet unexplored aspects of the client's relationship with the perpetrator.

WANTING TO RESCUE THE CLIENT: ADVOCACY, CHARITY, AND ADOPTION

Working with deeply injured people is both an honor and a burden, which give texture and depth to the therapist's professional identity. In the trauma field, one encounters many poignant situations of children, young adults, and older citizens who have been harmed so needlessly and who struggle so diligently to rise up again. Among these, there are a few whose personal attributes or character are so compelling that the therapist becomes caught in the fantasy of rescuing them by offering money, food, clothing, or scholarship to college; going with clients to court or Social Security to stand up for them publicly; joining them on an advocacy tour to schools and colleges; or, in the case of children, becoming their foster parent or even adopting them. This is not to say that helping clients find resources, fill out forms, and win court cases is inappropriate; the concern is whether the therapist is filled with the desire for rescue. The consensus of the professional literature is that these fantasies are countertransference reactions that should not be acted upon, however well meaning the therapist or well deserved the client. Interestingly, the risk of acting out these rescue fantasies is well distributed across young and older therapists, for what the young lack in experience, the older have in resources.

When these fantasies are evoked primarily from personal issues in the therapist's life (e.g., frustration with family members, loss of confidence in work skills, psychiatric illness), then supervision, personal psychotherapy, and self-care strategies are warranted. However, rescue fantasies more often are evoked by the therapist's interaction with the client and/or reflect unexpressed details of the client's trauma story. In these situations, the appearance of a rescue fantasy should first be explored as an expression of a trauma schema: some not yet revealed detail that is now close to the surface. Usually, this detail concerns the perpetrator because the rescue fantasy, similar to the retaliatory fantasy, serves largely to diminish awareness of the power of the perpetrator.

As discussed in Chapter 8, "Conducting Ongoing Treatment: Decoding the Trauma Schema in Current Behaviors," rescue is not a part of a trauma schema, because trauma by definition means the absence of rescue. The rescue, in the rescue fantasy, concerns a current threat: lack of money, no home, or inability to manage a court date. The deep-seated hope for the therapist is that by helping the client now, somehow a part of the client's trauma in the past will be undone, made up for, or rectified. The therapist may be filled with these thoughts about trauma clients: "They are *owed*." "They *deserve*." "Now it is *their turn*." The therapist may feel that if he or she did not help now, but rather stood on the side and let the client fall again, this inaction would be intolerable. The rescue fantasy serves to forestall the therapist's experience as a bystander, but displaced onto a current situation. The rescue fantasy is therefore more likely to be evoked when the client communicates to the therapist that the current challenge is indistinguishable from the past traumatic event, and the therapist also has not made this distinction.

> A male white therapist had been working with a 55-year-old black woman who had been arrested for several failure-to-appear charges secondary to a

ticket for an unregistered vehicle that had been parked on her lawn. She had severe diabetes, and while being processed in the local police station, the officers refused to allow her to take her insulin, whereupon she became panicked and may have had symptoms secondary to her diabetes. She struggled to leave the station, and they restrained her. After she was booked and eventually released, she failed to appear twice at scheduled court dates because of her terrifying fear that if she showed up she would again be held against her will. The police force was known in the community as being particularly unsympathetic to its black population.

The therapist became activated by this situation and decided to help out his client by accompanying her to her next scheduled court date. He met her very early in the morning and stood in line with her at the local courthouse, in a long line of minority citizens. He felt like he was her bodyguard; he felt like he was protecting her from an unfair and prejudiced court system, police force, and even society. He had fleeting thoughts that by standing in this line with his client, he was partly making amends for 350 years of slavery in America. He was a bit hypervigilant; he was prepared to stand up for her in court. When they appeared before the judge, the matter was resolved quickly and respectfully, his client being asked merely to pay the proper fine, which she did. The therapist slowly became aware that although he had done her a favor by helping her get to the court and resolving this matter, he had become caught up in a larger fantasy. He realized that she did have other family members who also could have accompanied her.

In the next session, the therapist explored the possibility that his client had had other previous situations with white people who had either protected or harmed her. With little hesitation, his client shared that when she was age 13, she had been held against her will by a group of teenage boys in the basement of her school, where they sexually assaulted her. Afterward, she was too afraid to return to her school. The principal, a white male, took an interest in her, came to her house one morning, and personally escorted her to school. After hearing her story, he identified and expelled the boys.

The client subsequently benefited by being able to process her memories of this incident and other traumatic events in her childhood. Nevertheless, she remained grateful to the therapist for helping her out with her failure-to-appear charges.

HAVING TO BE THERE: EMERGENCIES AND PHONE CALLS

The triggering of a trauma schema cannot be predicted; it does not erupt on a convenient schedule, such as once a week during the psychotherapy session. Trauma clients can experience emergencies at any time and place. Having experienced a real emergency in the original trauma, the client is primed to frame each obstacle he or she encounters as another form of emergency. Because these current emergencies are often over comparatively small things, clients' calls for help are largely viewed as histrionic or exaggerated, which intensifies the clients' sense of abandonment or of being perceived as deficient.

Typically, in the original traumatic emergency, no one came to help out. Therefore, each time the client announces that he or she is in an emergency in the present, the schema that no one will come to help out is activated. This is why so often the clients' calls for help occur at times when the therapist is least likely to be able to help. There are two parts to this scenario: the emergency and the calling for help. The calling for help is most often over the phone, to the therapist's system of coverage after hours. More recently, calls for help come over the Internet via e-mails. Each client has a different time frame within which he or she will expect the call to be answered. Most often, the return call is too late, consolidating the client's schema that the rescuers are too slow, are too incompetent, or have betrayed them.

One approach to this issue is for therapists to make themselves available by phone, which is one component of dialectical behavior therapy (Linehan 1993), for example. From a trauma perspective, not infrequently clients' calls for help in emergencies will not be responded to in time. Therefore, it is incumbent upon therapists to know how to handle this situation effectively. If not, either therapists succumb to being available and spend too much time on the phone with clients, to which the therapists develop a simmering resentment and fatigue, or they dissemble and promise to be available but act in a passive-aggressive manner by not returning the calls on time, making excuses why they did not get back to clients, or having other intermediaries make contact with clients. Their avoidant and not quite honest maneuvers begin to take on the shape of the clients' original perpetrators' betrayals, lies, and obfuscations. These therapist behaviors are eventually confronted by clients and serve to undermine the strength of the treatment relationship.

A therapist should set a policy about returning phone calls or e-mails that is comfortable, and then when the client experiences the therapist as being purposefully unavailable and a gap is created, the therapist should proceed with managing the gap as described in Chapter 9.

Therapists who have occasionally gone to special meetings for clients, or given clients money, car rides, clothing, or toys for their children, typically learn that although these acts were helpful to their clients in the moment, soon afterward the need arises again. Their good will is never enough. In fact, as one client exclaimed, "You've put salt in my wound," because by offering material help once, but not in an ongoing way, the therapist merely highlighted the client's helplessness. Rather than focusing on making emergencies go well, the trauma-centered psychotherapist will understand that calling for help, for any reason, is not a neutral activity for traumatized individuals and that it will usually express an important trauma schema, which will ensure that the situation will go poorly. However, at the same time, it will provide the therapist another opportunity to learn more about details of the traumatic experience that the client has not yet revealed.

A 22-year-old client called the therapist's office on a Saturday evening at approximately 11:30 P.M. and left the following voicemail message: "Dr. L, please call me immediately. I know it's late, but I don't know where I am. It's dark, and (*inaudible*) beat me up because I wouldn't let him have sex with me (*cries*). I'm scared. I don't know what to do. Please call me." The next message was left at around 3:00 A.M.: "Thanks a lot for not calling me back. You are never around, and I was almost raped while you are sleeping all soft and sound in your big house. You don't care. I'm quitting. This is ridiculous." The therapist retrieved these messages in the late morning on Sunday. The client had left similar messages before and had a long history of disrupted relationships and violent outbursts. Their next appointment was scheduled for Thursday. The therapist decided to return the phone call on Monday morning from her office.

> THERAPIST: Hi, Mora, how are you doing?
> MORA: Not so good; rough weekend.
> THERAPIST: I gathered that from your messages.
> MORA: You didn't call me back.
> THERAPIST: You are upset that I didn't call you back.
> MORA: Right.
> THERAPIST: That's got to be upsetting given all the times in your life when you were in need of help—being molested by that neighbor for instance—and you'd call out for your mother and she never came.
> MORA: Ignored me.
> THERAPIST: She let it all happen, and it caused a lot of harm to you.
> MORA: Yeah.
> THERAPIST: Sounds like you got scared Saturday night.
> MORA: It was bad. I didn't like the dark.
> THERAPIST: What about the dark?
> MORA: It was dark.
> THERAPIST: I'm wondering if that was particularly scary because you've been in the dark before? I don't remember you telling me about anytime—
> MORA: Rodney.
> THERAPIST: Rodney who?
> MORA: Rodney was a boyfriend of my mother's and one time when I was about 8 or so, he asked me if I wanted to go over to his mother's house. "She's got a big house!" he said, so I wanted to go, but when we got there, he tied me up and kept me all night.
> THERAPIST: It was dark.
> MORA: (*Cries.*) Yes.

THERAPIST: You were only 8. What did he do to you?

MORA: He had sex with me…all night.

THERAPIST: That's terrible. I wish someone could have been there to stop that.

MORA: Nobody did.

THERAPIST: Nobody did. And what happened Saturday night?

MORA: I got a cab.

THERAPIST: So that was different than the time with Rodney.

MORA: Yeah.

THERAPIST: I am glad that it was different. I'd like to talk more about what happened with Rodney in our session on Thursday. You hadn't told me about that one.

MORA: All right.

THERAPIST: Take care.

MORA: Thanks for calling.

The therapist did not attempt to rectify their miscommunication or address the client's anger or threat to quit, but rather followed the recommended procedure for handling the gap by listening for new information that might provide a clue to an unrevealed memory. This emerged in the reference to "dark," and the traumatic memory about Rodney came to light. The therapist did not notice the link between the client's reference on the phone to her "big house" and that of Rodney's mother's "big house," which probably points to an important detail in her trauma story. Nevertheless, the therapist was successful in keeping the therapy on track in identifying and exploring this client's traumatic past. In follow-up sessions, the therapist continued to work with the client on recognizing to what extent her current behavioral problems are reflections of pervasive trauma schemas.

STUDY QUESTIONS

17.1 T/F Trauma therapists should not have to expect high levels of stress in their work.

17.2 T/F Trauma-centered psychotherapy is based on the model of the therapist as a good-enough parent.

17.3 T/F The most effective way of handling compassion fatigue is to have the competence to handle the gap when it occurs in the therapeutic encounter.

17.4 T/F In trauma-centered psychotherapy, doubt about the accuracy of the client's story is the sign of a major problem in the relationship.

17.5 T/F In the therapeutic relationship, the therapist should hold the discrepancy between supporting the client's version of the facts and the possibility that what the client remembers is inaccurate.

17.6   T/F   The task and norms of psychotherapy and the law are basically the same.

17.7   Why are self-care strategies such as slowing down the trauma inquiry or not getting as much into the details *not* recommended in trauma-centered psychotherapy?

17.8   What is the major cause of a therapist's retaliatory fantasies against the client's perpetrator?

17.9   A strong desire to rescue the client by providing special or extra resources is often the sign of what unexplored issue in the client's traumatic experience?

17.10   T/F   Clients' calls for help often occur at times when they know or expect the therapist will not to be able to respond.

17.11   T/F   Therapists should do whatever they can to be available to their clients, in case an emergency arises.

17.12   T/F   The therapist's inconsistency in helping the client is likely to support the client's trauma schemas of his or her caretakers' neglect, betrayal, or false promises.

CHAPTER 18

Limits to the Trauma-Centered Approach

There are a number of circumstances in which trauma-centered psychotherapy may not be recommended. First, the required conditions may not exist: other less complex treatments may be effective, the therapist may not feel comfortable or confident with the approach, or the institution within which the treatment is taking place may not support direct trauma work. Second, objective assessment is required, as in independent forensic examinations. Here the interactive, supportive, and exploratory nature of trauma-centered psychotherapy will interfere with the need for objectivity. Third, certain clients, such as young children, may not have the verbal skills and cognitive development or capacity to engage in discussions about their traumatic events. Although there are ways to accommodate the method to these populations, generally, other methods are recommended.

WHEN OTHER TREATMENTS ARE EFFECTIVE

The most obvious limit to the trauma-centered approach is that the therapist may not feel it is needed. In many instances, trauma-centered psychotherapy may not be the treatment of first choice. Many traumatized individuals overcome their hardships on their own without requiring in-depth uncovering and processing of their traumatic experiences. An increasing number of treatment models are available that offer effective treatment with either no or minimal review of the trauma (Follette et al. 2015;

Ford and Russo 2006; Shapiro 1995). Some therapists use a resiliency model that encourages clients to strengthen themselves rather than a pathology model that seeks to repair the injury itself. Other therapists are impressed with the progressive knowledge base about the neurobiology of trauma and may wish to use medications as the major intervention for symptoms of the disorder. Although from the trauma-centered perspective, these methods accept a degree of avoidance, it is possible that under certain circumstances avoidance and even denial may have therapeutic effects. It is usually wise for the most parsimonious treatments to be used first, and if they are effective, then there may be no need to use the trauma-centered approach. When and if these more oblique approaches do not succeed, then trauma-centered psychotherapy should be considered.

WHEN THE THERAPIST IS NOT COMFORTABLE

The second limitation of the trauma-centered approach is that it is not for the faint-hearted therapist. The therapist should have achieved a degree of comfort and competence in the method to have success using it. Requisite skills include resiliency in being exposed to others' traumatic experiences, ability to listen closely and engage emotionally in a client's experiences, and most importantly ability to inquire dispassionately into distressing areas of a client's life and witness the pain caused by that inquiry. Like doctors in general and surgeons in particular, trauma therapists should be able to tolerate the pain caused by their interventions. Therapists should also be able to manage the intense strains, countertransference, and fatigue caused by the work.

We have been training therapists in trauma-centered work for more than 30 years, and we know that it is possible to successfully train clinicians to do this work. We have found that it takes approximately 2 years for clinicians to master the method. However, a proportion of these trainees go on to do other types of therapeutic work, even though they have successfully mastered these techniques. They do so because of personal preferences for other types of work. An interest in doing trauma-centered work may match certain personalities and preferences of therapists. Trauma-centered psychotherapy is not a method for all clients or for all therapists.

WHEN THERE IS INSUFFICIENT INSTITUTIONAL SUPPORT

Another limitation to doing trauma-centered work is that given the shift in the culture within mental health and indeed society at large, there is not always support for this work among colleagues or directors of the agencies, hospitals, or training programs within which therapists practice. Concerns over privacy, confidentiality, and mandatory reporting abound regarding direct inquiries into traumatic experience. Clinical concerns that trauma work will destabilize clients cause inpatient facilities to delay the work until the client gets into outpatient settings; outpatient settings to delay the work until the client can have the safety of the inpatient setting; and substance abuse programs to delay the work until sobriety is under control. Individual clinicians attempting to do this work may sense this lack of support, adding to the inherent burdens of conducting trauma-centered psychotherapy. The situation is much improved in designated trauma centers or clinics, because referring agencies are fully aware that trauma work is conducted by clinicians specifically trained and supervised for that purpose, and clinic staff can support one another. Such institutional and collegial support is therefore very helpful, and perhaps essential.

Although clinicians interested in doing trauma-centered work are encouraged to educate and advocate within their institutions for colleagues' support, these efforts are often not successful. It usually takes time before the benefits of trauma-centered work become evident to institution staff, who too often are chasing their clients' displaced acting-out behaviors. Unfortunately, the ongoing instability of their clients may make institutions more wary of trauma work, when ironically addressing the underlying trauma schemas is likely to help reduce the unstable behavior.

WHEN AN INDEPENDENT FORENSIC EVALUATION IS REQUESTED

Another important limitation of trauma work lies in the tension between the legal system and psychotherapy. Trauma-centered psychotherapy takes place in a relatively private, personal arena in which truth and fantasy, disbelief and hope can coexist. Trauma schemas by definition are distorted perceptions of the world. Traumatic experience usually occurs while the client is in a state of overwhelming arousal, hardly a situation that can be relied upon for accuracy. Psychotherapy is a territory in which objective reality and personal reality are interwoven and mutually valued. In contrast, the legal system is designed to sort out fact from fiction and to make decisions based on not shreds of evidence but a *preponderance* of evidence.

The easy situation would be for the psychotherapist to remain in his or her office and conduct the trauma-centered work for the psychological benefit of the client. However, because trauma involves injury and is often the product of an interaction between an accused perpetrator and an injured victim, legal involvement is very common. As the therapist's expertise grows, he or she is increasingly asked to testify in court in support of clients, to conduct forensic evaluations for or against an injured party, or to consult in cases as an expert witness (Simon 2003). Often therapists overestimate the value of their testimony as they embrace a position of advocacy for the victims of trauma.

Herein lies the limitation, as ironic as any: What has the therapist witnessed? From a legal perspective, the entire contents of a psychotherapy session or course of treatment involve *hearsay* (Simon 2003). Cross-examining attorneys relish confronting the overly confident therapist on the lack of real evidence in their views (opinions) of a client's trauma: "Have you conducted an independent investigation of the incident? Have you interviewed all the relevant parties? Have you talked with the accused?" The answer in most cases is a meekly uttered "no."

Trauma-centered psychotherapy is a method of treatment, not justice, and of healing, not the determination of fact. The enthusiasm and certainty with which therapists can become infused cannot hold up to the fact that memories are approximations and can be false or incomplete, beliefs are deeply self-serving and biased, and people can lie. Many of the traumatic events clients have suffered occurred long ago, many have not been reported until recently, and for most there is no physical evidence that they occurred. As a result, the therapist's first forays into the public arena and especially the courts are often eye-opening. Not only are the bases for the therapist's opinions dismissed as hearsay, but often the opposing attorney presents information or evidence about which the therapist is unaware because the client has not mentioned it.

In court, the trauma-centered psychotherapist usually has credibility in two areas: 1) in describing the current symptoms and resulting diagnoses of the client, based on direct observation of the client in sessions (this is not hearsay), any tests that have been administered, and review of information from other medical sources, and 2) as a character witness, in having an opinion as a credible professional in the community that the client is of good character and is telling the truth. Paradoxically, the trauma-centered psychotherapist is often more likely to have a positive effect on the client's case by looking into the eyes of the jury or judge and saying with confidence that the client is telling the truth than by trying to prove that the details the client has told the therapist are true because of some knowledge the therapist has about trauma or psychology.

Furthermore, the very process of conducting a trauma inquiry without appearing to lead the client by suggestion is often challenged, and rightly so. In a purely forensic situation, in which the examiner is not the therapist and attempts to carefully word each question so as not to lead or suggest to the client, and in which the examination is often videotaped, a semblance of objectivity can be attained. However, in a psychotherapy context, especially a trauma-centered one, the requirement for the therapist to be engaged and to inquire directly about the trauma cannot be viewed as objective or as having no suggestive elements. The situation is similar in assessing suicidality: concerns that asking a client directly "Are you suicidal?" may in fact be suggestive and cause them to report being suicidal have been overruled by the clinical utility of knowing whether the client is thinking of killing himself or herself. The difference is that in the assessment of suicidality, the stakes concern the client only. In a trauma context, the truth value of a reported abuse also has consequences for the accused perpetrator, whose rights must be protected as well.

Despite this limitation, which should not be minimized, sometimes the client's answers to questions within psychotherapy allow him or her to more fully report the details of abuse in a manner that public officials or juries find credible. In these situations, the results of the trauma-centered psychotherapeutic interview can be helpful in a legal setting, but *because of the inherent credibility of the client*, not the objectivity of the trauma-centered method. It is important that therapists understand this limitation.

WHEN WORKING WITH YOUNG CHILDREN

The principles and techniques of trauma-centered psychotherapy can be applied in individual work with children but are subject to the various limitations that children present, depending on their age. Generally, for children up to age 16, the advantages of treating them in a family therapy context are significant (see Chapter 15, "Trauma-Centered Couples and Family Psychotherapy"). Because trauma schemas are relational, the intimate relations among family members will be the major source of triggers of disturbed behaviors. Being an empathic therapist who is not responsible for the daily discipline of the child may lead to a close personal alliance with the child, but infrequently improves the relations between the child and his or her parents or family members. In some cases, individual therapy may increase the child's feelings that the parents are unsympathetic.

When individual therapy is indicated for a child, treatment is based on age. Generally, preschool children (ages 0–5) are too young to participate effectively in a verbal process that focuses on their traumatic experiences. Supportive play therapy is usually helpful in providing them an arena outside of their family where they can feel attended to and can get to know someone who is interested in and helpful to their parents and family as a whole. In some cases, the child is capable of engaging in trauma-centered play, or artwork, or discussion.

Latency-age children (ages 5–12) generally have limited capacities to tolerate focusing on the trauma or psychological issues for more than brief periods of time. Also, they may generate a host of distracting issues and behaviors or desires to play that are difficult for therapists to restrain and that impede the effectiveness of the treatment. In such cases, *trauma-centered play therapy* may be an effective option, in which a child's needs for movement and play can be integrated with a focus on his or her traumatic experience. However, this treatment requires specialized skills and training that are beyond the scope of this book. Readers interested in these approaches are referred to Gil and Terr (2010), Goodyear-Brown (2009), and Johnson (2014).

For latency-age children who do have some capacity to address their memories and for whom a family therapy context is not indicated or available, *trauma-focused cognitive behavioral therapy* (TF-CBT) (Cohen et al. 2006) and the *attachment, self-regulation, and competency model* (Blaustein and Kinniburgh 2010) are well established and effective approaches. These approaches, when extended into a longer-term psychotherapy, can be enhanced by applying the principles and techniques of trauma-centered psychotherapy described in this book. Foremost among these are the methods used to open up the narrative line, with the goal of achieving a more detailed narrative than is commonly achieved in the relatively condensed TF-CBT format. In the TF-CBT format, generally two to six sessions are devoted to the preparation of a trauma narrative (often in the form of a book). In a trauma-centered psychotherapy, many more sessions can be devoted to this task.

Most adolescents (ages 13–18), especially those older than 15, are quite capable of participating in the standard verbal format of trauma-centered psychotherapy presented in this book. As in any treatment for adolescents, attending to the sensitive issues regarding confidentiality between the adolescent and his or her parents, particularly around recreational drug use and sexual activity, is important. (This is a reason for a family therapy context for treatment of adolescent children, where this issue is less complex because everyone is in the room together.)

STUDY QUESTIONS

18.1 T/F Trauma-centered psychotherapy is the treatment of choice over other forms of trauma treatment.

18.2 T/F Trauma-centered psychotherapy should be used by clinicians who feel comfortable doing in-depth trauma inquiries.

18.3 T/F Therapists using trauma-centered psychotherapy should assess whether their institution supports this approach and, if not, find ways to gain that support through education and advocacy.

18.4 What are the two bases of credibility of a trauma-centered therapist in court?

18.5 T/F Trauma-centered psychotherapists are capable of determining the truthfulness of the client's trauma narrative.

18.6 T/F Aspects of trauma-centered psychotherapy can be considered suggestive to the client.

18.7 For traumatized clients ages 0–5, which treatment is recommended? (Check any that apply.)

_____ Supportive play therapy
_____ Trauma-centered play therapy
_____ Work with their caretakers
_____ No treatment but close monitoring of their condition

18.8 For traumatized clients ages 5–12, which treatment is recommended? (Check any that apply.)

_____ Supportive play therapy
_____ Trauma-centered play therapy
_____ Trauma-focused cognitive behavioral therapy
_____ Trauma-centered family therapy

CHAPTER 19

Conclusion

In this book we have described a rigorous method of conducting a trauma inquiry that applies the evidence-based knowledge of imaginal exposure, cognitive restructuring, and desensitization within a traditional psychotherapeutic context. Trauma-centered psychotherapy as presented here follows a set of general assumptions and principles and is therefore a *perspective* on trauma treatment rather than a new or independent method of treatment. The process we outline is intended to be useful to therapists of any theoretical persuasion, using a wide range of therapeutic methods, when the necessity of conducting an in-depth trauma inquiry arises.

We have found that collecting a general account of a person's trauma narrative is usually not sufficient to produce either the depth or the rapidity of symptom relief and personal healing that trauma treatment can achieve. Attending to the minute forms of avoidance that occur throughout the trauma inquiry does indeed improve clinical outcomes, and mastering these specific techniques will result in greater confidence and capacity in the therapist.

This book is intended particularly for those clinicians who harbor the desire to frame their work in the context of psychotherapy, where the relationship between client and therapist is nurtured and attended to over a lengthy period of time. There are many benefits from a longer-term psychotherapy relationship, for both client and therapist, and the trauma inquiry will be only one aspect of this work. Although clinical improvement can be gained through time-limited therapeutic interventions, psychotherapy remains a format through which the fullness of a person's journey through life can be examined and shared with a trusted guide.

The discussion and debate within the health field as to the relative merits of targeted and manualized interventions versus supportive psychotherapy and counseling are certain to continue in the years to come. The former have largely been developed within academic settings and have more often been supported by empirical studies, whereas the latter continue to be more widely practiced by many if not most clinicians and counselors. This book does not take a stand in this debate but rather attempts to integrate what each approach has to offer.

For people who have been severely traumatized, the process of psychotherapy can be a significant factor in their personal repair. We have seen this many times, in ways that are not captured by the disruptions of symptoms or behavioral anomalies, but lie more within the profound nuances of caring, mature relationships. We have also seen that without an organized and detailed inquiry into their traumatic events, the subtle effects of avoidance often permeate the therapeutic relationship, and the impact of the therapy on the client's posttraumatic stress disorder is lessened or eliminated.

Thus, we hope there is a role for this book in bridging the gap between the traditional forms of psychotherapy and the targeted and manualized approaches to trauma treatment. Each form of encounter has much to offer, and we have attempted to bring the best of each to bear here. Our clients deserve no less.

STUDY QUESTIONS

19.1   What component of trauma-centered psychotherapy seems most challenging for you as a clinician?

19.2   What is your opinion regarding the value of delving deeply into the details of another person's traumatic experience? Do you feel that it is essential to the client's recovery or unnecessary if he or she finds other means of building resilience and learning how to regulate emotions?

References

Adams K: The Way of the Journal. Denver, CO, Sidran Press, 1997

American Psychiatric Association: Diagnostic and Statistical Manual of Mental Disorders, 3rd Edition. Washington, DC, American Psychiatric Association, 1980

American Psychiatric Association: Diagnostic and Statistical Manual of Mental Disorders, 4th Edition. Washington, DC, American Psychiatric Association, 1994

American Psychiatric Association: Diagnostic and Statistical Manual of Mental Disorders, 5th Edition. Arlington, VA, American Psychiatric Association, 2013

Babington A: Shell Shock: A History of the Changing Attitudes to War Neurosis. London, Pen & Sword, 1990

Baker PJ: The Geneva Protocol. London, P.S. King & Son, 1925

Bateman A, Fonagy P: Mentalization-Based Treatment for Borderline Personality Disorder: A Practical Guide. New York, Oxford University Press, 2006

Beebe GW, Apple JW: Psychological breakdown in relation to stress and other factors, in Variation in Psychological Tolerance to Ground Combat in World War II, Final Report. Washington, DC, National Academy of Sciences, 1958, pp 88–131

Blanchard EB, Kolb LC, Pallmeyer TP, et al: A psychophysiological study of post traumatic stress disorder in Vietnam veterans. Psychiatr Q 54(4):220–229, 1982 7187510

Blaustein ME, Kinniburgh KM: Treating Traumatic Stress in Children and Adolescents: How to Foster Resiliency Through Attachment, Self-Regulation, and Competency. New York, Guilford, 2010

Bloom S: Creating Sanctuary. New York, Routledge, 1997

Bonnano G: The Other Side of Sadness. New York, Basic Books, 2010

Bremner JD: Alterations in brain structure and function associated with post-traumatic stress disorder. Semin Clin Neuropsychiatry 4(4):249–255, 1999 10553030

Briere J, Scott C: Principles of Trauma Therapy. Thousand Oaks, CA, Sage, 2006

Centers for Disease Control and Prevention: World Trade Center Health Program. Atlanta, GA, Centers for Disease Control and Prevention, 2012

Children's Bureau: Child Maltreatment in 2010. Washington, DC, U.S. Department of Health and Human Services, 2010

Cloitre M, Cohen L, Koenen K: Treating Survivors of Childhood Abuse. New York, Guilford, 2006

Cohen B, Barnes M, Rankin A: Managing Traumatic Stress Through Art. Lutherville, MD, Sidran, 1995

Cohen JA, Mannarino AP, Deblinger E: Treating Trauma and Traumatic Grief in Children and Adolescents. New York, Guilford, 2006

Courtois C: Healing the Incest Wound. New York, WW Norton, 1988

Courtois C, Ford J: Treatment of Complex Trauma. New York, Guilford, 2013

Craemer M, Forbes D, Phelps A, et al: Treating Traumatic Stress: Conducting Imaginal Exposure in PTSD (manual and video). Heidelberg West, Australia, Australian Centre for Posttraumatic Mental Health, 2004

Dalenberg C: Countertransference and the Treatment of Trauma. Washington, DC, American Psychological Association, 2000

Dershowitz A: The Abuse Excuse: And Other Cop-Outs, Sob Stories, and Evasions of Responsibility. Boston, MA, Little, Brown, 1994

Edwards VJ, Holden GW, Felitti VJ, et al: Relationship between multiple forms of childhood maltreatment and adult mental health in commmunity respondents: Results from the ACE Study. Am J Psych 160:1453–1460, 2003 12900308

Erichsen JE: On Railway Spine and Other Injuries of the Nervous System. Philadelphia, PA, Henry C Lea Publishers, 1867

Fabrizio B: Placebo Effects: Understanding the Mechanisms in Health and Disease. London, Oxford University Press, 2008

Fairbairn WRD: Nature and significance of war neuroses. BMJ 1(4284):183–186, 1943 20784682

Figley C: Helping Traumatized Families. San Francisco, CA, Jossey-Bass, 1989

Figley C: Compassion Fatigue. New York, Brunner/Mazel, 1995

Foa E, Rothbaum B: Treating the Trauma of Rape. New York, Guilford, 1998

Foa E, Hembree EA, Rothbaum O: Prolonged Exposure Therapy for Posttraumatic Stress Disorder: Emotional Processing of Traumatic Experiences. London, Oxford University Press, 2007

Foa E, Keane T, Friedman M, et al: Effective Treatments for Posttraumatic Stress Disorder, 2nd Edition. New York, Guilford, 2009

Follette VM, Briere J, Rozelle D, et al (eds): Mindfulness-Oriented Interventions for Trauma: Integrating Contemplative Practices. New York, Guilford, 2015

Ford JD, Russo E: Trauma-focused, present-centered, emotional self-regulation approach to integrated treatment for posttraumatic stress and addiction: trauma adaptive recovery group education and therapy (TARGET). Am J Psychother 60(4):335–355, 2006 17340945

Friedman MJ, Keane T, Resick P (eds): Handbook of PTSD: Science and Practice. New York, Guilford, 2007

Friedman M, Resick P, Bryant R, et al: Considering PTSD for DSM-5. Depress Anxiety 28(9):750–769, 2011 21910184

Gil E, Terr L: Working With Children to Heal Interpersonal Trauma. New York, Guilford, 2010

Goldenberg I, Goldenberg H: Family Therapy: An Overview. Belmont, CA, Wadsworth, 2000

Gonzales L: Surviving Survival: The Art and Science of Resilience. New York, WW Norton, 2012

Goodyear-Brown P: Play Therapy With Traumatized Children. New York, Wiley, 2009

Haber LF: The Poisonous Cloud: Chemical Warfare in the First World War. London, Oxford University Press, 1986

Hagen M: Whores of the Court: The Fraud of Psychiatric Testimony and the Rape of American Justice. New York, Regan Books, 1997

Harris M: Trauma Recovery and Empowerment. New York, Free Press, 1998

Herman J: Father-Daughter Incest. Cambridge, MA, Harvard University Press, 1981

Herman J: Trauma and Recovery. New York, Basic Books, 1992

Hersey J: Hiroshima. New York, Knopf, 1985

Institute of Medicine: Treatment of Posttraumatic Stress Disorder: An Assessment of the Evidence. Washington, DC, Institute of Medicine of the National Academies, 2007

Janoff-Bulman R: Shattered Assumptions: Towards a New Psychology of Trauma. New York, Free Press, 1992

Jayaraman N, Bruno K: Trading in disaster: World Trade Center scrap lands in India. CorpWatch February 6, 2002. Available at: http://www.corpwatch.org/articlc.php?id=1608. Accessed October 15, 2013.

Johnson D: The therapeutic use of ceremonies and rituals in posttraumatic stress disorder, in Encyclopedia of Trauma. Edited by Figley C. New York, Guilford, 2012, pp 573–575

Johnson D: Trauma-centered developmental transformations, in Trauma-Informed Drama Therapy: Transforming Clinics, Classrooms, and Communities. Edited by Sajnani N, Johnson D. Springfield, IL, Charles C Thomas, 2014, pp 68–92

Johnson D, Lubin H: Group psychotherapy for the symptoms of posttraumatic stress disorder, in Group Psychotherapy for Psychological Trauma. Edited by Klein RH, Schermer VL. New York, Guilford, 2000, pp 141–169

Johnson DR, Feldman S, Lubin H: Critical interaction therapy: couples therapy in combat-related posttraumatic stress disorder. Fam Process 34(4):401–412, 1995 8674521

Johnson D, Lubin H, Rosenheck R, et al: The impact of the homecoming reception on the development of posttraumatic stress disorder: the West Haven Homecoming Stress Scale (WHHSS). J Trauma Stress 10(2):259–278, 1997 9136091

Johnson D, Lahad M, Gray A: Creative therapies for adults, in Effective Treatments for PTSD, 2nd Edition. Edited by Foa E, Keane T, Friedman M, et al. New York, Guilford, 2009, pp 479–490

Johnson SM: Emotionally Focused Couple Therapy for Trauma Survivors. New York, Guilford, 2002

Jones E, Wessely S: War syndromes: the impact of culture on medically unexplained symptoms. Med Hist 49(1):55–78, 2005 15730130

Jones E, Wessely S: Psychological trauma: a historical perspective. Psychiatry 5(7):217–220, 2006

Jones TF: Mass psychogenic illness: role of the individual physician. Am Fam Physician 62(12):2649–2653, 2655–2656, 2000 11142471

Kardiner A: The Traumatic Neuroses of War. Washington, DC, National Research Council, 1941

Keane T, Fairbank JA, Caddell JM, et al: Implosive (flooding) therapy reduces symptoms of posttraumatic stress disorder in Vietnam combat veterans. Behav Ther 20(2):245–260, 1989

Kernberg O: Severe Personality Disorders: Psychotherapeutic Strategies. New Haven, CT, Yale University Press, 1984

Kessler RC, Sonnega A, Bromet E, et al: Posttraumatic stress disorder in the National Comorbidity Study. Arch Gen Psych 52:1048–1060, 1995 7492257

Klein RH, Schermer VL: Group Psychotherapy for Psychological Trauma. New York, Guilford, 2000

Kulka RA, Schlenger WE, Fairbank JA, et al: Trauma and the Vietnam War Generation: Report of Findings From the National Vietnam Veterans Readjustment Study. New York, Brunner/Mazel, 1990

Lifton R: Home From the War: Vietnam Veterans Neither Victims nor Executioners. New York, Touchstone Press, 1973

Linehan M: Cognitive-Behavioral Treatment of Borderline Personality Disorder. New York, Guilford, 1993

Lombardi K: Death by dust: the frightening link between the 9/11 toxic cloud and cancer. Village Voice, November 21, 2006

Lubin H, Johnson D: Use of ceremony in multiple family therapy for psychological trauma, in Action Therapy With Families and Groups. Edited by Wiener D, Oxford L. Washington, DC, American Psychological Association, 2003, pp 75–102

Lubin H, Johnson D: Trauma-Centered Group Psychotherapy for Women. New York, Taylor & Francis, 2008

Malchiodi CA, Perry B: Creative Interventions With Traumatized Children, 2nd Edition. New York, Guilford, 2014

Masferrer R: The Gulf War syndrome: is it really a new disorder? Barrow Quarterly 13(4):13–27, 1997

Masterson J: The Narcissistic and Borderline Disorders. New York, Brunner/Mazel, 1981

McCann L, Pearlman L: Psychological Trauma and the Adult Survivor: Theory, Therapy, and Transformation. New York, Brunner/Mazel, 1990

Mendelsohn M, Herman J, Schatzow E, et al: The Trauma Recovery Group: A Guide for Practitioners. New York, Guilford, 2011

Milgram S: Obedience to Authority: An Experimental View. New York, Harper & Row, 1974

Monson C, Fredman SJ: Cognitive-Behavioral Conjoint Therapy for PTSD. New York, Guilford, 2012

Myers CS: A contribution to the study of shell shock. Lancet 1:316–320, 1915

Nordstrom B: The History of Sweden. Westport, CT, Greenwood, 2002

O'Brien T: The Things They Carried. Boston, MA, Houghton-Mifflin, 1990

Ochberg F: Post-Traumatic Therapy and Victims of Violence. New York, Brunner/Mazel, 1988

Ochberg FM: The counting method for ameliorating traumatic memories. J Trauma Stress 9(4):873–880, 1996 8902753

Paris J: Social Factors in the Personality Disorders. Cambridge, UK, Cambridge University Press, 1996

Pearlman L, Saakvitne K: Trauma and the Therapist: Countertransference and Vicarious Traumatization in Psychotherapy With Incest Victims. New York, WW Norton, 1995

Power J: Lee's Miserables. Chapel Hill, University of North Carolina Press, 1998

Putkowski J, Sykes J: Shot at Dawn. London, Pen & Sword, 1999

Putnam F: Diagnosis and Treatment of Multiple Personality Disorder. New York, Guilford, 1989

Pynoos RS, Steinberg AM, Layne CM, et al: DSM-V PTSD diagnostic criteria for children and adolescents: a developmental perspective and recommendations. J Trauma Stress 22(5):391–398, 2009 19780125

Ready DJ, Thomas KR, Worley V, et al: A field test of group based exposure therapy with 102 veterans with war-related posttraumatic stress disorder. J Trauma Stress 21(2):150–157, 2008 18404634

Resick P, Schnicke M: Cognitive Processing Therapy for Rape Victims. Newbury Park, CA, Sage, 1993

Saakvitne K, Gamble S, Pearlman L, et al: Risking Connection: A Training Course for Working With Survivors of Childhood Abuse. Lutherville, MD, Sidran Press, 2000

Sajnani N, Johnson D (eds): Trauma-Informed Drama Therapy: Transforming Clinics, Classrooms, and Communities. Springfield, IL, Charles C Thomas, 2014

Schauer M, Neuner F, Ebert T: Narrative Exposure Therapy. Cambridge, MA, Hogrefe, 2011

Schnurr PP, Green B (eds): Trauma and Health: Physical Health Consequences of Exposure to Extreme Stress. Washington, DC, American Psychological Association, 2004

Selvini Palazzoli M, Boscolo L, Burt EV, et al: Paradox and Counterparadox. New York, Jason Aronson, 1978

Shapiro F: Eye Movement Desensitization and Reprocessing. New York, Guilford, 1995

Shay J: Achilles in Vietnam: Combat Trauma and the Undoing of Character. New York, Simon & Schuster, 1995

Shay J: Odysseus in America: Combat Trauma and the Trials of Homecoming. New York, Scribner, 2002

Simon R (ed): Posttraumatic Stress Disorder in Litigation: Guidelines for Forensic Assessment. Washington, DC, American Psychiatric Publishing, 2003

Sloan DM, Marx BP, Bovin MJ, et al: Written exposure as an intervention for PTSD: a randomized clinical trial with motor vehicle accident survivors. Behav Res Ther 50(10):627–635, 2012 22863540

Spiegel H, Spiegel D: Trance and Treatment: Clinical Uses of Hypnosis. Washington, DC, American Psychiatric Publishing, 2004

U.S. Department of Justice: National Crime Victimization Survey, 2006–2010. Washington, DC, U.S. Department of Justice, 2011

van der Kolk BA: Psychological Trauma. Washington, DC, American Psychiatric Press, 1987

van der Kolk BA: The history of trauma in psychiatry, in Handbook of PTSD: Science and Practice. Edited by Friedman M, Keane T, Resick PA. New York, Guilford, 2010, pp 21–37

van der Kolk BA, Hostetler A, Herron N, et al: Trauma and the development of borderline personality disorder. Psychiatr Clin North Am 17:715–730, 1994 7533284

Weathers FW, Keane TM: The Criterion A problem revisited: controversies and challenges in defining and measuring psychological trauma. J Trauma Stress 20(2):107–121, 2007 17427913

Weathers F, Blake D, Schnurr P, et al: Clinician-Administered PTSD Scale for DSM-5. White River Junction, VT, National Center for PTSD, 2014

Wilson J, Lindy J: Countertransference in the Treatment of Posttraumatic Stress Disorder. New York, Guilford, 1994

Yehuda R: Psychobiology of Posttraumatic Stress Disorder. New York, Wiley, 2006

Young A: The Harmony of Illusions: Inventing Posttraumatic Stress Disorder. Princeton, NJ, Princeton University Press, 1995

Answers to Study Questions

PREFACE

P.1   Match the items:

A. Trauma schema   ___ the objective event

B. Traumatic experience   ___ emotions experienced during the traumatic event

C. Traumatic memory   ___ what the client perceived during the event

D. Traumatic event   ___ how the trauma has impacted the client's view of the world

E. Neurotic schema   ___ pattern of behavior and thinking arising out of major personal relationships

F. Primary emotions   ___ what the client remembers now about the trauma

G. Secondary emotions   ___ emotions arising from appraisal of the trauma after the event

Answers: D, F, B, A, E, C, G

P.2   What is the difference between neurotic schemas and trauma schemas?

Answer: Neurotic schemas are patterns of perception of self and others derived from childhood experiences that maintain interpersonal coherence and connection in the presence of conflict. Trauma schemas are patterns of perception derived from a break in this fundamen-

tal connection to others and the world as a result of overwhelming fear or shame.

CHAPTER 1: THE DEVELOPING CULTURAL CONTEXT OF TRAUMA-CENTERED PSYCHOTHERAPY

1.1   What are the four main explanatory causes for PTSD?

Answer: Character weakness, social oppression, physical causes, and overwhelming fear or shame.

1.2   When should an individual's experience of trauma be contained, and when should it be expressed?

Answer: This is for each individual and society to determine, but generally a balance between the two should be maintained, where both containment and expression are allowed as appropriate to serve the needs of the individual and society.

1.3   What was the difference in the profession's view of trauma prior to 1960 and after 1990?

Answer: Prior to 1960, trauma was viewed as deeply buried in the unconscious, requiring strong measures to access it. After 1990, trauma was viewed as near the surface and often too easily accessible, requiring more preparation and more careful approaches to avoid evoking flooding of emotion or retraumatization.

1.4   Why are treatments such as sodium amytal and hypnosis not used often now for the treatment of PTSD?

Answer: Methods based on imaginal exposure have been found to be equally reliable and effective, without requiring the intensity of sodium amytal or hypnosis, which were used when trauma was viewed as deeply buried in the client's unconscious.

1.5   Describe these conditions:

     A.   Railway spine
     B.   Tropical asthenia
     C.   Shell shock

D. Gas hysteria
E. War neurosis

Railway spine: Physical pain and anxiety symptoms after railroad accidents in the 1800s.
Tropical asthenia: Name for disabling conditions shown by returning soldiers from the Spanish American War.
Shell shock: Name for disabling conditions shown by returning soldiers from World War I.
Gas hysteria: Mass retreats of soldiers from World War I battlefields when they believed they had been gassed, confusing anxiety symptoms with gas poisoning.
War neurosis: Name for anxiety and psychosomatic disorders shown by returning soldiers from World War II, influenced by psychoanalytic ideas.

1.6   Attribution to physical causes for PTSD tended to follow what developments?

Answer: New scientific discoveries such as bacteria or neuroscience, or new technologies such as railroads, large cannons, nerve gas, or brain scanning.

1.7   Why is there a conflict between evidence for exposure therapy and physical causes?

Answer: The physical causes hypothesis would suggest that the impairments are relatively chronic and stable, whereas exposure therapy is based on the idea that symptoms are due to conditioning that can be ameliorated with new learning.

1.8   Why does PTSD present itself so often as a physical malady?

Answer: Stress and anxiety are experienced in many parts of the body, and natural tendencies toward avoidance are supported by the belief that one has a medical condition.

1.9   Do you think that the diagnosis and treatment of PTSD as a medical condition contributes to an avoidance of dealing with the sources of social oppression in our society?

Answer: There are many ways of viewing this issue. Hopefully, the greater knowledge gained about the physical aspects of PTSD will

not draw attention away from the need to address social contributions to abuse, neglect, and community violence.

CHAPTER 2: AXIOMS OF TRAUMA-CENTERED PSYCHOTHERAPY

2.1 What are the four axioms of trauma-centered psychotherapy?

Answer:

Trauma schemas arise in order to reduce the primary emotions of fear and shame.

Both client and therapist will be participating in avoidance to some degree all the time.

The client's trauma narrative is always incomplete.

Trauma schemas are relational.

2.2 What is the major reason for avoidance?

Answer: Reexperiencing the fear or shame of the original traumatic experience.

2.3 What are common forms of avoidance in the therapy session?

Answer: Delaying the trauma inquiry, warming-up by talking about other topics first, and attending to an immediate crisis instead of the trauma inquiry.

2.4 If the narrative is always incomplete, what is it that is not included? Why should this matter?

Answer: What remains unsaid is the next most upsetting detail. This matters because the client will be thinking about what is next, and the therapist should not attribute the client's behavior completely to what he or she has just said. Therefore, the therapist should indicate awareness that the client has more to say.

2.5 If the client goes home and becomes upset after the session, what might this mean?

Answer: The client was upset by a detail from his or her traumatic memories that was not expressed in the session and/or was missed by the therapist.

2.6 Why do people tend to view their traumatic events in relational terms?

Answer: Our basic assumptions of safety include being protected by others around us. Thus, anger and distress tend not to be directed toward impersonal forces that have no agency, but instead to those people who are charged with protecting us but who failed.

2.7 Who are the most likely people to be blamed for impersonal traumatic events and why?

Answer: People who are expected to care for and protect us: authorities, family members, friends, and health care professionals.

CHAPTER 3: ESTABLISHING THE TRAUMA-CENTERED FRAME

3.1 Why is it important to establish a trauma-centered frame?

Answer: Because this provides a mutual understanding of the purpose of the treatment that will allow the therapist to refuse to join in the client's attempts at avoidance. The frame helps to keep the treatment focused on the trauma.

3.2 What is the rationale for conducting a trauma-centered psychotherapy?

Answer: Imaginal exposure to reminders of the trauma has been demonstrated to be the most effective form of trauma treatment.

3.3 What are some effective ways of establishing the frame?

Answer: During the first contact with the client, directly address the trauma-centered frame. Have direct references to trauma and trauma treatment in the office environment. Include mention of trauma and the nature of trauma treatment in the written forms used by the therapist.

CHAPTER 4: PRINCIPLES OF TRAUMA-CENTERED PSYCHOTHERAPY

4.1 What are the three main principles of trauma-centered psychotherapy?

Answer: Immediacy, engagement, and emotionality.

4.2   Does the principle of immediacy conflict with establishing safety in the therapeutic encounter? If not, why?

Answer: No, it does not, because the anticipatory anxiety experienced by many trauma clients will be reduced once the trauma inquiry is begun. The therapist's confidence in attending to the real problem and not colluding with the avoidance will give the client a feeling of trust that the therapist is competent.

4.3   How can a neutral stance by the therapist make the trauma client feel uncomfortable?

Answer: Because the traumatized client is likely to attribute the disinterest or distance of the bystander in the therapist's neutral stance, evoking memories of any bystanders in the traumatic experience.

4.4   What are the main elements of the therapist's engagement?

Answer: The therapist 1) maintains a strongly held gaze on the client; 2) remains aware of posture to avoid moving slightly away from the client when hearing traumatic material; 3) uses experience-near questioning in which the therapist imagines being present with the client in the traumatic event and asks questions about what is happening; and 4) shows some degree of affective response to the horrors of the client's experiences.

4.5   Why is it important that trauma-centered clinicians feel comfortable with expressions of strong emotion from their clients?

Answer: Because traumatized clients are deeply upset by their experiences and have generally suppressed the expression of their fears and distress. They anticipate that others will be unable to listen to or tolerate their distress and therefore fear that they will overwhelm others if they fully express themselves.

4.6   Does the trauma-centered approach discourage teaching clients affect regulation skills before engaging in the trauma inquiry? Explain your answer.

Answer: No. Therapists are welcome to use whatever methods and techniques they have found helpful in preparing clients for trauma-centered work, as long as these activities are not serving the avoidance of beginning the work.

CHAPTER 5: THE FOUR MAIN TECHNIQUES

5.1   What are the four main techniques of trauma-centered psychotherapy?

Answer: Getting the details, decoding current behavior, introducing discrepancy, and disclosing the perpetrator.

5.2   What is the difference between chronological/horizontal inquiry and detailed/vertical inquiry?

Answer: Chronological inquiry follows the natural timeline of an event, taking the client from beginning to end of the traumatic experience. Vertical inquiry holds at a given point in time and explores additional details of the moment, including sensory perceptions of the internal and external environment, thoughts and feelings of the victim, and fears of anticipated actions by the perpetrator.

5.3   What is the most important reason to get the details of a traumatic experience?

Answer: The experiences of horror, helplessness, and fear are usually located in minute details that are covered up, euphemized, or simply labeled. Without accessing the experience of fear or shame, the client's traumatic distress cannot be desensitized.

5.4   Define the technique of decoding.

Answer: Decoding is pointing out the overlap between current perceptions and behaviors and past trauma schemas. Decoding helps the client appreciate how his or her past traumatic experiences continue to exert an influence on current relationships.

5.5   What are the most likely elements to be decoded in this short narrative by a client who had previously experienced a trauma:

> "My boss was really enraged with Bob, so much so that he grabbed him by his shirt, no collar, and yelled at him, so I came over and told him to release Bob's collar and calm down. It was crazy, like there was foam coming out of his mouth or something, and Bob just took it and sat down in his chair. My boss looked at him with contempt and then spit into Bob's wastebasket and stormed off. I was really upset. Bob just whimpered."

Answer: The therapist should ask the client if any of these elements occurred during his or her own trauma: a collar, foam from the mouth, just taking it, spitting into something, and whimpering.

5.6   Introducing discrepancy means pointing out to the client the differences between which things?

Answer: Between the past and the present, and between the perpetrator (then) and the person challenging him or her (now).

5.7   Why is it common for people not to mention the perpetrator in trauma narratives?

Answer: Fear of the perpetrator; the perpetrator is no longer alive or near; avoidance of the memories because the mention of the perpetrator will bring up the event; not wanting to upset others.

5.8   What are the three main ways of disclosing the perpetrator?

Answer: Naming the perpetrator often, reframing the trauma as an act of the perpetrator, and describing the appearance and behavior of the perpetrator in detail.

5.9   Fill in the blanks:

Answer:

> **"Mr. Smith held Vivien down on the bed and raped her" is a <u>RE-FRAMING</u> of "Vivien experienced a sexual assault by a Mr. Smith."**
>
> **"Tell me more about how Mr. Smith looked at that moment when he was on top of you" is using the technique of <u>DESCRIBING</u>.**

CHAPTER 6: THE FIRST SESSION

6.1   What is the main goal of the first session?

Answer: To get enough details to establish the trauma-centered frame and demonstrate the competence and resolve of the therapist.

6.2   What written aids are helpful in the first session?

Answer: Traumatic life events questionnaire and structured interview.

6.3   Halfway through the first session, the client says, "I don't feel that comfortable talking in such detail about what happened to me....It's a bit much for me now. Can we talk about other things going on in

my life and get back to the trauma next time?" Which is the best response from the therapist, from a trauma-centered perspective?

   A. I can understand your concern, and we should go at your pace,
so certainly we can get back to it next time.

   B. As you are aware, this is a treatment for your trauma, so I'm afraid
that we have to keep working on it.

   C. What feelings just came up for you to make you feel like it is too
much?

   D. As we talked about before, this process is likely to bring up painful memories, and you don't have to continue, but no matter what
we do, we will return to this point, and I'm ready to help you with
it. (*Looks quietly at client.*)

**Answer: D. As we talked about before, this process is likely to bring
up painful memories, and you don't have to continue, but no matter
what we do, we will return to this point and I'm ready to help you with
it. (*Looks quietly at client.*)**

CHAPTER 7: CONTINUING THE TRAUMA HISTORY

7.1   Match the appropriate items.

A. Not agreeing	___ "I'm not sure I get what you are saying here."
B. Not understanding	___ "That is amazing, but tell me more about what happened in the boat."
C. Not accepting closure	___ "How could he have jumped that high?"

Answers: B, C, A

7.2   Match the appropriate items.

A. Bumps	___ The client pauses because he or she is upset.
B. Jumps	___ The client uses the phrase "sexual assault."
C. Stops	___ The client clears his or her throat and becomes flushed while speaking.
D. Bridges	___ The client skips a few minutes of time in the narrative.

E. Labels   ___ The client comments on an aspect
                             of the city in which the event took
                             place.

Answers: C, E, A, B, D.

7.3   Name the seven techniques useful in getting the details of the trau-
       matic memories.

**Answer: Looking around, zooming in, slowing down, repeating, back-
ing up, pausing, and using present tense.**

7.4   What are the five layers of a trauma schema?

**Answer: Fear or shame, pain, sensory elements, anticipated actions,
and lack of rescue.**

7.5   Name which layer is being represented in the following statements:

A. "I know things will be worse in the future."
B. "I don't believe it when people tell me they will help."
C. "I can't stand the smell of boxwood."
D. "I can get a headache at almost any time."
E. "There's no way to describe it."

Answers:

A. **Anticipated actions**
B. **Lack of rescue**
C. **Sensory elements**
D. **Pain**
E. **Fear**

7.6   What is the major function of formulating the client's trauma schemas?

**Answer: The target of trauma-centered psychotherapy is the altera-
tion of the client's trauma schemas, which are all that are left from the
original event. It is essential for the therapist to have a deep understanding of these fundamental misperceptions in order to be able to
help the client decode current behaviors and work toward differentiating the past from the present.**

CHAPTER 8: CONDUCTING ONGOING TREATMENT

8.1   What are the two main components of this phase of treatment?

Answer: Imaginal exposure and cognitive restructuring.

8.2   Fill in the blanks:

Answer: In decoding, one identifies the <u>TRIGGER,</u> then points out the <u>LINKS</u> between that and an element of the traumatic experience, noting the <u>SIMILARITIES</u> between the past event and the current situation, and then emphasizes the <u>DIFFERENCES</u> between the past and the present and between the perpetrator and the challenger.

CHAPTER 9: THE GAP

9.1   Define the gap.

Answer: The gap is a disruption in the continuity of the therapeutic relationship caused by the client's trauma schema being applied to that relationship. In the gap, the client experiences the therapist as a perpetrator, bystander, or collaborator in a current situation that the client feels is injurious to him or her and that the therapist feels is untrue or greatly overblown. The gap is an expected event within trauma-centered psychotherapy that provides opportunities to explore new details of the client's traumatic memories.

9.2   T/F   The rise of the gap in the therapeutic relationship indicates that the therapist has made a mistake in the trauma inquiry.

Answer: False.

9.3   What are the four roles in the usual trauma schema?

Answer: Victim, perpetrator, bystander, and collaborator.

9.4   Why is the role of the rescuer not present in a trauma schema?

Answer: Because there was no rescuer in the original traumatic event, or else it would not have been traumatic. If anyone did come to help, it was after the traumatic event had occurred.

9.5   Why is the experience of the gap so stressful for the therapist?

Answer: Therapists are trained to be empathic and feel competent in understanding their clients. The gap is the absence of the empathic bridge and understanding between the client and therapist, which most therapists will experience as a failure on their part, if not accused of failing by the client.

9.6   What are the five steps of a response to the gap?

Answer: Restating the problem, linking to the trauma, acknowledging harm, pointing out the discrepancy, and recognizing the failure to prevent the trauma.

9.7   T/F   When responding to the gap, it is important not to imply that the current complaint by the client is baseless because it is a displacement from a past trauma.

Answer: True.

9.8   How does trauma interfere with the process of normal mourning?

Answer: In normal mourning, the person identifies with the lost person or object and gradually comes to realize that that person or object is gone. Trauma leads to identification with the perpetrator as a result of the fear, and until that identification can be loosened through desensitization, mourning cannot begin.

CHAPTER 10: LONG-TERM PROCESS IN TREATMENT

10.1   T/F   In long-term work, new details of the past traumas are rarely disclosed.

Answer: False.

10.2   T/F   In long-term work, the traumatic events are mentioned in every session.

Answer: True.

10.3   T/F   In long-term work, clients learn how to employ the techniques of trauma-centered treatment themselves.

Answer: True.

10.4 T/F In long-term work, the therapist generally discourages the client from finding ways of repairing his or her losses, because this would support denial that the trauma occurred.

Answer: False.

10.5 T/F In treatment checkups, it is not necessary to ask the client again about his or her traumas.

Answer: False.

10.6 T/F The process of reparation involves engaging the client not only in positive activities but also in activities that are meaningfully linked to the suffering and experiences the client has had.

Answer: True.

CHAPTER 11: HANDLING THE EDGES

11.1 T/F Dissociative reactions in treatment are not generally harmful, and the best strategy is to wait them out.

Answer: True.

11.2 T/F When a client is threatening violence, the therapist should not attempt to control or eliminate the behavior at first, but rather should try to connect the behavior to a past traumatic experience.

Answer: True.

11.3 T/F Clients' disruptive behaviors outside of the session are often a way of communicating a new detail of their traumatic experience.

Answer: True.

11.4 T/F Trauma-centered psychotherapy is possible even when the client has no direct memories of abuse.

Answer: False.

CHAPTER 12: WORKING WITH CLIENTS WITH DISSOCIATIVE IDENTITY DISORDER

12.1   What is the difference between primary and secondary personalities?

Answer: An assumption in trauma-centered psychotherapy is that all of the primary personalities were present at the original traumatic event. Secondary personalities arise later in response to new threats to the person, including the trauma inquiry itself.

12.2   T/F   It is possible for new alters to emerge in treatment in response to the trauma inquiry.

Answer: True.

12.3   What are the common primary personalities?

Answer: Innocent child, witness figure, protective figure, acting-out figure, host personality.

12.4   T/F   The therapist should at all times maintain a neutral, slightly disinterested stance toward any dramatic presentations of the personalities.

Answer: True.

12.5   T/F   In trauma-centered work with clients with dissociative identity disorder, the therapist works to integrate the client's dissociated identities.

Answer: False.

12.6   What is the major challenge to trauma-centered psychotherapy in working with clients with dissociative identity disorder?

Answer: Conducting the trauma inquiry and getting the details of the original traumatic event are impeded by shifting among personalities and strong avoidance from the fragmented personality system.

Chapter 13: Working With Clients With Borderline Personality Disorder

13.1 Is it necessary to believe that borderline personality disorder is caused by trauma in order to do trauma-centered psychotherapy with these clients? Why or why not?

Answer: No, but the client must have experienced traumatic events in order to do trauma-centered psychotherapy. The therapist should be able to explain the association or link between early childhood trauma and the expression of borderline symptoms, either as causative or as exacerbatory.

13.2 What are the major challenges to trauma-centered psychotherapy with clients who have borderline personality disorder?

Answer: Clients will resist having their problems explained by trauma and will resist providing details. They will be in the gap with the therapist often, experiencing the therapist as abandoning or betraying them. They will blame their acting out on the trauma work and tell other professionals so. They will quit the treatment and then reengage only if the trauma work is suspended.

13.3 T/F It is important to establish the trauma-centered frame and collect an initial detailed trauma history as quickly as possible with clients who have borderline personality disorder.

Answer: True.

13.4 T/F It is fair to say that the therapist will experience being in the gap with the client who has borderline personality disorder often during the treatment.

Answer: True.

13.5 T/F The client with borderline personality disorder is most likely to cast the therapist in the role of victim in the trauma schema.

Answer: False.

13.6   T/F   The therapist should explain the relationship between border-line personality disorder and trauma often during the treatment in order to concretize and externalize the client's condition, as a way of building an alliance with the client to engage in the trauma-centered work.

Answer: True.

13.7   What is the role of the reparative dream in working with clients who have borderline personality disorder?

Answer: Supporting the reparative dream provides hope, reframes clients' suffering as a basis for a future career or contribution, and distances the therapeutic process from the immediate crisis.

CHAPTER 14: TRAUMA-CENTERED GROUP PSYCHOTHERAPY

14.1   When should the client be referred to trauma-centered group therapy?

Answer: When the client or the therapist determines that working more intensely on interpersonal aspects of the client's trauma schemas in the presence of other clients with similar and different experiences will be helpful. This usually occurs after the initial stages of trauma-centered work have been completed.

14.2   T/F   The group setting itself might trigger clients who were traumatized in group environments.

Answer: True.

14.3   T/F   Clients are not likely to be triggered by the stories of other group members.

Answer: False.

14.4   T/F   It is possible to conduct trauma-centered therapy in structured or unstructured groups, and in time-limited and open-ended groups.

Answer: True.

14.5   T/F   Each group member should describe his or her major traumatic events in the first group meeting.

Answer: True.

14.6   T/F   Groups provide greater opportunities for introducing discrepancy, because each group member can share his or her own unique experience that will vary from the client's.

Answer: True.

14.7   T/F   It is not necessary to inform the group members in the beginning about possible dissociative reactions and how they will be dealt with.

Answer: False.

CHAPTER 15: TRAUMA-CENTERED COUPLES AND FAMILY PSYCHOTHERAPY

15.1   Why is it likely that trauma-centered therapy with the client's partner or family will be helpful?

Answer: Trauma schemas are most often applied in the client's intimate relationships, distorting and straining them, and evoking behaviors in the others that mimic those of the original perpetrator. Family or couples therapy can be very useful in disentangling these distortions.

15.2   T/F   Quite often, family members think that they know about the trauma, when in fact they have not been told most of the details.

Answer: True.

15.3   T/F   Quite often, the roles of the trauma schema (victim, perpetrator, bystander, collaborator) are being played out among family members without their awareness.

Answer: True.

15.4   What are the main goals of trauma-centered family treatment?

Answer: To identify and share the specific traumas, to share the details of each trauma with the family, to learn how the trauma schemas are influencing current behaviors, and to collectivize family members' relationship with the trauma.

15.5   T/F   It is not necessary for the therapist to be active and maintain control of the family or couples sessions.

Answer: False.

15.6   T/F   The therapist should never meet individually with any family member, because that would make other family members feel the therapist was aligning with another member.

Answer: False.

15.7   T/F   Circular questioning is asking a question to a family member that he or she has the authority to answer.

Answer: False.

15.8   T/F   In third-party questioning, the therapist discusses the behavior of a family member with another member, while the first person is present.

Answer: True.

15.9   Why is it so important to externalize the perpetrator in trauma-centered family therapy?

Answer: Because the client's trauma schema often infiltrates the family interactions, such that other family members are cast in the role of perpetrator, causing resentment and anger, which mimics the original behavior of the perpetrator, thereby conflating past and present outside the awareness of family members.

CHAPTER 16: ADJUNCTIVE METHODS

16.1   When might a therapist suggest a written narrative approach to a client?

Answer: If the client indicates an interest in writing or journaling, and if the standard trauma inquiry seems too abstract for the client.

16.2 T/F In the two-story method, each story should be written to be as credible as possible.

Answer: True.

16.3 T/F In the two-story method, the goal is to tolerate the ambiguity of not knowing for certain the truth of the traumatic experience.

Answer: True.

16.4 What is the main rationale for using the mailbox method?

Answer: The mailbox provides a playful and distanced way of dialoguing with significant people in the client's life. The power of writing and receiving letters offers an immediacy that can open up a client's expressive range.

16.5 T/F In the two-dimensional grid, the goal is for the client to identify and express the moments of greatest distress in his or her traumatic memories.

Answer: True.

16.6 T/F In the two-dimensional grid, the client moves forward or backward in time, and zooms inward or outward in proximity, from the first picture.

Answer: True.

16.7 What are the advantages of the therapist participating in the conversational art method?

Answer: By participating, the therapist joins the conversation just as in verbal therapy, where the therapist can influence the flow of the client's thought process, identify avoidant behaviors, and introduce graduated levels of imaginal exposure.

16.8 T/F The purpose of the technique of harming the picture is to flood the client with emotion.

Answer: False.

16.9 T/F   The aim of perpetrator portraits supports the goal of disclosing the perpetrator.

Answer: True.

16.10 T/F   The use of photographs and videotaping often increases the vividness of the client's recall of his or her experiences, and therefore aids in the desensitization process.

Answer: True.

16.11 What reasons do clients have to desire to dispose of their autobiographical materials?

Answer: They may feel a sense of accomplishment in the processing of their traumas, and they may wish to symbolically "graduate" or "move on" and to put their perpetrator "to rest."

16.12 Why is the use of the telephone usually more comfortable for the therapist in role-playing with the client?

Answer: Because the therapist does not have to play another character and can remain himself or herself in the role-play on the telephone.

16.13 How does use of the memory box address the client's avoidance?

Answer: The use of the ironic label "Do Not Open" names the act of avoidance and thereby undermines it, while at the same time respecting the client's desire to not talk about the memory.

CHAPTER 17: STRAINS ON THE THERAPIST

17.1 T/F   Trauma therapists should not have to expect high levels of stress in their work.

Answer: False.

17.2 T/F   Trauma-centered psychotherapy is based on the model of the therapist as a good-enough parent.

Answer: False.

17.3 T/F The most effective way of handling compassion fatigue is to have the competence to handle the gap when it occurs in the therapeutic encounter.

Answer: True.

17.4 T/F In trauma-centered psychotherapy, doubt about the accuracy of the client's story is the sign of a major problem in the relationship.

Answer: False.

17.5 T/F In the therapeutic relationship, the therapist should hold the discrepancy between supporting the client's version of the facts and the possibility that what the client remembers is inaccurate.

Answer: True.

17.6 T/F The task and norms of psychotherapy and the law are basically the same.

Answer: False.

17.7 Why are self-care strategies such as slowing down the trauma inquiry or not getting as much into the details *not* recommended in trauma-centered psychotherapy?

Answer: Because these strategies interfere with the work of trauma-centered psychotherapy, as opposed to self-care strategies that help the therapist outside of sessions.

17.8 What is the major cause of a therapist's retaliatory fantasies against the client's perpetrator?

Answer: Insufficient attention to the client's feelings and perceptions of his or her perpetrator, and not enough time spent working on disclosing the perpetrator in the therapy sessions.

17.9 A strong desire to rescue the client by providing special or extra resources is often the sign of what unexplored issue in the client's traumatic experience?

Answer: The client's feelings at the time of the trauma of being ignored, unprotected, not believed, or betrayed by people who should have been able to help him or her.

17.10 T/F   Clients' calls for help often occur at times when they know or expect the therapist will not to be able to respond.

Answer: True.

17.11 T/F   Therapists should do whatever they can to be available to their clients, in case an emergency arises.

Answer: False.

17.12 T/F   The therapist's inconsistency in helping the client is likely to support the client's trauma schemas of his or her caretakers' neglect, betrayal, or false promises.

Answer: True.

CHAPTER 18: LIMITS TO THE TRAUMA-CENTERED APPROACH

18.1   T/F   Trauma-centered psychotherapy is the treatment of choice over other forms of trauma treatment.

Answer: False.

18.2   T/F   Trauma-centered psychotherapy should be used by clinicians who feel comfortable doing in-depth trauma inquiries.

Answer: True.

18.3   T/F   Therapists using trauma-centered psychotherapy should assess whether their institution supports this approach and, if not, find ways to gain that support through education and advocacy.

Answer: True.

18.4   What are the two bases of credibility of a trauma-centered therapist in court?

Answer: The observations of the client's symptoms and behaviors in the therapy sessions, and opinions about their personal character; not determinations of fact.

18.5   T/F   Trauma-centered psychotherapists are capable of determining the truthfulness of the client's trauma narrative.

Answer: False.

18.6   T/F   Aspects of trauma-centered psychotherapy can be considered suggestive to the client.

Answer: True.

18.7   For traumatized clients ages 0–5, which treatment is recommended? (Check any that apply.)

Answer:

> **_X_Supportive play therapy**
> **_____Trauma-centered play therapy**
> **_X_Work with their caretakers**
> **_____No treatment but close monitoring of their condition**

18.8   For traumatized clients ages 5–12, which treatment is recommended? (Check any that apply.)

Answer:

> **_____Supportive play therapy**
> **_X_Trauma-centered play therapy**
> **_X_Trauma-focused cognitive behavioral therapy**
> **_X_Trauma-centered family therapy**

CHAPTER 19: CONCLUSION

19.1   What component of trauma-centered psychotherapy seems most challenging for you as a clinician?

Answers will vary.

19.2   What is your opinion regarding the value of delving deeply into the details of another person's traumatic experience? Do you feel that it is essential to the client's recovery or unnecessary if he or she finds other means of building resilience and learning how to regulate emotions?

Answers will vary.

Consent to Treatment

David Read Johnson, Ph.D.

Hadar Lubin, M.D.

I, the undersigned, agree to enter treatment/evaluation at the _____. I have been given a copy of the privacy policy, and the procedures have been explained to me to my satisfaction. I understand that all information about me will be held in strictest confidence by my clinician.

I understand that the benefits from psychotherapy will result from the collaboration between my clinician and me and that the results are not guaranteed. I understand that I am welcome to discuss how my treatment is going at any time with my clinician and his or her supervisor, whose identity I have been apprised of. I understand that I have the right to terminate my treatment at any time, for any reason.

I understand that a significant part of my treatment will involve discussing the details of events that were abusive, neglectful, stressful, and/or traumatic, because of their relevance to my condition. I understand that doing so may be difficult, may evoke emotions, and/or may upset me and that it is not my clinician's intent to cause me distress but rather to lower my distress through a process of desensitization, in which I will become less upset when I remember what happened to me. I understand that I can stop or delay the work on my traumatic events at any time and that I am encouraged to talk with my clinician about the process of the trauma treatment at any time.

I have been informed how to reach my clinician after business hours and what procedures to follow if I have an urgent request or need. I also understand that I must cancel my appointment 24 hours in advance or I will be charged for the appointment.

Therefore, I authorize _____ to provide treatment/evaluation for my condition.

Client _____

Clinician_____

Date_____

Traumatic Life Events Questionnaire

David Read Johnson, Ph.D.

Hadar Lubin, M.D.

TRAUMATIC LIFE EVENTS QUESTIONNAIRE

Please check off the appropriate boxes below, and then give this form to your therapist.

Did you or people close to you experience or witness any of these events as a child or an adult?	Were you bothered by this at the time?		Are you bothered by this now?	
Natural disaster				
☐ Flood	☐ yes	☐ no	☐ yes	☐ no
☐ Hurricane/tornado	☐ yes	☐ no	☐ yes	☐ no
☐ Fire	☐ yes	☐ no	☐ yes	☐ no
☐ Earthquake	☐ yes	☐ no	☐ yes	☐ no
Accidents				
☐ Medical/surgical error	☐ yes	☐ no	☐ yes	☐ no
☐ Motor vehicle accident	☐ yes	☐ no	☐ yes	☐ no
☐ Plane crash	☐ yes	☐ no	☐ yes	☐ no
☐ Drowning	☐ yes	☐ no	☐ yes	☐ no
☐ Explosion	☐ yes	☐ no	☐ yes	☐ no
☐ Chemical/gas leak	☐ yes	☐ no	☐ yes	☐ no
☐ Building collapse	☐ yes	☐ no	☐ yes	☐ no
Illness				
☐ Unexpected death of loved one	☐ yes	☐ no	☐ yes	☐ no
☐ Serious medical illness	☐ yes	☐ no	☐ yes	☐ no
☐ Serious mental illness	☐ yes	☐ no	☐ yes	☐ no
Neglect/humiliation				
☐ Being denied food or water	☐ yes	☐ no	☐ yes	☐ no
☐ Left alone for long periods	☐ yes	☐ no	☐ yes	☐ no
☐ Put in dangerous situations	☐ yes	☐ no	☐ yes	☐ no
☐ Verbally humiliated or ignored	☐ yes	☐ no	☐ yes	☐ no
☐ Forced to perform humiliating actions	☐ yes	☐ no	☐ yes	☐ no
☐ Insulted/treated as worthless	☐ yes	☐ no	☐ yes	☐ no
☐ Teased/bullied	☐ yes	☐ no	☐ yes	☐ no

Did you or people close to you experience or witness any of these events as a child or an adult?	Were you bothered by this at the time?		Are you bothered by this now?	

Control

☐ Being locked in a room/closet	☐ yes	☐ no	☐ yes	☐ no
☐ Controlled use of phone	☐ yes	☐ no	☐ yes	☐ no
☐ Being stalked	☐ yes	☐ no	☐ yes	☐ no
☐ Controlled contact with others	☐ yes	☐ no	☐ yes	☐ no
☐ Controlled possessions	☐ yes	☐ no	☐ yes	☐ no
☐ Forced to take drugs or alcohol	☐ yes	☐ no	☐ yes	☐ no

Physical punishment

☐ Being hit, kicked, thrown, dragged, or tied up	☐ yes	☐ no	☐ yes	☐ no
☐ Being bruised, burned, cut, or given broken bones	☐ yes	☐ no	☐ yes	☐ no
☐ Witnessed violence on other family members	☐ yes	☐ no	☐ yes	☐ no

Unwanted sexual contact

☐ Forced intercourse (oral, anal, or vaginal)	☐ yes	☐ no	☐ yes	☐ no
☐ Forced masturbation	☐ yes	☐ no	☐ yes	☐ no
☐ Forced to watch pornography	☐ yes	☐ no	☐ yes	☐ no
☐ Being fondled against will	☐ yes	☐ no	☐ yes	☐ no
☐ Forced to perform sexual acts in front of others	☐ yes	☐ no	☐ yes	☐ no
☐ Being filmed or videotaped	☐ yes	☐ no	☐ yes	☐ no
☐ Being prostituted	☐ yes	☐ no	☐ yes	☐ no

Assault and robbery

☐ Victim of robbery	☐ yes	☐ no	☐ yes	☐ no
☐ Assaulted with a weapon	☐ yes	☐ no	☐ yes	☐ no
☐ Threatened to be killed	☐ yes	☐ no	☐ yes	☐ no
☐ Beaten up	☐ yes	☐ no	☐ yes	☐ no
☐ Kidnapped/held hostage	☐ yes	☐ no	☐ yes	☐ no
☐ Witnessed a murder/assault	☐ yes	☐ no	☐ yes	☐ no

Did you or people close to you experience or witness any of these events as a child or an adult?	Were you bothered by this at the time?		Are you bothered by this now?	

Stigma and prejudice (harm due to any of the following)

☐ Race	☐ yes	☐ no	☐ yes	☐ no
☐ Gender	☐ yes	☐ no	☐ yes	☐ no
☐ Age	☐ yes	☐ no	☐ yes	☐ no
☐ Ethnic or national identity	☐ yes	☐ no	☐ yes	☐ no
☐ Income	☐ yes	☐ no	☐ yes	☐ no
☐ Sexual orientation	☐ yes	☐ no	☐ yes	☐ no
☐ Religion	☐ yes	☐ no	☐ yes	☐ no
☐ Nonconventional family	☐ yes	☐ no	☐ yes	☐ no

War

☐ Served in a combat zone	☐ yes	☐ no	☐ yes	☐ no
☐ Treated the wounded	☐ yes	☐ no	☐ yes	☐ no
☐ Was fired upon	☐ yes	☐ no	☐ yes	☐ no
☐ Close-hand combat	☐ yes	☐ no	☐ yes	☐ no
☐ Prisoner of war	☐ yes	☐ no	☐ yes	☐ no
☐ Friendly fire	☐ yes	☐ no	☐ yes	☐ no

Other events

☐ Miscarriage/stillbirth	☐ yes	☐ no	☐ yes	☐ no
☐ Abortion	☐ yes	☐ no	☐ yes	☐ no
☐ Foster or residential care	☐ yes	☐ no	☐ yes	☐ no
☐ Removed from home by the state	☐ yes	☐ no	☐ yes	☐ no
☐ Homeless/lived on streets	☐ yes	☐ no	☐ yes	☐ no
☐ Subject of lawsuit	☐ yes	☐ no	☐ yes	☐ no
☐ Being falsely accused	☐ yes	☐ no	☐ yes	☐ no
☐ Arrest/imprisonment	☐ yes	☐ no	☐ yes	☐ no
☐ Hospitalized against will	☐ yes	☐ no	☐ yes	☐ no
☐ Being embezzled/ blackmailed	☐ yes	☐ no	☐ yes	☐ no
☐ Spouse/partner had an affair	☐ yes	☐ no	☐ yes	☐ no
☐ Unexpected demotion or loss of job	☐ yes	☐ no	☐ yes	☐ no
☐ Identity theft	☐ yes	☐ no	☐ yes	☐ no

Thank you.

Appendix C

Clinical Interview for Assessment of Trauma History

David Read Johnson, Ph.D.

Hadar Lubin, M.D.

This interview is designed to identify potentially traumatic events in your client's life. Each area of trauma is assessed in Part A with a general question. If the client answers positively, then ask him or her to describe it to you in more detail. If the client answers in the negative, then ask several more detailed questions to probe further. When a traumatic event is uncovered or described, in whatever category, then shift to a separate set of questions (Part B) and a detailed elicitation of the event and the client's reactions to it. [Note that this is not a diagnostic interview that will result in assessing symptoms of posttraumatic stress disorder.]

PART A: ASSESSMENT OF EVENTS

Introductory Statement to Client

Now I am going to ask you about personal experiences that for one reason or another have been bad, unfortunate, or frightening to you, such as losing someone close to you, being physically or sexually mistreated, or being seriously injured. Some people can talk about these experiences without much trouble, and others find them very difficult to talk about. Some of these experiences may even have been kept secret for years. I am interested in finding out about these experiences, because they often have important effects on a person's life, and understanding them may help me treat you in the best possible way. May I begin?

I. General Screening Question

Looking back on your life, from childhood to present, has anything happened that you found to be extremely frightening, upsetting, unfortunate, or traumatic? (If client seems unsure:) For example, terrible events that involve death, injury, accidents, physical pain, sexual mistreatment, or natural disasters?

- If yes: Say, **Tell me what happened.** (Go to Part B.)
- If no: Continue to Section II.

II. Loss

Sometimes over the course of a person's life, one has to deal with losing something or someone very valuable, such as the loss of a child; the sudden loss of income, job, or home; or being arrested. Do you recall whether anything like this ever happened to you?

- If yes: Say, **Tell me what happened.** (Go to Part B.)
- If no: Ask the following questions:
  - Did you ever have a miscarriage, stillbirth, or abortion?
  - Did you ever live in a foster home or residential care?
  - Were you ever homeless or removed from your home?
  - Were you ever falsely accused, subject of a lawsuit, arrested, or imprisoned?
  - Were you ever hospitalized against your will, embezzled, or blackmailed, or have you ever had your identity stolen?
  - Were you ever fired from your job, or did you ever lose your home or a lot of your income?
  - Did a spouse or partner ever have an affair that you discovered?

III. Disasters, Accidents, Illness, or Combat

Sometimes people have to live through serious illness, accidents, military combat, natural disasters, or unexpected death of a loved one. Do you recall whether anything like that ever happened to you, your family, or someone close to you?

- If yes: Say, **Tell me what happened.** (Go to Part B.)
- If no: Ask the following questions:
  - **Did you ever experience a natural disaster such as a flood, hurricane, fire, or earthquake?**
  - **Did you ever experience or witness a medical error, motor vehicle accident, plane crash, drowning, explosion, chemical leak, or building collapse?**
  - **Did you ever experience an unexpected death of a loved one or have a serious medical or mental illness?**
  - **Did you ever serve in a combat zone?**
  - **If so, were you ever fired upon by enemy or exposed to friendly fire, or did you engage in close-hand combat, treat the wounded, or become a prisoner of war?**

IV. Physical Abuse

Sometimes people get spanked a lot, get hit or physically punished, or are mistreated in other ways while growing up. People also can get beat up, mugged, or threatened with weapons during their adult life. Do you recall whether anything like that ever happened to you?

- If yes: Say, **Tell me what happened.** (Go to Part B.)
- If no: Ask the following questions:
  - **How were you punished as a child?**
  - **Were you ever hit, kicked, thrown, dragged, or tied up?**
  - **Were you ever bruised, burned, cut, or given broken bones?**
  - **Did you ever witness violence between other family members?**
  - **Were you ever the victim of a robbery or kidnapping, or assaulted with a weapon, threatened to be killed, or beaten up?**

V. Emotional Abuse and Neglect

Sometimes, either while growing up or as adults, people feel as if they can't do anything right in other people's eyes; they are often put down, yelled at, humiliated, or told they are no good. People can also be denied food, be left alone, or be overly controlled. Do you recall whether anything like that ever happened to you?

- If yes: Say, **Tell me what happened.** (Go to Part B.)
- If no: Ask the following questions:

- Have you been denied food or water, put in dangerous situations, or left alone for a long time?
- Have you been humiliated, ignored, bullied, insulted, or forced to perform humiliating actions?
- Have you been locked in a room or forced to take drugs or alcohol against your will?
- Has someone controlled your use of the phone, contact with others, or your possessions?

VI. Sexual Abuse

Sometimes people have sexual experiences that make them uncomfortable, cause them to get upset, or were forced upon them. Do you recall whether anything like that ever happened to you either in childhood or as an adult?

- If yes: Say, **Tell me what happened.** (Go to Part B.)
- If no: Ask the following questions:
    - **Did you have any sexual experiences before age 15?**
    - **Were you ever fondled or forced to watch pornography, masturbate, or have intercourse (oral, anal, or vaginal) against your will, including while dating?**
    - **Were you ever photographed or filmed, or forced to perform sexual acts in front of others?**
    - **Were you ever prostituted?**
    - **Did you ever have sexual contact with a relative?**

VII. Stigma and Prejudice

Sometimes people are discriminated against or harmed because of some personal or social characteristic, like race, gender, age, or sexual orientation. Do you recall whether anything like that ever happened to you either in childhood or as an adult?

- If yes: Say, **Tell me what happened.** (Go to Part B.)
- If no: Ask the following questions:
    - **Were you ever discriminated against or harmed in any way because of your race, gender, age, or ethnic identity?**
    - **Were you ever discriminated against or harmed because of your low income, sexual orientation, religion, or living in a nonconventional family?**

PART B: WHEN AN EVENT IS ANSWERED IN THE AFFIRMATIVE

Ask the client to tell you what happened in as much detail as possible. As the client describes the event, slow him or her down, and intersperse the questions listed below, where relevant. Notice when the client glosses over important moments with a catch phrase or a leap in chronology. If it becomes evident that this event was not traumatic (e.g., client witnessed minor accident, client feels guilty when masturbating alone), then you can return to the main interview and continue questioning.

During Trauma

- When did the event occur?
- How old were you?
- How long did the event last? How often did it occur?
- Who was the perpetrator?
- How sudden or unpredictable was it?
- What was your level of fear, horror, shame, disgust, anger?
- How helpless did you feel at the time?

Immediately Posttrauma

- After the event, how did you cope? (for example, withdrawal, panic, denial, anger, self-injury, secrecy)
- To what extent do you feel somehow responsible for the event?
- Was there any physical injury?
- How did others (family, spouse, professionals, police) respond to you?
- What treatment or support did you receive?

Present

- What impact has this event had on your (emotional, work, social, family) life?
- To what extent are your memories of this event still bothering you today?
- How are your memories still bothering you?

To therapist: Return to the main interview to continue questioning about other traumatic events.

Index

*Page numbers printed in **boldface** type refer to tables or figures.*